CONSUMER GUIDE®

PRESCRIPTION
DRUGS

**With the compliments
of
Home Health Handbook**

11150 W. Olympic Boulevard, Suite 650, Los Angeles, CA 90064

NOTE: Neither the Editors of CONSUMER GUIDE® and PUBLICATIONS INTERNATIONAL, LTD. nor the consultant or publisher takes responsibility for any possible consequences from any treatment, action, or application of medication or preparation by any person reading or following the information in this publication. The publication of this material does not constitute the practice of medicine, and this publication does not attempt to replace your physician or your pharmacist. The consultant and publisher advise the reader to check with a physician before administering or consuming any medication or using any health care device.

Every effort has been made to assure that the information in this publication is accurate and current at time of printing. However, new developments occur almost daily in drug research, and the consultant and publisher suggest that the reader consult a physician or pharmacist for the latest available data on specific products. All trade names of drugs used in the text of this publication are capitalized.

Contents

What do you know about the drugs you take? Do you know
how they work, what side effects they are likely to cause, and
whether you can safely drink alcohol or take other drugs while
using them? The more you know about your prescription drugs,
the lower your risk of suffering allergic reactions, an overdose,
or other drug-induced problems and the greater the probability
that the drug will help you.

Your prescription shouldn't be a mystery to you; you should be
able to read and understand it. That way, you can be sure your
pharmacist has given you the correct drug and the correct
instructions for taking it. Here you'll find an easy-to-use guide
to reading your prescription and talking to your pharmacist, a
useful discussion of generic substitutions, and helpful
information on how much of a drug to buy and how to store it
properly.

To get the best results from the drugs you take, you must
administer them correctly. Proper administration can help save
you money, too. These simple guidelines show you how to use
liquids, creams, and ointments without waste. You'll even find
tips on how to warm ear drops and how to make swallowing
tablets and capsules easier.

A side effect is any effect other than the one for which you took
the drug. Some side effects are serious and demand your
doctor's attention; others may be expected, unavoidable, and of
little consequence. But which are which? Here you'll find out
how to tell the difference, as well as how to alleviate or avoid
some of the most common minor side effects.

You know you're taking a diuretic, but what does a diuretic do?
How does a vaccine work? This primer on the basic action of
drugs will help you understand how your medications work.
You'll discover how your antiulcer medication protects your
stomach, why you probably shouldn't be taking decongestants
if you have high blood pressure, and why antibiotics won't cure
your cold.

Drug Profiles

Here, arranged alphabetically, are profiles of the most frequently prescribed drugs in the United States. The drug profile provides information on the uses, ingredients, dosage forms, and equivalent products of a drug. It tells you who should be extra careful when taking the drug and who should not be taking the medication at all. It lists both the minor and major side effects associated with a drug. It also tells you if it's better to take a drug with meals or on an empty stomach; what you can do to avoid or minimize dizziness, light-headedness, or other unwanted side effects caused by the drug; and whether a drug may interfere with other medications you might be taking. The information in a drug profile is vital to your comfort and safety and to the success of your treatment.

Introduction

The right drug for the right patient in the right dose by the right route at the right time. This rule sums up the decisions made when your doctor gives you a prescription. You've helped make those decisions by giving a complete medical history; you've informed your doctor of any previous allergic reactions you've suffered, any other drugs you may be taking, and any chronic health problems you may have. Once you leave your doctor's office, prescription in hand, you have still more to do as a responsible patient.

You must know how to administer the medication you will be taking. You must understand and comply with your dosage schedule. You must know what to do should side effects occur. You must recognize the signals that indicate the need to call your doctor. All too often, patients leave their doctor's office without a full understanding of the drug therapy they're about to start, with the result that they do not comply fully with their doctor's prescription. They may stop taking the medication too soon because it doesn't seem to work or because they feel better or because it causes bothersome side effects. They may take the drug improperly or at the wrong time or too often. They may continue drinking alcohol or taking other drugs, perhaps not even realizing that such things as cold pills, oral contraceptives, aspirin, and vitamins could affect the action of the prescribed drug. The end result may be that they do not get better; perhaps they will get worse, or they may suffer a dangerous overdose.

PRESCRIPTION DRUGS provides the information you need to take drugs safely. Along with general information on reading a prescription and buying, storing, and using drugs, it provides an introduction to the action of drugs—how drugs work to stop infection, lower blood pressure, or relieve pain. Then it provides detailed information on hundreds of the most commonly prescribed drugs. The information in the drug profiles includes how to alleviate certain side effects, whether you should take the drug on an empty stomach or with meals, whether the drug is likely to affect your ability to drive, and whether you can substitute a less expensive generic drug for a prescribed trade name medication. You will discover which side effects are common to some medications and which are danger signals that require immediate attention from your physician.

Of course, this book is not a substitute for consulting your doctor and pharmacist. They are your primary reference sources on the use of drugs. To assure that you receive the best health care possible, however, you too must be informed and knowledgeable about the drugs you use.

Filling Your Prescription

While you're having your prescription filled, you should make sure you understand your dosage schedule, what kinds of precautions to take to prevent or reduce side effects, whether you should restrict your diet or drinking habits while taking the drug, which side effects are expected or unavoidable, and which side effects signal a need for a doctor's attention. Your first step in filling your prescription is reading what your doctor has written.

Reading Your Prescription

You do not have to be a doctor, nurse, or pharmacist to read a prescription. As a health-conscious consumer, you *can* and *should* learn how. After all, the prescription describes the drug you will be taking. You should understand what your doctor has written on the prescription blank to be sure the label on the drug container you receive from your pharmacist coincides with the prescription.

Prescriptions are not mysterious; they contain no secret messages. Many of the symbols and phrases doctors use on prescriptions are simply abbreviated Latin words—holdovers from the days when doctors actually wrote in Latin. For example, "gtt" comes from the Latin word *guttae,* which means drops, and "bid" is a shortened version of *bis in die,* Latin for twice a day. By becoming familiar with these abbreviations, you'll be able to read and understand your prescription.

The accompanying chart lists the symbols and abbreviations most commonly used on prescriptions. Use it as a guide to read the sample prescriptions illustrated in this chapter as well as any prescriptions you receive from your doctor.

Common Abbreviations and Symbols Used in Writing Prescriptions

Abbreviation	Meaning	Derivation and Notes
A_2	both ears	*auris* (Latin)
aa	of each	*ana* (Greek)
ac	before meals	*ante cibum* (Latin)
AD	right ear	*auris dextra* (Latin)
AL	left ear	*auris laeva* (Latin)
AM	morning	*ante meridiem* (Latin)
AS	left ear	*auris sinistra* (Latin)
bid	twice a day	*bis in die* (Latin)
$\overline{C}$	100	—
$\overline{c}$	with	*cum* (Latin)

Abbreviation	Meaning	Derivation and Notes
Cap	let him take	*capiat* (Latin)
caps	capsule	*capsula* (Latin)
cc or cm³	cubic centimeter	30 cc equals one ounce
disp	dispense	—
dtd#	give this number	*dentur tales doses* (Latin)
ea	each	—
ext	for external use	—
gtt	drops	*guttae* (Latin)
gt	drop	*gutta* (Latin)
h	hour	*hora* (Latin)
HS	bedtime	*hora somni* (Latin)
M ft	make	*misce fiat* (Latin)
mitt#	give this number	*mitte* (Latin)
ml	milliliter	30 ml equals one ounce
O	pint	*octarius* (Latin)
O₂	both eyes	*oculus* (Latin)
OD	right eye	*oculus dexter* (Latin)
OJ	orange juice	—
OL	left eye	*oculus laevus* (Latin)
OS	left eye	*oculus sinister* (Latin)
OU	each eye	*oculus uterque* (Latin)
pc	after meals	*post cibum* (Latin)
PM	evening	*post meridiem* (Latin)
po	by mouth	*per os* (Latin)
prn	as needed	*pro re nata* (Latin)
q̄	every	*quaque* (Latin)
qd	once a day	*quaque die* (Latin)
qid	four times a day	*quater in die* (Latin)
qod	every other day	—
s	without	*sine* (Latin)
Sig	label as follows	*signa* (Latin)
sl	under the tongue	*sub lingua* (Latin)
SOB	shortness of breath	—
sol	solution	—
ss	one-half	*semis* (Latin)
stat	at once, first dose	*statim* (Latin)
susp	suspension	—
tab	tablet	—
tid	three times a day	*ter in die* (Latin)
top	apply topically	—
ung or ungt	ointment	*unguentum* (Latin)
UT	under the tongue	—
ut dict	as directed	*ut dictum* (Latin)
x	times	—

The first sample prescription is for Fiorinal analgesic and sedative. The prescription tells the pharmacist to give you 24 capsules (#24), and it tells you to take one capsule (caps i) every four hours ($\bar{q}$4h) as needed (prn) for pain. The prescription indicates that you may receive five refills (5x), that the label on the drug container should state the name of the drug (yes), and that the pharmacist may substitute (substitution) a less expensive equivalent product.

Look at the second prescription. It shows you will receive 100 (dtd C) tablets of Lanoxin heart drug, 0.125 mg. You will take three tablets at once (iii stat), then two (ii) tomorrow morning (AM), and one (i) every ($\bar{q}$) morning (AM) thereafter with ($\bar{c}$) orange juice (OJ). You will receive the specific brand noted (dispense as written); you may receive refills as needed (prn); and the name of the drug will be on the package ($\sqrt{}$).

Do remember to check the label on the drug container. If the information on the label is not the same as on the prescription, question your pharmacist. Make doubly sure that you are receiving the right medication and the correct instructions for taking it.

Talking to Your Pharmacist

Once you have read the prescription, the directions may seem clear enough, but will they seem clear when you get home? For example, the prescription for Fiorinal analgesic and sedative tells you to take one capsule every four hours as needed. How many capsules can you take each day—four, six, more? The phrase "as needed" is not clear, and unless you understand what it means, you don't know how much medication you can take per day. What if your prescription instructs you to take "one tablet four times a day"? What does four times a day mean? For some antibiotics, it may mean one tablet every six hours

---

John D. Jones MD
Anytown, U.S.A.

DEA# 123456789   PHONE# 123-4567

NAME *Your Name*   AGE **47**
ADDRESS *Anytown, U.S.A.*   DATE **5/10/89**

℞   *Fiorinal*
      #24
      Sig: caps i $\bar{q}$ 4h prn pain

REFILLS **5x**   DISPENSE AS WRITTEN
LABEL **yes**   *John D. Jones, M.D.*
                                     SUBSTITUTION

CONSUMER GUIDE®

around the clock. For other medications, it may mean one tablet in the morning, one at noon, one in the early evening, and one at bedtime. For still others, it may mean one tablet every hour for the first four hours after you get up in the morning. Don't leave the pharmacy with unanswered questions; ask your pharmacist for an explanation of any confusing terms on your prescription.

Your pharmacist is a valuable resource in your health care. He or she should have a record of all the prescription drugs you receive in order to detect any possible life-threatening drug interactions. The pharmacist will be able to tell you if your therapy may be affected by smoking tobacco, eating certain foods, or drinking alcohol. He or she can tell you what to expect from the medication and about how long you will have to take it. Of course, people's treatments vary tremendously, but you should know whether you will have to take medication for five to ten days (for example, to treat a mild respiratory infection) or for a few months (for example, to treat a kidney infection). Your pharmacist should also tell you how many refills you may have and whether you may need them.

Your pharmacist should advise you of possible side effects and describe their symptoms in terms you can understand. For example, your pharmacist can tell you if the drug is likely to cause nausea or drowsiness. The pharmacist should also tell you which side effects require prompt attention from your physician. For example, one of the major side effects of the drug Zyloprim is a blood disorder. One of the first symptoms of a blood disorder is a sore throat. Your pharmacist should tell you to consult your physician if you develop a sore throat.

Your pharmacist should also explain how to take your medicine. You should know whether to take the drug before or after a meal or along

---

John D. Jones MD
Anytown, U.S.A.

DEA# 123456789   PHONE# 123-4567

NAME _Your Name_   AGE _55_
ADDRESS _Anytown, U.S.A._   DATE _5/23/89_

R͟x   Lanoxin 0.125
         dtd C
         Sig: iii stat, ii tomorrow AM,
            then i q̄ AM c̄ OJ

                              John D. Jones, M.D.
                              DISPENSE AS WRITTEN

REFILLS _prn_
LABEL _✓_
                              _____
                              SUBSTITUTION

with it. The time at which you take a drug can make a big difference, and the effectiveness of each drug depends on following the directions for its use. Your pharmacist should describe what "as needed," "as directed," and "take with fluid" mean. You may take water but not milk with some drugs. With other drugs, you should take milk.

Here is a quick checklist of questions to ask about your prescription:
- What is the name of the drug and what is it supposed to do?
- How, when, and for how long should it be taken?
- What foods, drinks, activities, or other medications should I avoid while taking this drug?
- Are there any side effects; can I avoid them; and what do I do if they occur?

Over-the-Counter Drugs

Drugs that can be purchased without a prescription are referred to as over-the-counter (OTC) drugs and are sold in a wide variety of settings, such as drug and grocery stores and hotel lobbies. There are no legal requirements or limitations on who may buy or sell them.

Products sold OTC contain amounts of active ingredients considered to be safe for self-treatment by consumers when labeling instructions are followed.

Many people visit a doctor for ailments that can be treated effectively by taking nonprescription drugs. Actually, prescriptions are sometimes written for such drugs. Your pharmacist will be able to recommend appropriate use of OTC drugs.

If your pharmacist recommends that you not take certain OTC drugs, follow the advice. OTC drugs may affect the way your body reacts to the prescription drugs you are taking. For instance, people taking tetracycline antibiotic should avoid taking antacids or other iron-containing products at the same time; their use should be separated by at least two hours. Antacids and iron interfere with the body's absorption of tetracycline. Be sure you know what you are taking.

Generic Drugs

"Generic" means not protected by trademark registration. The generic name of a drug is usually a shortened form of its chemical name. Any manufacturer can use the generic name when marketing a drug. Thus, many manufacturers make a drug called tetracycline.

Usually, a manufacturer uses a trade name as well as a generic name for a drug. A trade name is registered, and only the manufacturer who holds the trademark can use the trade name when marketing a drug. For example, only Lederle Laboratories can call their tetracycline product Achromycin, and only The Upjohn Company can use the trade name Panmycin. Most trade names are capitalized in print and usually include the register symbol ® after them.

Many people think that drugs with trade names are made by large manufacturers and that generic drugs are made by small manufacturers. But, in fact, a manufacturer may market large quantities of a drug under a trade name and also sell the base chemical to several other companies, some of which sell the drug generically and some of which sell it under their own trade names. For example, the antibiotic ampicillin is the base for over two hundred different products. However, all ampicillin is produced by only a few dozen drug companies.

Generic drugs are generally priced lower than their trademarked equivalents, largely because they are not as widely advertised. Not every drug is available generically, however, and not every generic is significantly less expensive than its trademarked equivalent. For certain drugs, it's inadvisable to "shop around" for a generic equivalent. Although the Food and Drug Administration has stated that there is no evidence to suspect serious differences between trade name and generic drugs, differences have been shown between brands of certain drugs. This is especially true for the various digoxin and phenytoin products. It is, therefore, important to discuss with your doctor or pharmacist the advantages or disadvantages of any particular product.

However, for other drugs, consumers may be able to save as much as 40 percent. For example, one hundred tablets of Inderal (40 mg) may cost $22 to $25. One hundred tablets of the generic equivalent product may cost about $18 — a savings of $4 to $7. Motrin anti-inflammatory may cost $20 per 100 tablets, but if bought generically, the drug may cost as little as $12 per 100 tablets — again, a savings of about $8 per prescription.

All states have some form of substitution law that allows pharmacists to fill prescriptions with the least expensive equivalent product. However, your doctor can authorize the use of a specific brand by signing on the appropriate line or otherwise noting this on the prescription form (see sample prescriptions). You should be aware that certain patients can sometimes respond in different ways to various equivalent products, and your doctor may have good reasons for being specific. Discuss this with your doctor.

How Much to Buy

On a prescription, your doctor specifies exactly how many tablets or capsules or how much liquid medication you will receive. If you must take a drug for a long time, however, or if you are very sensitive to drugs, you may want to purchase a different quantity.

The amount of medication to buy depends on several factors. The most obvious is how much money you have or, for those who have a comprehensive insurance program, how much the insurance company will pay for each purchase. These factors may help you decide how much medication to buy. But you must also consider the kind of medication you will be taking.

Medication to treat heart disease, high blood pressure, diabetes, or a thyroid condition may be purchased in large quantity. Patients with such chronic conditions take medication for prolonged periods, and chances are, they will pay less per tablet or capsule by purchasing large quantities of drugs. Generally, the price per dose decreases with the amount of the drug purchased. In other words, a drug that generally costs six cents per tablet may cost four or five cents per tablet if you buy 100 at a time. Many doctors prescribe only a month's supply of a drug even if the drug will be taken for a long time. If you wish to buy more, check with your pharmacist. It is also important to make sure that you have enough medication on hand to cover vacation travel and long holidays. Serious side effects could occur if you miss even a few doses of such drugs as propranolol, prednisone, or clonidine.

On the other hand, if you have been plagued with annoying side effects or have had allergic reactions to some drugs, ask your pharmacist to dispense only enough medication on initial prescriptions to last a few days or a week. This will allow you to determine whether the drug agrees with you. Pharmacists cannot take back prescription drugs once they have left the pharmacy. You may have to pay more by asking the pharmacist to give you a small amount of the drug, but at least you will not be paying for a supply of medication you cannot take. Be sure you can get the remainder of the prescribed amount of the drug if it does agree with you. With some drugs, after you have received part of the intended amount, you cannot receive more without obtaining another prescription.

Storing Your Drugs

Before you leave the pharmacy, find out how you should store your drug. If drugs are stored in containers that do not protect them from heat or moisture, they may lose potency.

You can safely store most prescription drugs at room temperature and out of direct sunlight. Even those drugs dispensed in colored bottles or containers that reflect light should be kept out of direct sunlight.

Some drugs require storage in the refrigerator. The statement "keep in the refrigerator," however, does not mean that you can keep the drug in the freezer. If frozen and thawed, sugar-coated tablets may crack, and some liquid medications may separate into layers that cannot be remixed.

Other drugs cannot be stored in the refrigerator. For example, some liquid cough suppressants will thicken as they become cold and will not pour from the bottle. Some people keep nitroglycerin tablets in the

Definitions of Ideal Storage Temperatures

Cold	Any temperature under 46°F (8°C)
Refrigerator	Any cold place where the temperature is between 36°-46°F (2°-8°C)
Cool	Any temperature between 46°-59°F (8°-15°C)
Room temperature	Temperature usually between 59°-86°F (15°-30°C)
Excessive heat	Any temperature above 104°F (40°C)

refrigerator because they believe the drug will be more stable. Nitroglycerin, however, should not be stored in the refrigerator.

Many people keep prescription drugs and other medications in the bathroom medicine cabinet, but this is one of the worst places to keep drugs. Small children can easily climb onto the sink and reach drugs stored above it. Also, the temperature and humidity changes in the bathroom may adversely affect prescription drugs.

Keep all drugs away from children. Do not keep unused prescription medications. Flush any leftover medication down the toilet or pour it down the sink; wash and destroy the empty container. Regularly clean out your medicine cabinet and discard all drugs you are no longer using. These drugs can be dangerous to your children, and you might be tempted to take them in the future if you develop similar symptoms. Though similar, the symptoms may not be due to the same disease, and you may complicate your condition by taking the wrong medication.

Administering Medication Correctly

You must use medication correctly to obtain its full benefit. If you administer drugs improperly, you may not receive their full therapeutic effects. Furthermore, improper administration can be dangerous. Some drugs may become toxic if used incorrectly.

Liquids

Liquids may be used externally on the skin; they may be placed into the eye, ear, nose, or throat; or they may be taken internally.

Before taking or using any liquid medication, look at the label to see if there are any specific directions, such as shaking the container before measuring the dose. If a liquid product contains particles that settle to the bottom of the container, it must be shaken before you use it. If you don't shake it well each time, you may not get the correct amount of the active ingredient. Likewise, as the amount of liquid remaining in the bottle becomes smaller, the drug will become more concentrated. You will be getting more of the active ingredient with each dose. The concentration may even reach toxic levels.

When opening the bottle, point it away from you. Some liquid medications may build up pressure inside the bottle; the liquid could spurt out quickly and stain your clothing.

If the medication is intended for application on the skin, pour a small quantity onto a cotton pad or a piece of gauze. Do not use a large piece of cotton or gauze as it will absorb the liquid and much will be wasted. Don't pour the medication into your cupped hand; you may spill some of it. If you're using it on only a small area, you can spread the medication with your finger or a cotton-tipped applicator. Never dip cotton-tipped applicators or pieces of cotton or gauze into the bottle of liquid, as this might contaminate the rest of the medication.

Liquid medications that are to be swallowed must be measured accurately. When your doctor prescribes one teaspoonful of medication, he is thinking of a 5 milliliter medical teaspoon. The teaspoons you have at home may hold anywhere from 2 milliliters to 10 milliliters of liquid. If you use one of these to measure your medication, you may get too little or too much with each dose. Ask your pharmacist for a medical teaspoon or for one of the other plastic devices for accurately measuring liquid medications. Most of these cost only a few cents, and they are well worth their cost to assure accurate dosages. These plastic measuring devices have another advantage. While many children balk at medication taken from a teaspoon, they often seem to enjoy taking it from a special spoon.

Capsules and Tablets

If you find it difficult to swallow a tablet or capsule, rinse your mouth with water, or at least wet your mouth, first. Then place the tablet or capsule on the back of your tongue, take a drink of water, and swallow.

If you cannot swallow a tablet or capsule because it is too large or because it "sticks" in your throat, empty the capsule or crush the tablet into a spoon and mix it with applesauce, soup, or even chocolate syrup. But BE SURE TO CHECK WITH YOUR PHARMACIST FIRST. Some tablets and capsules must be swallowed whole.

On the other hand, some capsules that contain beads are made to be opened and the contents sprinkled onto food. These capsules are called *sprinkles.* They are useful for children and for persons who have difficulty swallowing whole capsules. Theo-Dur sprinkles are used in this manner. Once again, however, be sure to ask your pharmacist if your medication should be taken in this way.

If you have trouble swallowing a tablet or capsule and do not wish to mix the medication with food, ask your doctor to prescribe a liquid drug preparation or a chewable tablet instead, if one is available.

Examples of Drugs that Must be Swallowed Whole

Donnatal Extentabs	Naldecon	Tagamet
E-Mycin	Ornade	Trinalin
Isordil Tembids		

Examples of Drugs that Should be Used Quickly (within 12 Hours) if Crushed or Opened

Compazine	Mellaril	Stelazine
Elavil	Phenergan	Tofranil
Etrafon	Sinequan	Triavil
Haldol		

Sublingual Tablets

Some drugs, such as nitroglycerin, are prepared as tablets that must be placed under the tongue. To take a sublingual tablet properly, place the tablet under your tongue, close your mouth, and hold the saliva in your mouth and under your tongue as long as you can before swallowing. If you have a bitter taste in your mouth after five minutes, the drug has not been completely absorbed. Wait five more minutes before drinking water. Drinking water too soon may wash the medication into the stomach before it has been absorbed thoroughly.

Eye Drops and Eye Ointments

Before administering eye drops or ointments, wash your hands. Then lie down or sit down and tilt your head back. Using your thumb and forefinger, gently and carefully pull your lower eyelid down to form a pouch.

If you're applying eye drops, lay your second finger alongside your nose and apply gentle pressure to your nose. This will close off a duct that drains fluid from the eye. If you don't close off this duct, the drops are likely to drain away too soon. Hold the dropper close to the eyelid without touching it. Place the prescribed number of drops into the pouch. Do not place the drops directly on the eyeball; you may blink and lose the medication. Close your eye and keep it shut for a few moments. Do not wash or wipe the dropper before replacing it in the bottle. Tightly close the bottle to keep out moisture, then store the bottle as directed.

To administer an ointment to the eye, squeeze a one-quarter to one-half inch line of ointment into the pouch formed as above and close your eye. Roll your eye a few times to spread the ointment. As long as you do not squeeze the ointment directly onto the eyeball, you should feel no stinging or pain.

Be sure the drops or ointments you use are intended for the eye (manufacturers must sterilize all products intended for use in the eye). Also, check the expiration date of the drug on the label or container. Do not use a drug product after that date, and never use any eye product that has changed color. If you find that the medication contains particles that weren't there when you bought it, do not use it.

Ear Drops

Ear drops must be administered so that they fill the ear canal. To administer ear drops properly, tilt your head to one side, turning the affected ear upward. Grasp the earlobe and gently pull it upward and back to straighten the ear canal. When administering ear drops to a child, gently pull the child's earlobe downward and back. Fill the dropper and place the prescribed number of drops (usually a dropperful) in the ear, but be careful to avoid touching the ear canal. The dropper can be easily contaminated by contact with the ear canal.

Keep your ear tilted upward for five to ten seconds while continuing to hold the earlobe. Then gently insert a small piece of clean cotton into the ear to be sure the drops do not escape. Do not wash or wipe the dropper after use; replace it in the bottle and tightly close the bottle to keep out moisture.

You may warm the bottle of ear drops before administering the medication by rolling the bottle back and forth between your hands to bring the solution to body temperature. Do not place the bottle in boiling water. The ear drops may become so hot that they will cause pain when placed in the ear, and boiling water can loosen or peel off the label and possibly destroy the medication.

CONSUMER GUIDE®

Nose Drops and Sprays

Before using nose drops and sprays, gently blow your nose if you can. To administer nose drops, fill the dropper, tilt your head back, and place the prescribed number of drops in your nose. Do not touch the dropper to the nasal membranes. This will prevent contamination of the medicine when the dropper is returned to the container. Keep your head tilted for five to ten seconds and sniff gently two or three times.

Do not tilt your head back when using a nasal spray. Insert the sprayer into the nose, but try to avoid touching the inner nasal membranes. Sniff and squeeze the sprayer at the same time. Do not release your grip on the sprayer until you have withdrawn it from your nose; this will prevent nasal mucus and bacteria from entering the plastic bottle and contaminating its contents. After you have sprayed the prescribed number of times in one or both nostrils, gently sniff two or three times.

Unless your doctor has told you otherwise, nose drops and sprays should not be used for more than two or three days at a time. If they have been prescribed for a longer period, do not administer nose drops or sprays from the same container for more than one week. Bacteria from your nose can easily enter the container and contaminate the solution. If you must take medication for more than a week, purchase a new container. Never allow anyone else to use your nose drops or spray.

Inhalers

Aerosol inhalers are used for asthma and other breathing disorders; they assure that a drug gets deep into the lungs where it is most effective. The medication is contained in a pressurized canister that has a mouthpiece attached to it. The drug is actually inhaled into the lungs.

The inhaler must be used properly for maximum benefit. Shake the canister well immediately before using it. Hold the inhaler about two inches from your open mouth and tilt your head back slightly. Next, exhale fully but don't force it. Bring the inhaler to your mouth, close your mouth around the mouthpiece, then breathe in deeply and slowly for four to five seconds while simultaneously depressing the top of the canister fully. Then hold your breath for five to ten seconds after inhaling to allow the drug to settle in the lungs. If another inhalation is prescribed, wait two to five minutes before repeating the procedure.

Clean the inhaler under warm running water at least once a day. Because the contents of the inhaler are pressurized, do not store inhalers near heat or open flame.

Rectal Suppositories

A rectal suppository may be used to relieve the itching, swelling, and pain of hemorrhoids or as a laxative. Regardless of the reason for their use, all rectal suppositories are inserted in the same way.

In extremely hot weather, a suppository may become too soft to handle properly. If this happens, place the suppository inside the refrigerator or in a glass of cool water until firm. A few minutes is usually sufficient. Before inserting a suppository, remove any aluminum wrappings. Rubber finger coverings or disposable rubber gloves may be worn when inserting a suppository, but they are not necessary unless your fingernails are extremely long and sharp.

To insert a suppository, lie on your left side and push the suppository, pointed end first, into the rectum as far as is comfortable. You may feel like defecating, but lie still until the urge has passed. If you cannot insert a suppository, or if the process is painful, coat the suppository with a thin layer of petroleum jelly or mineral oil.

Manufacturers of many suppositories that are used in the treatment of hemorrhoids suggest that the suppositories be stored in the refrigerator. Be sure to ask your pharmacist if the suppositories you have purchased should be stored in the refrigerator.

Vaginal Ointments and Creams

Most vaginal products contain complete instructions for use. If a woman is not sure how to administer vaginal medication, she should ask her pharmacist.

Before using any vaginal ointment or cream, read the directions. They will probably tell you to attach the applicator to the top of the tube and squeeze the tube from the bottom until the applicator is completely filled. Then lie on your back with your knees drawn up. Hold the applicator horizontally or pointed slightly downward and insert it into the vagina as far as it will go comfortably. Press the plunger down to empty the cream or ointment into the vagina. Withdraw the plunger and wash it in warm, soapy water. Rinse it thoroughly and allow it to dry completely. Once it is dry, return the plunger to its package.

Vaginal Tablets and Suppositories

Most packages of vaginal tablets or suppositories include complete directions for use, but you may wish to review these general instructions.

Remove any foil wrapping. Place the tablet or suppository in the applicator that is provided. Lie on your back with your knees drawn up. Hold the applicator horizontally or tilted slightly downward, and insert it into the vagina as far as it will go comfortably. Depress the plunger slowly to release the tablet or suppository into the vagina. Withdraw the applicator and wash it in warm, soapy water. Rinse it and let it dry completely. Once it is dry, return the applicator to its package.

Unless your doctor has told you otherwise, do not douche within the two to three weeks before or after you use vaginal tablets or suppositories.

Throat Lozenges and Discs

Lozenges are made of crystalline sugar; discs are not. Both contain medication that is released in the mouth to soothe a sore throat, to reduce coughing, or to treat laryngitis. Neither should be chewed; they should be allowed to dissolve in the mouth. After the lozenge or disc has dissolved, try not to swallow or drink any fluids for awhile.

Throat Sprays

To administer a throat spray, open your mouth wide and spray the medication as far back as possible. Try not to swallow — hold the spray in your mouth as long as you can and do not drink any fluids for several minutes. Swallowing a throat spray is not harmful. If you find that your throat spray upsets your stomach, don't swallow it; simply spit it out.

Topical Ointments and Creams

Most ointments and creams have only local effects — that is, they affect only the area on which they are applied. Most creams and ointments (especially steroid products, such as hydrocortisone, Lidex, Mycolog, Synalar, Valisone) should be applied to the skin as thinly as possible. A thin layer is as effective as a thick layer, and some steroid-containing creams and ointments can cause toxic side effects if applied too heavily.

Before applying the medication, moisten the skin by immersing it in water or by dabbing the area with a clean, wet cloth. Blot the skin dry and apply the medication as directed. Gently massage it into the skin until it has disappeared. You should feel no greasiness after applying a cream. After applying an ointment, the skin will feel slightly greasy.

If your doctor has not indicated whether you should receive a cream or an ointment, ask your pharmacist for the one you prefer. Creams are greaseless and will not stain your clothing. Creams are best to use on the scalp or other hairy areas of the body. If, however, your skin is dry, ask for an ointment. Ointments help keep the skin soft for a longer period.

If your doctor tells you to place a wrap on top of the skin after the cream or ointment has been applied, you may use a wrap of transparent plastic film like that used for wrapping food. A wrap will hold the medication close to the skin and help keep the skin moist so that the drug can be absorbed. To use a wrap correctly, apply the cream or ointment as directed, then wrap the area with a layer of transparent plastic film. Be careful to follow your doctor's directions. If he or she tells you to leave the wrap in place for a certain length of time, do not leave it in place longer. If you keep a wrap on the skin too long, too much of the drug may be absorbed, which may cause side effects. Do not use such a wrap without your doctor's approval and never on a weeping (oozing) lesion.

Aerosol Sprays

Many topical items are packaged as pressurized aerosol sprays. These sprays usually cost more than the cream or ointment form of the same product. On the other hand, they are useful on very tender or hairy areas of the body where it is difficult to apply a cream or ointment.

Before using an aerosol, shake the can. Hold it upright four to six inches from the skin. Press the nozzle for a few seconds, then release.

Never use an aerosol around the face or eyes. If your doctor tells you to use the spray on a part of your face, apply it to your hand and then rub it into the area. If you get it in your eyes or on a mucous membrane, it can be very painful and may damage your eyes.

Aerosol sprays may feel cold when they are applied. If this sensation bothers you, ask your pharmacist or doctor whether another form of the same product is available.

Transdermal Patches

Transdermal patches allow for controlled, continuous release of medication. They are convenient and easy to use. For best results, apply the patch to a hairless or clean-shaven area of skin, avoiding scars and wounds. Choose a site (such as the chest or upper arm) that is not subject to excessive movement. It is okay to bathe or shower with the patch in place. In the event that the patch becomes dislodged, discard and replace it. Replace a patch by applying a new unit before removing the old one. This will allow for uninterrupted drug therapy. By changing the site of application each time, skin irritation will be minimized. If redness or irritation does develop at the application site, consult your physician. Some people are sensitive to the materials used to make the patches.

Coping with Side Effects

Drugs have certain desirable effects—that's why they are taken. The desirable effects of a drug are known as the drug's activity or therapeutic effects. Drugs, however, have undesirable effects as well. Undesirable effects are called side effects, adverse reactions, or, in some cases, lethal effects. An adverse reaction is any undesirable effect of a drug. It can range from minor side effects to toxic or lethal reactions.

Common Minor Side Effects

Side Effect	Management
Blurred vision	Avoid operating machinery
Decreased sweating	Avoid working or exercising in the sun
Diarrhea	Drink lots of water; if diarrhea lasts longer than 3 days, call your doctor
Dizziness	Avoid operating machinery
Drowsiness	Avoid operating machinery
Dry mouth	Suck on candy or ice chips, or chew gum
Dry nose and throat	Use a humidifier or vaporizer
Fluid retention	Avoid adding salt to foods
Headache	Remain quiet; take aspirin or acetaminophen*
Insomnia	Take last dose of the drug earlier in the day*; drink a glass of warm milk at bedtime; ask your doctor about an exercise program
Itching	Take frequent baths or showers or use wet soaks
Nasal congestion	If necessary, use nose drops*
Palpitations (mild)	Rest often; avoid tension; do not drink coffee, tea, or cola; stop smoking
Upset stomach	Take the drug with milk or food*

*Consult your doctor first.

Some side effects are expected and unavoidable, but others may surprise the doctor as well as the patient. Unexpected reactions may be due to a person's individual response to the drug.

Side effects may fall into one of two major groups—those that are obvious and those that cannot be detected without laboratory testing. The discussion of a drug should not be restricted to its easily recognized side effects; other, less obvious side effects may also be harmful.

If you know a particular side effect is expected from a particular drug, you can relax a little. Most expected side effects are temporary and need not cause alarm. You'll merely experience discomfort or inconvenience for a short time. For example, you may become drowsy after taking an antihistamine or develop a stuffy nose after taking reserpine or certain other drugs that lower blood pressure. Of course, if you find minor side effects especially bothersome, you should discuss them with your doctor, who may be able to prescribe another drug or at least assure you that the benefits of the drug far outweigh its side effects. Sometimes, side effects can be minimized or eliminated by changing your dosage schedule or taking the drug with meals. Consult your doctor or pharmacist before making such a change.

Many side effects, however, signal a serious—perhaps dangerous—problem. If these side effects appear, you should consult your doctor immediately. The following discussion should help you determine whether your side effects require attention from your physician.

OBVIOUS SIDE EFFECTS

Some side effects are obvious to the patient; others can be discerned only through laboratory testing. We have divided our discussion according to the body parts affected by the side effects.

Ear

Although a few drugs may cause loss of hearing if taken in large quantities, hearing loss is uncommon. Drugs that are used to treat problems of the ear may cause dizziness, and many drugs produce tinnitus, a sensation of ringing, buzzing, thumping, or hollowness in the ear. Discuss with your doctor any problem with your hearing or your ears if it persists for more than three days.

Eye

Blurred vision is a common side effect of many drugs. Drugs such as digitalis may cause you to see a "halo" around a lighted object (a television screen or a traffic light), and other drugs may cause night blindness. Indocin anti-inflammatory (used in the treatment of arthritis) may cause impaired vision. Librax antianxiety drug makes it difficult to accurately judge distance while driving and makes the eyes sensitive to sunlight. While the effects on the eye caused by digitalis and Indocin are dangerous signs of toxicity, the effects caused by Librax are to be expected. In any case, if you have difficulty seeing while taking drugs, contact your doctor.

Gastrointestinal System

The gastrointestinal system includes the mouth, esophagus, stomach, small and large intestines, and rectum. A side effect that affects the gastrointestinal system can be expected from almost any drug. Many drugs produce dry mouth, mouth sores, difficulty in swallowing, heartburn, nausea, vomiting, diarrhea, constipation, loss of appetite, or abnormal cramping. Others cause bloating and gas or rectal itching.

Examples of Drugs that May Cause Ulcers

aspirin	Indocin	prednisone
Clinoril	Medrol	

Diarrhea can be expected after taking many drugs. Drugs can create localized reactions in intestinal tissue — usually a more rapid rate of contraction, which leads to diarrhea. Diarrhea caused by most drugs is temporary.

Diarrhea, however, can also signal a problem. For example, some antibiotics may cause severe diarrhea. When diarrhea is severe, the intestine may become ulcerated and begin bleeding. If you develop diarrhea while taking antibiotics, contact your doctor.

Diarrhea produced by a drug should be self-limiting; that is, it should stop within three days. During this time, do not take any diarrhea remedy; drink liquids to replace the fluid you are losing. If diarrhea lasts more than three days, call your doctor.

Examples of Drugs that May Cause Diarrhea

Aldactazide	Flagyl	oral contraceptives
Aldactone	Haldol	Ornade
Aldomet	Inderal	penicillins
aminophylline	Indocin	Pronestyl
ampicillin	Keflex	sulfa drugs
Benadryl	K-Lyte	Tagamet
Clinoril	Lanoxin	Talwin Nx
Coumadin	Minipress	tetracycline
Dyazide	Minocin	Tofranil
erythromycin	oral antidiabetics	Zyloprim

As a side effect of drug use, constipation is less serious and more common than diarrhea. It occurs when a drug slows down the activity of the bowel. Drugs such as Librax slow down bowel activity. Constipation also occurs when drugs absorb moisture in the bowel. It may occur if a drug acts on the nervous system and decreases nerve impulses to the intestine — an effect produced, for example, by a drug such as Aldomet antihypertensive. Constipation produced by a drug may last several days, and you may help relieve it by drinking at least eight glasses of water a day. Do not take laxatives unless your doctor directs you to do so. If constipation continues for more than three days, call your doctor.

Examples of
Drugs that May Cause Constipation

Aldomet	Compazine	Librium
Aldoril	Dilantin	Mellaril
Benadryl	Dyazide	Minipress
Bentyl	Flagyl	Percodan
Catapres	Haldol	Stelazine
Clinoril	Inderal	Valium

Circulatory System

Drugs may speed up or slow down the heartbeat. If a drug slows the heartbeat, you may feel drowsy and tired or even dizzy. If a drug accelerates the heartbeat, you probably will experience palpitations (thumping in the chest). You may feel as though your heart is skipping a beat occasionally, and you may have a headache. For most people, none of these symptoms indicates a serious problem. If, however, they bother you, consult your doctor, who may adjust the dosage of the drug or prescribe other medication.

Some drugs cause edema (fluid retention). When edema forms, fluid from the blood collects outside the blood vessels. Ordinarily, edema is not serious. But if you are steadily gaining weight or have gained more than two or three pounds a week, talk to your doctor.

Examples of Drugs that May Cause Fluid Retention*

Clinoril	Mellaril	prednisone
Compazine	Motrin	Premarin
Elavil	Nalfon	Stelazine
Librax	Naprosyn	sulfa drugs
Librium	Norpace	Tolectin
Medrol	oral contraceptives	Triavil

*Indicated by a weight gain of two or more pounds a week.

Drugs may increase or decrease blood pressure. When blood pressure decreases, you may feel drowsy and tired; you may become dizzy and even faint, especially if you rise suddenly from a reclining position. When blood pressure increases, you may feel dizzy, have a headache or blurred vision, or hear ringing or buzzing in your ears. If you develop any of these symptoms, call your doctor.

Nervous System

Drugs that act on the nervous system may cause drowsiness or stimulation. If a drug causes drowsiness, you may become dizzy or your coordination may be impaired. If a drug causes stimulation, you may become nervous or have insomnia or tremors. Neither drowsiness nor stimulation is cause for concern for most people. When you are drowsy, however, you should be careful around machinery and avoid driving. Some drugs cause throbbing headaches, and others produce tingling in the fingers or toes. These symptoms are generally expected and should disappear in a few days to a week. If they don't, call your doctor.

Examples of Drugs that May Cause Dizziness

Aldactazide	Enduron	Nitrostat
Aldactone	Flagyl	Norpace
Aldomet	Keflex	oral antidiabetics
Ativan	Lomotil	Ornade
Benadryl	Medrol	Tagamet
Bentyl	Minipress	Tofranil
Clinoril	Nitro-Bid	Triavil

Respiratory System

Side effects common to the respiratory system include stuffy nose, dry throat, shortness of breath, and slowed breathing. A stuffy nose and dry throat usually disappear within a few days, but you may use nose drops (consult your doctor first), throat lozenges, or a warm salt-water gargle to relieve them. Shortness of breath is a characteristic side effect of some drugs (for example, Inderal antiarrhythmic). Shortness of breath may continue, but it is not usually serious. Barbiturates or drugs that promote sleep may retard respiration. Slowed breathing is expected, and you should not be concerned as long as your doctor knows about it.

Skin

Skin reactions include rash, swelling, itching, and sweating. Itching, swelling, and rash frequently indicate a drug allergy; you should not continue to take a drug if you have developed an allergy to it. Do, however, consult your doctor before stopping the drug. Some drugs increase sweating; others decrease it. Drugs that decrease sweating may cause problems in hot weather when the body must sweat to reduce body temperature.

If you have a minor skin reaction not diagnosed as an allergy, ask your pharmacist for a soothing cream. Your pharmacist may also suggest that you take frequent baths and dust the sensitive area with a suitable powder.

Another type of skin reaction is photosensitivity (or phototoxicity or sun toxicity) — that is, unusual sensitivity to the sun. Tetracyclines can cause photosensitivity. If, after taking such a drug, you remain exposed to the sun for a brief period of time, say 10 or 15 min-

Examples of
Drugs that May Cause a Mild Rash

Aldactazide	Dyazide	penicillins
Aldactone	Elavil	Pronestyl
Aldoril	Enduron	Stelazine
ampicillin	Haldol	Tagamet
Ativan	Indocin	Tofranil
Benadryl	Librax	Triavil
Catapres	Librium	Valium
Clinoril	Lomotil	Zyloprim

utes, you may receive a severe sunburn. You do not have to stay indoors while taking these drugs, but you should be fully clothed while outside and should use a protective sunscreen while in the sun. Ask your pharmacist to help you choose a protective lotion. Furthermore, you should not remain in the sun too long. Since these drugs may be present in the bloodstream after you stop taking them, you should continue to take these precautions for two days after therapy with these drugs has been completed.

Examples of
Drugs that May Cause Photosensitivity

Bactrim	hydrochlorothiazide	sulfa drugs
Compazine	oral antidiabetics	tetracycline
Enduron	Phenergan	Tofranil

SUBTLE SIDE EFFECTS

Some side effects are difficult to detect. You may not notice any symptoms at all, or you may notice only slight ones. Laboratory testing may be necessary to confirm the existence of such side effects.

Kidneys

If a drug reduces the kidneys' ability to remove chemicals and other substances from the blood, these substances begin to accumulate in body tissues. Over a period of time, this accumulation may cause vague symptoms such as swelling, fluid retention, nausea, headache, or weakness. Obvious symptoms, especially pain, are rare.

Liver

Drug-induced liver damage may result in fat accumulation. Often, liver damage occurs because the drug changes the liver's ability to metabolize other substances. Liver damage may be quite advanced before it produces any symptoms; therefore, periodic tests of liver function are recommended during therapy with certain drugs.

Blood

A great many drugs affect the blood and the circulatory system but do not produce noticeable symptoms for some time. If a drug lowers the level of sugar in the blood, for example, you probably will not have any symptoms for several minutes to an hour. If symptoms develop, they may include tiredness, muscular weakness, and perhaps palpitations or tinnitus (ringing or buzzing in the ears). Low blood levels of potassium produce dry mouth, thirst, and muscle cramps.

Examples of
Drugs that May Cause Blood Disorders*

Aldactazide	oral contraceptives	steroids
Dyazide	Orinase	Tagamet
Elavil	Stelazine	Tofranil
Hygroton	sulfa drugs	Tolinase

*Indicated by a sore throat that doesn't go away in one or two days.

Some drugs decrease the number of red blood cells, which carry oxygen and nutrients throughout the body. If you have too few red blood cells, you have anemia; you may appear pale and feel tired, weak, dizzy, and perhaps hungry.

Some drugs decrease the number of white blood cells, which combat bacteria. Having too few white blood cells increases susceptibility to infection and may prolong illness. If a sore throat or a fever begins after you begin taking a drug and continues for a few days, you may have an infection and too few white blood cells to fight it. Call your doctor.

MANAGEMENT OF SIDE EFFECTS

Consult the drug profiles to determine whether the side effects you are experiencing are minor (relatively common and usually not serious) or major (rare but important signs that something is amiss in your drug therapy). If your side effects are minor, you may be able to compensate for them simply. (See table on page 21 for suggestions.) However, consult your doctor if you find minor side effects particularly annoying.

If you experience any major side effects, contact your doctor immediately. Your dosage may need adjustment, or you may have a sensitivity to the drug. Perhaps you should not be taking the drug at all.

Types of Drugs

Prescription drugs fall into a number of groups according to conditions for which they are prescribed. In the following pages we will provide you with a better understanding of the types of medications that are prescribed for different conditions. We'll describe the intended actions of drugs and the therapeutic effects you can expect from different types of common medications.

ANTI-INFECTIVES

Antibiotics

Antibacterials are used to treat many bacterial infections. Antibiotics, a specific kind of antibacterial, can be derived from molds or produced synthetically. They have the ability to destroy or inhibit the growth of bacteria and fungi. When used properly, antibiotics are usually effective. Antibiotics, however, do not counteract viruses, the major cause of the common cold; using antibiotics in cold therapy is irrational.

To adequately treat an infection, antibiotics must be taken regularly for a specific period of time. If a patient does not take an antibiotic for the prescribed period, the infection may not be resolved, and microorganisms resistant to the antibiotic may appear. Antibiotics include aminoglycosides, cephalosporins, erythromycins, penicillins (including ampicillin and amoxicillin), and tetracyclines.

Antivirals

Antiviral drugs are used to combat virus infections. A new antiviral drug called Zovirax is being used in the management of herpes. Zovirax reduces the reproduction of the herpes virus in initial outbreaks, lessens the number of recurring outbreaks, and speeds the healing of herpes blisters. This antiviral drug, however, does not actually cure herpes.

Vaccines

Vaccines were used long before antibiotics. A vaccine contains weakened or dead disease-causing microorganisms, which activate the body's defense mechanisms to produce a natural immunity against a particular disease such as polio or measles. A vaccine may be used to alleviate or treat an infectious disease, but most commonly it is used to prevent a specific disease.

CONSUMER GUIDE®

Other Anti-infectives

Another group of drugs commonly used to treat infections, especially infections of the urinary tract, includes the synthetically produced sulfonamides and nitrofurantoins (Macrodantin).

Fungal infections are treated with *antifungals,* such as Mycostatin, which destroy and prevent the growth of fungi. Drugs called *anthelmintics* are used to treat worm infestations. A *pediculicide* is a drug used to treat a person infested with lice, and a *scabicide* is a preparation used to treat a person with scabies.

ANTINEOPLASTICS

Also referred to as chemotherapeutics, these drugs are used primarily in the treatment of cancer. These drugs are, without exception, extremely toxic and may cause serious side effects. To many cancer patients, however, the benefits of drug therapy far outweigh the risks involved. Cancer patients may be treated with one or several anticancer drugs. Treatment with more than one drug is called combination chemotherapy; it is used to produce a more effective result.

Some of the anticancer drugs currently available include methotrexate, cisplatin, tamoxifen, and interferon. Most anticancer drugs act by disrupting the growth of cancer cells. Others, like interferon, help to boost the immune system response, thus helping the body to "fight" the cancer. If you will be undergoing chemotherapy, it is important that you discuss in detail with your doctor the use of antineoplastic drugs and that you fully understand the medications you will be taking and the expectations of therapy.

CARDIOVASCULAR DRUGS

Antianginals

The chest pain known as angina occurs when there is an insufficient supply of blood, and consequently of oxygen, to the heart. Antianginal drugs cause a sudden drop in blood pressure and cause an increased amount of oxygen to enter certain parts of the heart. They are used to relieve or prevent angina. Nitroglycerin is the most frequently prescribed antianginal.

Antiarrhythmics

If the heart does not beat rhythmically or smoothly (a condition called arrhythmia), its rate of contraction must be regulated. Antiarrhythmic drugs, including Inderal, Norpace, Pronestyl, and quinidine sulfate, prevent or alleviate cardiac arrhythmias. Dilantin (phenytoin), most frequently used as an anticonvulsant in the treatment of epilepsy, can act as an antiarrhythmic agent when it is injected intravenously.

Anticoagulants

Drugs that prevent blood clotting are called anticoagulants, or blood thinners. Anticoagulants fall into two categories.

The first contains only one drug, heparin. Heparin must be given by injection, so its use is generally restricted to hospitalized patients.

The second category includes oral anticoagulants, principally derivatives of the drug warfarin. Warfarin may be used in the treatment of conditions such as stroke, heart disease, or abnormal blood clotting. It is also used to prevent the movement of a clot, which could cause serious problems. Use of warfarin after a heart attack is controversial. Some physicians believe that anticoagulants are not helpful beyond the first month or two following a heart attack.

Persons taking warfarin must avoid using many other drugs (including aspirin) because their interaction with the anticoagulant could cause internal bleeding. Patients taking warfarin should check with their pharmacist or physician before using any other medications, including over-the-counter products for coughs or colds. In addition, they must have their blood checked frequently by their physician.

Antihypertensives

Briefly, high blood pressure, or *hypertension,* is a condition in which the pressure of the blood against the walls of the blood vessels is higher than what is considered normal. High blood pressure is controllable. Keeping it under control can help prevent other diseases, such as coronary heart disease. Drugs that counteract or reduce high blood pressure can effectively prolong a hypertensive patient's life.

Several different drug actions produce an antihypertensive effect. Some drugs block nerve impulses that cause arteries to constrict; others slow the heart's rate and force of contraction; others reduce the amount of a certain hormone in the blood that causes blood pressure to rise. The mainstay of antihypertensive therapy is often a *diuretic,* a drug that reduces body fluids (see below). Examples of antihypertensive drugs include Aldomet, Aldoril, Catapres, Dyazide, Inderal, Lopressor, Minipress, and Tenormin.

Antilipidemics

Drugs used to treat atherosclerosis (hardening of the arteries) act to reduce the cholesterol and triglycerides (fats) in the blood that form plaques on the walls of the arteries. These drugs are generally prescribed only after dietary therapy and lifestyle changes have failed to lower blood cholesterol to a desirable level. Even then, however, dietary therapy must be continued.

Beta Blockers

Beta-blocking drugs block the response to nerve stimulation in order to slow the heart rate and reduce high blood pressure. They are used in the treatment of angina, hypertension, and arrhythmias. Propranolol (Inderal) and metoprolol (Lopressor) are examples of beta blockers.

Digitalis

Drugs derived from digitalis (for example, digoxin or Lanoxin) affect the heart rate but are not strictly antiarrhythmics. Digitalis slows the heart rate but increases the force of contraction. Thus, digitalis acts as both a heart depressant and a stimulant and may be used to regulate erratic heart rhythm or to increase heart output in heart failure.

Diuretics

Diuretic drugs, such as Aldactazide, Aldactone, Dyazide, Enduron, Esidrix, hydrochlorothiazide, HydroDIURIL, Hygroton, and Lasix, promote the loss of water and salt from the body. They also lower blood pressure by causing blood vessels to expand. Because many antihypertensive drugs cause the body to retain sodium and water, they are often used concurrently with diuretics. Most diuretics act directly on the kidneys, but there are different types of diuretics, each with different actions. Thus, therapy for high blood pressure can be individualized for each patient's specific needs.

Thiazide diuretics are the most popular water pills available today. They are generally well tolerated and can be taken once or twice a day. Thiazide diuretics are effective all day, whereas some diuretics have a shorter duration of action. Patients do not develop a tolerance for the antihypertensive effects of these drugs, so the drugs can be taken for long periods.

A major drawback to thiazide diuretics, however, is that they often deplete potassium. This depletion can be compensated for with a *potassium supplement,* such as K-Lor or Slow-K. Potassium-rich foods and liquids, such as bananas, apricots, and orange juice, can also be used to correct the potassium deficiency. *Salt substitutes* are also sources of potassium. Your doctor will direct you as to which source of potassium, if any, is appropriate for you.

Loop diuretics, such as Lasix, act more vigorously than thiazide diuretics. They promote more water loss but also deplete more potassium.

To remove excess water from the body but retain its store of potassium, manufacturers developed *potassium-sparing diuretics.* Potassium-sparing diuretics, such as Aldactone, are effective in the treatment of potassium loss, heart failure, and hypertension. Potassium-sparing diuretics have been combined with thiazide diuretics in medications such as Aldactazide and Dyazide. Such combinations enhance the antihypertensive effect and reduce the loss of potassium. They are among the most commonly used antihypertensive agents.

Vasodilators

Vasodilating drugs cause the blood vessels to widen. They are used in the treatment of stroke and diseases characterized by poor circulation.

CENTRAL NERVOUS SYSTEM DRUGS

Analgesics

Pain is not a disease but a symptom. Drugs used to relieve pain are called analgesics. We do not fully understand how most analgesics work. Whether they all act in the brain or whether some act outside the brain is not known. Analgesics may be *narcotic* or *nonnarcotic*.

Narcotics are derived from the opium poppy. They act on the brain to cause deep analgesia and often drowsiness. Narcotics relieve coughing spasms and are used in many cough syrups. Narcotics relieve pain and also give the patient a feeling of well-being. They also are addictive.

Many nonnarcotic pain relievers are commonly used. *Salicylates* are the most commonly used pain relievers in the United States today. The most widely used salicylate is aspirin. While aspirin does not require a prescription, many doctors may prescribe it to treat such diseases as arthritis.

The aspirin substitute acetaminophen (Tylenol and Phenaphen, for example) may be used in place of aspirin. It cannot, however, relieve inflammation caused by arthritis, and it is much more toxic if overdoses are taken. Ibuprofen, which is discussed in the section on anti-inflammatory drugs, is also frequently used to relieve pain.

A number of analgesics contain codeine or other narcotics combined with nonnarcotic analgesics, such as aspirin or acetaminophen —for example, Empirin Compound with Codeine, Fiorinal with Codeine, Phenaphen with Codeine, and Tylenol with Codeine. These analgesics are not as potent as pure narcotics, but frequently they are as effective. Because these medications contain narcotics, they have the potential for abuse and must therefore be used with caution.

Anorectics

Amphetamines are commonly used as anorectics, which are drugs used to reduce the appetite. These drugs quiet the part of the brain that causes hunger, but they also keep people awake, speed up the heart rate, and raise blood pressure. After two to three weeks, they lose their effectiveness.

Amphetamines stimulate most people, but they have the opposite effect on hyperkinetic children. Hyperkinesis (the condition of being highly overactive) is difficult to diagnose and define and must be treated by a specialist. When hyperkinetic children take amphetamines or the stimulant Ritalin, their activity slows down. Why amphetamines affect hyperkinetic children in this way is unknown. Most likely, they quiet these youngsters by selectively stimulating parts of the brain that ordinarily provide control of activity.

Anticonvulsants

Drugs such as phenobarbital can effectively control most symptoms of epilepsy. They selectively reduce excessive stimulation in the brain.

Anti-inflammatory Drugs

Inflammation, or swelling, is the body's response to injury; it causes pain, fever, redness, and itching. Common aspirin is one of the most effective anti-inflammatory drugs. Other drugs — Indocin, Motrin (ibuprofen), Nalfon, Naprosyn, and Tolectin — relieve inflammation, but none is more effective than aspirin. Steroids are also used to treat inflammatory diseases.

Gout, however, is one inflammatory disease that can be treated more effectively with other agents, such as probenecid *uricosuric,* colchicine antigout remedy, or Zyloprim antigout remedy. Gout is caused by excessive uric acid, which causes swelling and pain in the toes and joints. Probenecid stimulates excretion of the uric acid in urine; colchicine prevents swelling; and Zyloprim decreases the production of uric acid. Both probenecid and Zyloprim guard against attacks of gout; they do not relieve the pain of an attack as does colchicine.

When sore muscles tense up, they cause pain and inflammation. *Skeletal muscle relaxants* — Equagesic and Norgesic — can relieve these symptoms. Skeletal muscle relaxants often are given with an anti-inflammatory drug, such as aspirin. Some doctors believe that aspirin and rest alleviate the pain and inflammation of muscle strain more effectively than do skeletal muscle relaxants.

Antiparkinson Agents

Parkinson's disease is a progressive disease that is due to a chemical imbalance in the brain. Victims of Parkinson's disease have uncontrollable tremors, develop a characteristic stoop, and eventually become unable to walk. Drugs such as Cogentin anticholinergic and levodopa are used to correct the chemical imbalance and thereby relieve the symptoms of the disease. They are also used to relieve tremors caused by other drugs.

Local Anesthetics

Local anesthetics are another type of pain-relieving drug. Local anesthetics are applied directly to a painful area and relieve such localized pain as toothaches, earaches, and hemorrhoidal pain. Local anesthetics do not relieve major, generalized pain, and many people are allergic to them. Some local anesthetics, such as lidocaine, are also useful in the treatment of heart disease when given by intravenous or intramuscular injection because they restore the heartbeat to normal.

Sedatives

All drugs used in the treatment of anxiety or insomnia selectively reduce activity in the central nervous system. Drugs that have a calming effect include Atarax, barbiturates, Librium, Serax, Sinequan,

Tranxene, and Valium. Drugs to induce sleep in insomniacs include Dalmane and Durapam.

Tranquilizers

Psychotics usually receive *major tranquilizers* or *antipsychotic agents*. These drugs calm certain areas of the brain but permit the rest of the brain to function normally. They act as a screen that allows transmission of some nerve impulses but restricts others. The drugs most frequently used are *phenothiazines,* such as Mellaril and Stelazine.

Psychotic patients sometimes become depressed. In such cases, *antidepressants,* such as Elavil, or *monoamine oxidase inhibitors* are used to combat the depression.

Antidepressants may produce dangerous side effects and may interact with other drugs or foods. For example, monoamine oxidase inhibitors greatly increase blood pressure when taken with certain kinds of cheese or other foods or beverages.

DRUGS FOR THE EARS

For an ear infection, a physician usually prescribes an antibiotic and a steroid—for example, Cortisporin otic suspension. The antibiotic attacks infecting bacteria, and the steroid reduces inflammation and pain. Often, a local anesthetic, such as benzocaine or lidocaine, may be prescribed to relieve pain.

DRUGS FOR THE EYES

Almost all drugs that are used to treat eye problems can be used to treat disorders of other parts of the body as well.

Glaucoma is one of the major disorders of the eye—especially for people over age 40. It is caused by increased pressure within the eyeball. Although sometimes treated surgically, glaucoma often can be resolved—and blindness prevented—through the use of eye drops. Two drops frequently used are epinephrine and pilocarpine. Pilocarpine is a *cholinergic* drug. Cholinergic drugs act by stimulating the body's parasympathetic nerve endings. These are nerve endings that assist in the control of the heart, lungs, bowels, and eyes. Epinephrine is an *adrenergic* agent. Drugs with adrenergic properties have actions similar to those of adrenaline. Adrenaline is secreted in the body when one must flee from danger or resist attack or combat stress. Adrenaline increases the blood sugar level, accelerates the heartbeat, and dilates the pupils.

Antibiotics usually resolve eye infections. Steroids can be used to treat eye inflammations as long as they are not used for too long. Pharmacists carefully monitor requests for eye drop refills, particularly for drops that contain steroids, and may refuse to refill such medication until the patient has revisited the doctor.

GASTROINTESTINAL DRUGS

Anticholinergics

Anticholinergic drugs—for example, Bentyl—slow the action of the bowel and reduce the amount of stomach acid. Because these drugs slow the action of the bowel by relaxing the muscles and relieving spasms, they are said to have an *antispasmodic* action.

Antidiarrheals

Diarrhea may be caused by many conditions, including influenza and ulcerative colitis, and can sometimes occur as a side effect to drug therapy. Narcotics and anticholinergics are used in the treatment of diarrhea because they slow the action of the bowel. An antidiarrheal such as Lomotil combines a narcotic with an anticholinergic.

Antinauseants

Antinauseants reduce the urge to vomit. Perhaps the most effective antinauseants are *phenothiazine derivatives*, such as Compazine. Compazine antinauseant is often administered rectally (in suppository form) and usually alleviates acute nausea and vomiting within a few minutes to an hour.

Antihistamines are also commonly used to prevent nausea and vomiting, especially when those symptoms are due to motion sickness.

Antiulcer Medications

Antiulcer medications are prescribed to relieve the symptoms and promote the healing of a peptic ulcer. The *antisecretory* ulcer medication Tagamet works by suppressing the production of excess stomach acid. Another antiulcer drug, Carafate, works by forming a chemical barrier over an exposed ulcer — rather like a "bandage" — thus protecting the ulcer from stomach acid. These medications provide sustained relief of ulcer pain and also promote healing.

HORMONES

A hormone is a substance produced and secreted by a gland. Hormones stimulate body functions. Hormone drugs are given to mimic the effects of hormones naturally produced by the body.

Diabetic Drugs

Insulin, which is secreted by the pancreas, regulates the level of sugar in the blood and the metabolism of carbohydrates and fats.

Insulin's counterpart, *glucagon,* stimulates the liver to produce glucose, or sugar. Both insulin and glucagon must be present in the right amounts to maintain a proper blood sugar level in the body.

Treatment of diabetes (the condition in which the body is unable to supply and/or utilize insulin) may involve an adjustment of diet and/or the administration of insulin. Glucagon is given only in emergencies (for example, insulin shock when the blood sugar must be raised quickly).

Oral antidiabetic drugs, including Diabinese, Glucotrol, Micronase, Orinase, and Tolinase, induce the pancreas to secrete more insulin by acting on small groups of cells within the pancreas that make and store insulin. Oral antidiabetics are used by diabetics who cannot follow a diet program and do not need to use insulin. These drugs cannot be used by insulin-dependent (juvenile-onset) diabetics, who can only control their diabetes with injections of insulin.

Sex Hormones

Although the adrenal glands secrete small amounts of sex hormones, these hormones are produced mainly by the sex glands. *Estrogens* are the female hormones responsible for secondary sex characteristics, such as development of the breasts, maintenance of the lining of the uterus, and enlargement of the hips at puberty. *Testosterone* (also called androgen) is the corresponding male hormone. It is responsible for secondary sex characteristics, such as beard growth and enlargement of muscles. *Progesterone* is produced in females and prepares the uterus for pregnancy.

Testosterone causes retention of protein in the body, thereby producing an increase in muscle size. Athletes sometimes take drugs called anabolic steroids, similar to testosterone, for this effect, but such use of these drugs is dangerous. Anabolic steroids can adversely affect the heart, nervous system, and kidneys.

Most *oral contraceptives*, or birth control pills, combine estrogen and progesterone, but some contain only progesterone. The estrogen in birth control pills prevents egg production. Progesterone aids in preventing ovulation, alters the lining of the uterus, and thickens cervical mucus — processes which help to prevent conception. Oral contraceptives have many side effects; their use should be discussed with a doctor.

Premarin estrogen hormone is used to treat symptoms of menopause. Provera progesterone hormone is used for uterine bleeding and menstrual problems.

Steroids

The pituitary gland secretes *adrenocorticotropic hormone* (ACTH), which directs the adrenal glands to produce glucocorticoids, such as hydrocortisone and other steroids. Steroids help fight inflammation, and ACTH may be injected to treat inflammatory diseases.

Oral steroid preparations (for example, Medrol and prednisone) may also be used to treat inflammatory diseases, such as arthritis, and to treat poison ivy, hay fever, and insect bites.

Steroids also may be applied to the skin. Hydrocortisone and Lidex are topical (applied to the skin) steroid hormone preparations.

CONSUMER GUIDE®

Thyroid Drugs

Thyroid hormone was one of the first hormone drugs to be produced synthetically. Originally, thyroid preparations were made by drying the thyroid glands of animals and pulverizing them into tablets. Such preparations are still used today in the treatment of patients who have reduced levels of thyroid hormone production. However, a synthetic thyroid hormone (Synthroid) is also available.

Drugs, such as propylthiouracil, and radioactive-iodine therapy are used to slow down thyroid hormone production in patients who have excessive amounts of the hormone.

RESPIRATORY DRUGS

Allergy Medication

Antihistamines counteract the symptoms of an allergy by blocking the effects of histamine, a chemical released in the body that typically causes swelling and itching. For mild respiratory allergies such as hay fever, antihistamines like Benadryl can be used. Benadryl and other antihistamines are slow-acting. Injectable epinephrine, which is fast-acting, will often be prescribed for severe allergy attacks.

Antitussives

Antitussives control coughs. Dextromethorphan is a nonnarcotic medication that controls the cough from a cold. Another antitussive drug is the narcotic codeine. Most cough drops and syrups must be absorbed into the blood and must circulate through the brain before they act on a cough; they do not "coat" the throat and should be taken with a glass of water.

Bronchodilators

Bronchodilators (agents that relax airways in the lungs) and *smooth muscle relaxants* (agents that relax smooth muscle tissue, such as that in the lungs) are also used to improve breathing. Theophylline is commonly used to relieve the symptoms of asthma and pulmonary emphysema. Aminophylline is often given to patients with pulmonary emphysema or chronic bronchitis.

Decongestants

Decongestants constrict the blood vessels in the nose and sinuses in order to open up air passages. Decongestants can be taken by mouth or as nose drops or spray. Oral decongestants are slow-acting but do not interfere with the production of mucus or the movement of the cilia in the respiratory tract. They do increase blood pressure. Topical decongestants (nose drops or spray) provide almost immediate relief. They do not increase blood pressure as much as oral decongestants, but they do slow the movement of the cilia. People who use these topical products may also develop a tolerance for them. Consequently, they should not be used for more than a few days at a time.

Expectorants

Expectorants are used to change a nonproductive cough to a productive one (one that brings up phlegm). Expectorants are supposed to increase the amount of mucus produced. However, the effectiveness of some expectorants has been questioned. Drinking water or using a vaporizer or humidifier may be as effective in increasing mucus. Popular expectorant products include Phenergan expectorant.

TOPICAL DRUGS

Dry skin is a very common complaint. One way to treat it is to add moisture to the air with a humidifier. Another is to soak in water, blot the skin dry, and apply a lotion, cream, or oil in order to seal in the moisture.

Dermatologic problems, such as infection or inflammation, are also common ailments. Antibiotics are used to treat skin infections; steroids are used to treat inflammations.

Another common dermatologic problem is acne. Acne can be — and often is — treated with over-the-counter drugs, but it sometimes requires prescription medications. Over-the-counter drugs generally contain agents that open blocked skin pores. Antibiotics, such as the tetracyclines, erythromycin, or clindamycin, are used orally or applied topically to prevent pimple formation. *Keratolytics,* agents that soften the skin and cause the outer cells to slough off, are also sometimes prescribed. Tretinoin (Retin A), a skin irritant derived from vitamin A, is also used topically in the treatment of acne.

Isotretinoin, also related to vitamin A, is available in an oral form, called Accutane, and is used to treat severe cystic acne that has not responded to other treatment.

VITAMINS AND MINERALS

Vitamins and minerals are chemical substances vital to the maintenance of normal body function. Vitamin deficiencies do occur, but most people get enough vitamins and minerals in their diet. Serious nutritional deficiencies, such as pellagra and beriberi, must be treated by a physician. People who have an inadequate or restricted diet, those with certain disorders or debilitating illnesses, women who are pregnant or breast-feeding, and some others may benefit from taking supplemental vitamins and minerals. Even these people, however, should consult a doctor to see if a true vitamin deficiency exists.

Drug Profiles

On the following pages are drug profiles for the most commonly prescribed drugs in the United States. These profiles are arranged alphabetically.

A drug profile summarizes the most important information about a particular drug. By studying a drug profile, you will learn what to expect from your medication, when to be concerned about possible side effects, which drugs interact with the drug you are taking, and how to take the drug to achieve its maximum benefit. You may notice that some drugs have longer lists of side effects than do other drugs. This may sometimes indicate that one drug does indeed have the potential to cause a greater number of side effects than does another drug. On the other hand, an extensive listing of possible side effects may simply be a result of the drug having been on the market for a greater length of time and having been used by a greater number of people. In other words, the more people who take a particular drug and the longer it's been in use, the greater the chance that new side effects will be identified.

Each drug profile includes the following information:

Name. Most of the drugs profiled in this book are listed by trade name; those drugs commonly known or prescribed by their generic names (such as insulin, tetracycline, penicillin) are listed generically. All trade name drugs can be identified by an initial capital letter; generics, by an initial lower-case letter. The chemical or pharmacological class is listed for each drug after its name.

Manufacturer. The manufacturer of each trade name product is identified. "Various manufacturers" is listed for generic drugs; most generics are generally available from several different manufacturers.

Ingredients. The components of each drug product are itemized. Many drugs contain several active chemical components, all of which are included in this category.

Equivalent Products. Products with the same chemical formulation as the profiled drug, including both trade name and generic drugs, are listed as equivalent products. If your prescription is for a product that has equivalents, ask your physician to write your prescription using the generic name. This will enable your pharmacist to fill the prescription with the least expensive equivalent available. Remember, however, that not all drugs have equivalents and that your doctor may have a good reason for prescribing a specific trade name drug. For more information about generic and equivalent products, see the section on Generic Drugs, page 10.

Dosage Forms. The most common forms (i.e., tablets, capsules, liquid, suppositories) of each profiled drug are listed, along with the color of the tablets or capsules. Strengths or concentrations are also given. Colors for liquids and suppositories are not included.

Use. This category includes the most important and most common clinical uses for each profiled drug. Your doctor may prescribe a drug for a reason that does not appear in this category. This exclusion does not mean that your doctor has made an error. If the use for which you are taking a drug does not appear in this category, and if you have any questions concerning the reason for which the drug was prescribed, consult your doctor.

Minor Side Effects. The most common and least serious reactions to a drug are found in this category. Most of these side effects, if they occur, disappear in a day or two. Do not expect to experience these minor side effects, but if they occur and are particularly annoying, do not hesitate to seek medical advice. For advice on how to cope with or relieve some of these side effects, look to the "Comments" section.

Major Side Effects. Should the reactions listed as "Major Side Effects" occur, you should call your doctor. These reactions indicate that something may be going wrong with your drug therapy. You may have developed an allergy to the drug, or some other problem could have developed. Many drugs can cause blood disorders; anti-infective agents may suppress the growth of some infecting microorganisms while allowing others to proliferate wildly; some medications may cause peptic ulcers. If you experience a major side effect, it may be necessary to adjust your dosage or substitute a different drug in your treatment. Major side effects are less common than minor side effects, and you will probably never experience them, but if you do, consult your doctor immediately.

Contraindications. Some drugs are counterproductive when taken by people with certain conditions, i.e., they should not be taken by people with these conditions. These conditions are listed under "Contraindications." If the profiled drug has been prescribed for you and you have a condition listed in this category, consult your doctor.

Warnings. This category lists the precautions necessary for safe use of the profiled drug. For example, certain conditions, while not contraindicating use of the drug, do demand close monitoring. Pregnant women, children under 12, the elderly, people with liver or kidney disease, and those with heart problems must use many drugs cautiously. In some cases, these people will have to have frequent lab tests while taking drugs; in other cases, the doctor will monitor dosages carefully. The "Warnings" category also lists drugs that can interact with the profiled drug. Certain drugs are safe when used alone but may cause serious reactions when taken with other drugs or chemicals, or with certain foods. In this category, you'll also find out whether the profiled drug is likely to affect your ability to drive, whether you are likely to become tolerant to its effects, and whether any laboratory tests are included in the usual course of therapy with the drug. If you have any questions about the precautions, possible interactions, or recommended tests discussed in this category, be sure to consult your doctor or pharmacist.

Comments. While the information in the "Contraindications" and "Warnings" categories reflects that included in the official package inserts, the information in "Comments" is more general and concerns use of the profiled drug. For example, you'll find out if you can avoid

CONSUMER GUIDE®

stomach upset by taking the drug with meals or with milk or if you can avoid sleeplessness by taking a drug early in the day. You'll find out how to deal with certain side effects, such as dizziness or light-headedness or mouth dryness. You may also find out whether you should take the drug around the clock or only during waking hours. Other information included might concern supplemental therapy, such as drinking extra fluids while treating a urinary infection, wearing cotton panties while treating a vaginal infection, or using a protective sunscreen while taking a drug that increases your sensitivity to sunlight. "Comments" might also include information about the price of the drug, equivalent products, or methods of administering the drug. This kind of information should guide you in using the profiled drug. Never be reluctant to ask your doctor or pharmacist for further information about any drug you are taking.

**Accurbron bronchodilator (Merrell Dow Pharmaceuticals, Inc.),
see theophylline bronchodilator.**

Accutane acne preparation

Manufacturer: Roche Dermatologics
Ingredient: isotretinoin (13-*cis*-retinoic acid)
Dosage Form: Capsule: 10 mg (pink); 20 mg (maroon); 40 mg (yellow)
Use: Treatment of severe cystic acne
Minor Side Effects: Changes in skin color; conjunctivitis; dry lips and mouth; fatigue; headache; increased susceptibility to herpes simplex virus; increased susceptibility to sunburn; indigestion; inflammation of lips; muscle pain and stiffness; peeling of palms and soles; rash; swelling; thinning of hair
Major Side Effects: Abdominal pain; black stools; bruising; burning or tingling sensation of the skin; changes in menstrual cycle; dizziness; hives; increased susceptibility to bone changes; respiratory infections; severe diarrhea; skin infection; visual disturbances; weight loss
Contraindications: This drug should not be used by any woman who is, who thinks she is, or who intends to become, pregnant. Use of this drug in any amount for even short periods during pregnancy is associated with an extremely high risk of fetal abnormalities and spontaneous abortion. • You should receive both oral instructions and a patient information sheet with this drug; you may also be asked to sign a consent form prior to therapy. • This drug should not be used by women who are breast-feeding. Be sure your doctor knows if you are breast-feeding a baby. • This drug should not be used by people who are allergic to parabens (a preservative). Consult your doctor immediately if this drug has been prescribed for you and any of these conditions applies to you.
Warnings: This drug may increase blood fat levels (triglycerides, lipoproteins, cholesterol), especially in overweight or diabetic persons, in persons with increased alcohol intake, and in persons with a family history of high blood fat levels. Reduce or eliminate alcohol consumption while taking this medication. • This drug may cause you to become especially sensitive to the sun. Be sure to avoid sun exposure, and use an effective sunscreen when outdoors. • Because this drug is a form of vitamin A, do not continue to take vitamin A supplements while taking Accutane. • Inform your doctor if you wear contact lenses. This drug may reduce your tolerance to them. • This drug may interfere with blood transfusions. If you give or receive blood, make sure your doctor knows you are taking this drug.
Comments: During the course of treatment with this drug, occasionally there may be an apparent increase in skin lesions with crusting. This is usually not a reason to discontinue its use. • This drug may affect the results of blood and urine tests. If you are scheduled to have any such tests, remind your doctor that you are taking this drug. • This drug is usually used only after other acne treatments have failed. • This drug is most effective when taken with meals. • Do not crush or chew the capsules. • Store away from light.

acetaminophen with codeine analgesic

Manufacturer: various manufacturers
Ingredients: acetaminophen; codeine phosphate
Equivalent Products: Aceta with Codeine, Century Pharmaceuticals, Inc.; Capital with Codeine, Carnrick Laboratories, Inc.; Codap, Reid-Rowell; Empracet with Codeine, Burroughs Wellcome Co.; Myapap with Codeine, My-K Labs; Papadeine, Vangard Laboratories; Phenaphen with Codeine, A. H. Robins Company; Proval, Reid-Rowell; Tylenol with Codeine, McNeil Con-

sumer Products Co.; Ty-Pap with Codeine, Major Pharmaceuticals; Ty-Tab, Major Pharmaceuticals

Dosage Forms: Capsule (various dosages and colors; see Comments). Liquid (content per 5 ml teaspoon): acetaminophen, 120 mg and codeine, 12 mg. Tablet (various dosages and colors; see Comments)

Use: Symptomatic relief of mild to severe pain, depending on strength

Minor Side Effects: Constipation; difficulty in urinating; dizziness; drowsiness; dry mouth; flushing; light-headedness; nausea; rash; sweating; vomiting

Major Side Effects: Anxiety; bleeding or bruising; breathing difficulties; excitation; fatigue; jaundice; low blood sugar; palpitations; rapid or slow heartbeat; restlessness; sore throat; tremors; weakness

Contraindication: This drug should not be taken by people who are allergic to either acetaminophen or narcotic pain relievers. Consult your doctor immediately if this drug has been prescribed for you and you have such an allergy.

Warnings: This drug should be used cautiously by children under 12; by the elderly; by people who have heart or lung disease, blood disorders, asthma or other respiratory problems, epilepsy, head injuries, liver or kidney disease, colitis, gall bladder disease, thyroid disease, acute abdominal conditions, or prostate disease; and by pregnant or nursing women. Be sure your doctor knows if any of these conditions applies to you. • This drug may cause drowsiness; avoid tasks that require alertness. • To prevent oversedation, avoid the use of alcohol or other drugs that have sedative properties. • Because this product contains codeine, it has the potential for abuse and must be used with caution. It usually should not be taken for more than ten days. Tolerance may develop quickly; do not increase the dose without consulting your doctor.

Comments: The name of this drug is often followed by a number that refers to the amount of codeine present. Hence, #1 contains $\frac{1}{8}$ grain (gr) or 7.5 mg codeine; #2 has $\frac{1}{4}$ gr (15 mg); #3 has $\frac{1}{2}$ gr (30 mg); and #4 contains 1 gr (60 mg) codeine. • Notify your doctor if you develop signs of jaundice (yellow eyes or skin; dark urine). • Side effects caused by this drug may be somewhat relieved by lying down. • Avoid use of any other drugs that contain acetaminophen, codeine, or other narcotics. If you have questions about the contents of your medications, ask your doctor or pharmacist.

Aceta with Codeine analgesic (Century Pharmaceuticals, Inc.), see acetaminophen with codeine analgesic.

Achromycin V antibiotic (Lederle Laboratories), see tetracycline hydrochloride antibiotic.

Adalat antianginal (Miles Pharmaceutical), see Procardia antianginal.

Adapin antidepressant and antianxiety (Pennwalt Pharmaceutical Division), see Sinequan antidepressant and antianxiety.

Adsorbocarpine ophthalmic preparation (Alcon Laboratories, Inc.), see Isopto Carpine ophthalmic preparation.

Advil anti-inflammatory (Whitehall Laboratories, Inc.), see ibuprofen anti-inflammatory.

Aerolate bronchodilator (Fleming & Co.), see theophylline bronchodilator.

Akarpine ophthalmic preparation (Akorn, Inc.), see Isopto Carpine ophthalmic preparation.

AK-Spore H.C. Otic preparation (Akorn, Inc.), see Cortisporin Otic preparation.

AK-Spore ophthalmic antibiotic preparation (Akorn, Inc.), see Neosporin Ophthalmic antibiotic preparation.

Alatone diuretic and antihypertensive (Major Pharmaceuticals), see Aldactone diuretic and antihypertensive.

Aldactazide diuretic and antihypertensive

Manufacturer: Searle & Co.
Ingredients: spironolactone; hydrochlorothiazide
Equivalent Products: Spironazide, Henry Schein, Inc.; spironolactone with hydrochlorothiazide, various manufacturers (see Comments); Spirozide, Rugby Laboratories
Dosage Form: Tablet: spironolactone, 25 mg and hydrochlorothiazide, 25 mg (tan); spironolactone, 50 mg and hydrochlorothiazide, 50 mg (tan)
Uses: Treatment of high blood pressure; congestive heart failure; cirrhosis of the liver accompanied by edema or ascites or both; removal of tissue fluid
Minor Side Effects: Cramping; deepened voice; diarrhea; dizziness; drowsiness; dry mouth; fatigue; hairiness; headache; increased urination; itching; loss of appetite; nausea; rash; restlessness; sun sensitivity; vomiting
Major Side Effects: Blood disorders; blurred vision; breast enlargement (in both sexes); bruising; confusion; diabetes; difficulty in achieving erection; elevated blood sugar; elevated calcium; elevated potassium; elevated uric acid; fever; gout; impotence; irregular heartbeat; irregular menses; jaundice; low blood pressure; low potassium; low sodium; lupus erythematosus; muscle spasm; sore throat; stumbling; sudden weight gain; tingling in fingers and toes; weakness
Contraindications: This drug should not be taken by people who are allergic to either of its ingredients or to sulfa drugs. Consult your doctor immediately if this drug has been prescribed for you and you have such an allergy. • This drug should not be taken by people who have severe kidney disease, hyperkalemia (high blood levels of potassium), anuria (inability to urinate), or liver failure. Be sure your doctor knows if any of these conditions applies to you.
Warnings: This drug should be used with caution by people with certain liver diseases, by those about to undergo surgery, and by pregnant women and nursing mothers. Be sure your doctor knows if any of these conditions applies to you. • This drug interacts with colestipol hydrochloride, digitalis, lithium carbonate, oral antidiabetics, potassium salts, and steroids. If you are currently taking any drugs of these types, consult your doctor about their use. If you are unsure of the type or contents of your medications, ask your doctor or pharmacist. • In large doses, spironolactone has been shown to cause cancer in rats. This has not been shown to occur in humans. • Do not take potassium supplements while taking this drug. • This drug may cause diarrhea, stomach cramps, skin rash, thirst, lethargy, menstrual abnormalities, deepening of the voice, and breast enlargement. Notify your doctor if any of these effects occurs. • Because of its effects on water and salt balance in the body, people taking this drug should have routine blood tests. If you develop signs of an imbalance — dry mouth, thirst, weakness, confusion, muscle cramps, or lack of urine — call your doctor.

Comments: Unlike some diuretics, Aldactazide diuretic rarely causes potassium loss. Hence, the need for potassium supplements may be eliminated. • This drug causes frequent urination. Expect this effect; it should not alarm you. • When taking this drug, as with many drugs that lower blood pressure, you should limit your consumption of alcoholic beverages in order to prevent dizziness or light-headedness. • Persons taking digitalis in addition to this drug should watch carefully for symptoms of increased digitalis effects (e.g., nausea, blurred vision, palpitations) and notify their doctor immediately if symptoms occur. • Notify your doctor if you develop signs of jaundice (yellow eyes or skin; dark urine). • If you have high blood pressure, do not take any nonprescription item for weight control, cough, cold, or sinus problems without first checking with your doctor. Such items may include ingredients that can increase blood pressure. • A doctor probably should not prescribe this drug or other "fixed dose" combination products as the first choice in the treatment of high blood pressure. The patient should receive each of the individual ingredients singly, and if the response is adequate to the fixed dose contained in this product, it can then be substituted. The advantage of a combination product is increased convenience to the patient. • There are a few "generic brands" of spironolactone with hydrochlorothiazide. Consult your pharmacist; some of them are not generically equivalent to this drug. • This drug must be taken exactly as directed. Do not take extra doses or skip a dose without first consulting your doctor.

Aldactone diuretic and antihypertensive

Manufacturer: Searle & Co.
Ingredient: spironolactone
Equivalent Products: Alatone, Major Pharmaceuticals; spironolactone, various manufacturers
Dosage Form: Tablet: 25 mg (yellow); 50 mg (orange); 100 mg (peach)
Uses: Treatment of high blood pressure and low blood levels of potassium; removal of fluid from the tissues; diagnosis and treatment of primary hyperaldosteronism
Minor Side Effects: Cramping; diarrhea; dizziness; drowsiness; dry mouth; headache; increased urination; nausea; rash; restlessness; vomiting; weakness
Major Side Effects: Confusion; deepened voice; difficulty in achieving or maintaining an erection; elevated chloride; elevated potassium; breast enlargement (in both sexes); fever; hairiness; impotence; irregular heartbeat; irregular menses; low salt; postmenopausal bleeding; sudden weight gain; tingling in fingers and toes; uncoordinated movements
Contraindications: This drug should not be used by persons with anuria (inability to urinate), acute renal failure, significant impairment of renal function, or hyperkalemia (high blood levels of potassium). Be sure your doctor knows if any of these conditions applies to you.
Warnings: This drug should be used with caution by pregnant women, nursing mothers, and people with kidney disease. Be sure your doctor knows if any of these conditions applies to you. • In large doses, spironolactone has been shown to cause cancer in rats. This has not been shown to occur in humans. • When this drug is taken with potassium salts or other diuretics or antihypertensive agents, extreme caution should be used. If you are currently taking any drugs of these types, consult your doctor about their use. If you are unsure of the type or contents of your medications, ask your doctor or pharmacist. • This drug may cause diarrhea, stomach cramps, skin rash, thirst, lethargy, menstrual abnormalities, deepening of the voice, and breast enlargement. Notify your doctor if any of these effects occurs.
Comments: Unlike many diuretics, this drug does not cause potassium loss. Potassium supplements should be avoided unless your doctor prescribes them

for you. Most persons do not require extra potassium while taking this medication. • This drug causes frequent urination. Expect this effect; it should not alarm you. • While taking this drug, as with many drugs that lower blood pressure, you should limit your consumption of alcoholic beverages. Because this drug can cause dizziness and drowsiness, use caution when driving, operating machinery, or performing other tasks that require alertness. To avoid dizziness or light-headedness when you stand, contract and relax the muscles of your legs for a few moments before rising. Do this by pushing one foot against the floor while raising the other foot slightly, alternating feet so that you are "pumping" your legs in a pedaling motion. • Persons taking digitalis in addition to this drug should watch carefully for symptoms of increased digitalis effects (e.g., nausea, blurred vision, palpitations), and notify their doctor immediately if symptoms occur. • If you have high blood pressure, do not take any nonprescription item for weight control, cough, cold, or sinus problems without first checking with your doctor. Such items may include ingredients that can increase blood pressure. • Take this drug exactly as directed. Do not take extra doses or skip a dose without consulting your doctor first. • If this drug upsets your stomach, it may be taken with food or milk.

Aldomet antihypertensive

Manufacturer: Merck Sharp & Dohme
Ingredient: methyldopa
Equivalent Product: methyldopa, various manufacturers
Dosage Forms: Oral suspension (content per 5 ml teaspoon): 250 mg. Tablet: 125 mg; 250 mg; 500 mg (all are yellow)
Use: Treatment of high blood pressure
Minor Side Effects: Bloating; blurred vision; confusion; constipation; decreased sexual ability; diarrhea; dizziness; dry mouth; gas; headache; inflamed salivary glands; light-headedness; nasal congestion; nausea; sedation; sore tongue; tremors; vomiting; weakness
Major Side Effects: Anemia; breast enlargement (in both sexes); breathing difficulties; chest pain; dark urine; depression; distention; fever; fluid retention; insomnia; jaundice; liver disorders; liver and urine test abnormalities; loss of appetite; nightmares; numbness or tingling; reduction in number of white blood cells; severe, continuing stomach cramps; slow pulse; sore joints; unusual body movements
Contraindications: This drug should not be taken by people with active liver disease, such as acute cirrhosis or acute hepatitis, or by persons who have had liver reactions from this drug before. Be sure your doctor knows if you have such a condition. • This drug should not be taken by people who are allergic to it. Consult your doctor immediately if this drug has been prescribed for you and you have such an allergy.
Warnings: This drug should be used with extreme caution by persons who have had a stroke and by persons who have angina, heart disease, kidney disease, depression, Parkinson's disease, or a history of liver disease or dysfunction. Be sure your doctor knows if you have ever had any of these conditions. • You should receive liver function tests periodically as long as you are taking this drug in order to monitor its effects. • This drug should be used cautiously by women who may become pregnant, by pregnant women, and by nursing mothers. • This drug may interfere with lab tests. Be sure your doctor knows that you are taking this drug if you are going to have any tests done. Many patients taking this drug react positively to the Coombs' blood test, indicating destruction of red blood cells or allergy. Often the test is false positive, and no disorder is present, but you should have periodic blood tests as long as you are taking this drug. • Remind your doctor if you have been or are being treated for gout. •

This drug should be used with caution in conjunction with other antihypertensive drugs. • This drug should not be taken with amphetamines or decongestants. If you are currently taking any drugs of these types, consult your doctor about their use. Do not take any nonprescription item for weight control, cough, cold, or sinus problems without first checking with your doctor. Such items may include ingredients that can increase blood pressure. If you are unsure of the type or contents of your medications, ask your doctor or pharmacist. • This drug may interfere with blood transfusions. If you give or receive blood, be sure to tell the doctor you are taking this drug. • Do not discontinue taking this drug unless directed to do so by your doctor, because high blood pressure can return very quickly. • This drug may cause drowsiness, especially during the first few days of use; avoid tasks that require alertness, such as driving or operating machinery.

Comments: Mild side effects (e.g., nasal congestion) are noticeable during the first two weeks of therapy and become less bothersome after this period. • If you develop a fever or jaundice (yellow eyes or skin; dark urine) while taking this drug, call your doctor. • To avoid dizziness or light-headedness when you stand, contract and relax the muscles of your legs for a few moments before rising. Do this by pushing one foot against the floor while raising the other foot slightly, alternating feet so that you are "pumping" your legs in a pedaling motion. • Notify your doctor if any unexplained, prolonged general tiredness occurs; it may be a sign of a blood side effect. • Occasionally, tolerance to this drug may develop, usually between the second and third month of therapy. Your doctor can deal with this circumstance. • Take this drug exactly as directed. Do not take extra doses or skip a dose without first consulting your doctor. • Intake of alcoholic beverages should be limited while taking this drug to prevent dizziness and light-headedness.

Aldoril diuretic and antihypertensive

Manufacturer: Merck Sharp & Dohme
Ingredients: hydrochlorothiazide; methyldopa
Equivalent Product: methyldopa and hydrochlorothiazide, various manufacturers
Dosage Form: Tablet: Aldoril 15: hydrochlorothiazide, 15 mg and methyldopa, 250 mg (salmon); Aldoril 25: hydrochlorothiazide, 25 mg and methyldopa, 250 mg (white); Aldoril D30: hydrochlorothiazide, 30 mg and methyldopa, 500 mg (salmon); Aldoril D50: hydrochlorothiazide, 50 mg and methyldopa, 500 mg (white)
Use: Treatment of high blood pressure
Minor Side Effects: Bloating; breast swelling; constipation; cramping; decrease in sexual desire; diarrhea; dizziness; dry mouth; gas; headache; impotence; increased urination; light-headedness; loss of appetite; nasal congestion; nausea; sedation; slow pulse; sore tongue; sun sensitivity; tremors; vomiting
Major Side Effects: Anemia; blood disorders; blurred vision; breathing difficulties; bruising; chest pain; dark urine; depression; elevated blood sugar; fever; fluid retention; hyperuricemia (elevated uric acid in the blood); hypokalemia (low blood potassium); irregular heartbeat; jaundice; joint pain; liver disease; muscle spasm; nightmares; psychosis; rash; sore throat; stroke; tingling in fingers and toes; weakness
Contraindications: This drug should not be taken by people who are allergic to either of its components or to sulfa drugs. Consult your doctor immediately if this drug has been prescribed for you and you have such an allergy. If you are unsure of the type of contents of your medications, ask your doctor or pharmacist. • This drug should not be used by people with active liver disease (e.g.,

acute hepatitis or active cirrhosis) or severe kidney disease. Be sure your doctor knows if you have either of these conditions.

Warnings: This drug should be used with caution by persons who have had a stroke; by persons who have liver disease, anemia, depression, Parkinson's disease, allergies, asthma, or kidney diseases; and by persons who are on kidney machines. Be sure your doctor knows if any of these conditions applies to you. • Use of this drug may cause fever, lupus erythematosus, jaundice, liver disease, stroke, low white cell levels, low blood levels of potassium and sodium, calcium retention, diabetes, and gout. If you develop jaundice (yellow eyes or skin; dark urine) or body salt imbalance (characterized by thirst, dry mouth, muscle weakness, or cramps), call your doctor. • This drug may affect urine tests, lab tests, and thyroid tests. Be sure your doctor knows you are taking this drug before you undergo any testing. • This drug should be used with caution by pregnant women and nursing mothers. • This drug should be used cautiously with other blood pressure drugs; it also interacts with amphetamine, anesthetics, colestipol hydrochloride, curare, decongestants, digitalis, lithium carbonate, oral antidiabetics, and steroids. If you are currently taking any drugs of these types, consult your doctor about their use. If you are unsure about the type or contents of your medications, ask your doctor or pharmacist. • Many patients react positively to the Coombs' test, which is often done as part of blood transfusions. The positive reaction usually indicates an allergy or destruction of red blood cells. Often, however, the test is false positive and no disorder is present. Have periodic blood tests as long as you take this drug. • If you must have surgery, or are going to give or receive blood, be sure your doctor knows you are taking this drug.

Comments: While taking this drug, do not take any nonprescription item for weight control, cough, cold, or sinus problems without first checking with your doctor. Such items may contain ingredients that can increase blood pressure. • Mild side effects (e.g., nasal congestion) are most noticeable during the first two weeks of therapy and become less bothersome after this period. • While taking this product, you should limit your consumption of alcoholic beverages in order to prevent dizziness or light-headedness. • To avoid dizziness or light-headedness when you stand, contract and relax the muscles of your legs for a few moments before rising. Do this by pushing one foot against the floor while raising the other foot slightly, alternating feet so that you are "pumping" your legs in a pedaling motion. • This drug can cause potassium loss. Symptoms of potassium loss include dry mouth, thirst, and muscle cramps. To help avoid potassium loss, take this drug with a glass of fresh or frozen orange juice. You may also eat a banana each day. The use of a salt substitute helps prevent potassium loss. Do not change your diet, however, without consulting your doctor. Too much potassium may also be dangerous. • This drug may interfere with the treatment of diabetes. Be sure your doctor knows you are taking this drug. • Persons taking this product and digitalis should watch carefully for symptoms of increased digitalis effects (e.g., nausea, blurred vision, palpitations), and notify their doctor immediately if symptoms occur. • Remind your doctor if you have been or are being treated for gout if this drug is prescribed for you. • This drug may interfere with the measurement of blood uric acid. • A doctor probably should not prescribe this drug or other "fixed dose" products as the first choice in the treatment of high blood pressure. The patient should receive each ingredient singly, and if the response is adequate to the fixed dose contained in this product, it can then be substituted. The advantage of a combination product is increased convenience to the patient. • Take this product exactly as directed. Do not take extra doses or skip a dose without consulting your doctor first.

Allerest 12 Hour antihistamine and decongestant (Pharmacraft), see Ornade Spansules antihistamine and decongestant.

allopurinol antigout drug (various manufacturers), see Zyloprim antigout drug.

Alupent bronchodilator

Manufacturer: Boehringer Ingelheim
Ingredient: metaproterenol sulfate
Equivalent Product: Metaprel, Sandoz Pharmaceuticals
Dosage Forms: Inhaler (metered dose). Oral syrup (content per 5 ml teaspoon): 10 mg. Solution for inhalation: 0.6%; 5%. Tablet: 10 mg (white); 20 mg (white)
Use: For symptomatic treatment of asthma and bronchospasm associated with bronchitis and emphysema
Minor Side Effects: Bad taste in mouth; dizziness; dry mouth and throat; fear; headache; insomnia; nausea; nervousness; restlessness; sweating; tension; vomiting; weakness
Major Side Effects: Breathing difficulties; chest pain; confusion; difficulty in urinating; flushing; muscle cramps; palpitations; trembling
Contraindications: This drug should not be used by persons allergic to it or by persons with heart arrhythmias. Consult your doctor if this drug has been prescribed for you and you have either of these conditions.
Warnings: This drug must be used with caution by diabetics; by persons with high blood pressure, certain types of heart disease, or hyperthyroidism; and by pregnant or nursing women. Be sure your doctor knows if any of these conditions applies to you. • The inhaler forms of this drug should not be used by children under 12 years of age. The tablet form of this drug is not recommended for children under six years of age. • This drug has been shown to interact with monamine oxidase inhibitor antidepressants, antihistamines, beta blockers, and anesthetics. If you are currently taking any of these drugs, consult your doctor about their use. If you are unsure about the type or contents of your medications, ask your doctor or pharmacist. • Prolonged or excessive use of this drug may reduce its effectiveness. Take this drug as prescribed. Do not take it more often than prescribed without first consulting your physician. It may be necessary to temporarily stop using this drug for a short period to ensure its effectiveness.
Comments: If your symptoms do not improve, or if they worsen while taking this drug, or if dizziness or chest pain develop, contact your doctor. • Make sure you know how to use the inhaler properly. Ask your pharmacist for a demonstration and a patient instruction sheet. In addition, check the section entitled Administering Medications Correctly in this book to ensure that you are using the inhaler properly. • If more than one inhalation is prescribed, wait at least one full minute between inhalations for maximum effectiveness. • Store the inhaler away from heat and open flame. Do not puncture, break, or burn the container. • If stomach upset occurs while taking the tablets or solution, take the drug with food or milk. • To help relieve dry mouth, chew gum or suck on ice chips or hard candy.

Alzapam antianxiety and sedative (Major Pharmaceuticals), see Ativan antianxiety and sedative.

Amacodone analgesic (Trimen Laboratories, Inc.), see Vicodin analgesic.

amantadine HCl antiviral and antiparkinson (Rugby Laboratories), see Symmetrel antiviral and antiparkinson.

Amaril "D" decongestant and antihistamine (Vortech Pharmaceutical, Ltd.), see Naldecon decongestant and antihistamine.

Amcill antibiotic (Parke-Davis), see ampicillin antibiotic.

Amen progesterone hormone (Carnrick Laboratories, Inc.), see Provera progesterone hormone.

aminophylline bronchodilator

Manufacturer: various manufacturers

Ingredient: aminophylline

Equivalent Products: Amoline, Major Pharmaceuticals; Phyllocontin, The Purdue Frederick Company; Somophyllin, Fisons Corporation; Somophyllin-DF, Fisons Corporation; Truphylline, G & W Laboratories, Inc.

Dosage Forms: Liquid; Rectal solution; Suppository; Sustained-release tablet; Tablet (various dosages and colors)

Uses: To relieve and/or prevent bronchial asthma; treatment of symptoms of chronic bronchitis and emphysema

Minor Side Effects: Diarrhea; drowsiness; gastrointestinal disturbances (stomach pain, nausea, vomiting); headache; insomnia; irritability; loss of appetite; muscle twitches; nervousness or restlessness

Major Side Effects: Bloody or black, tarry stools; breathing difficulties; convulsions; flushing; high blood sugar; low blood pressure; palpitations; rapid or irregular heart rate

Contraindications: This drug should not be taken by people who are allergic to it or similar drugs or by those who have an active peptic ulcer. Consult your doctor immediately if this drug has been prescribed for you and either of these conditions applies.

Warnings: Excessive doses of this drug are toxic, so follow your doctor's dosage instructions exactly. • This drug should be used cautiously by pregnant women, the elderly, and people who have heart disease, thyroid disease, liver disease, high blood pressure, or a history of peptic ulcer. Be sure your doctor knows if any of these conditions applies to you. • Some children are unusually sensitive to aminophylline; this drug should be used cautiously by children. • This drug should be used cautiously in conjunction with lithium carbonate, propranolol, cimetidine, diazepam, chlordiazepoxide, certain antibiotics, ephedrine, high blood pressure drugs, certain sedatives, or other xanthines; if you are currently taking any drugs of these types, consult your doctor about their use. If you are unsure of the type or contents of your medications, ask your doctor or pharmacist. • While taking this drug, do not use any nonprescription item for asthma without first checking with your doctor. • Call your doctor if you develop severe stomach pain, vomiting, or restlessness; you may need to have your dosage changed.

Comments: While taking this drug, you may need to have periodic blood tests to determine the amount of drug in your system. The results are used to guide your dosing. Discuss this with your doctor. • While taking this drug, drink at least eight glasses of water daily. • Be sure to take your dose at exactly the right time. • If this drug upsets your stomach, it may be taken with food or milk. • Avoid drinking coffee, tea, cola drinks, cocoa, or other beverages that contain caffeine, and avoid eating large amounts of chocolate, since the side effects of aminophylline may be increased. • Do not crush or chew the sustained-release forms of this drug; swallow them whole. • Be sure your doctor knows if you smoke if you are taking this drug. Do not stop or start smoking without informing your doctor. • Aminophylline tablets, liquid, and rectal solution should be stored at room temperature in tightly closed containers. The suppositories should be stored in a cool place. This medication should never be frozen.

Amitril antidepressant (Parke-Davis), see amitriptyline antidepressant.

amitriptyline antidepressant

Manufacturer: various manufacturers
Ingredient: amitriptyline hydrochloride
Equivalent Products: Amitril, Parke-Davis; Elavil, Merck Sharp & Dohme; Emitrip, Major Pharmaceuticals; Endep, Roche Products Inc.
Dosage Form: Tablet: 10 mg; 25 mg; 50 mg; 75 mg; 100 mg; 150 mg
Use: Relief of depression
Minor Side Effects: Agitation; blurred vision; confusion; constipation; cramps; diarrhea; dizziness; drowsiness; dry mouth; fatigue; headache; heartburn; increased sensitivity to light; insomnia; loss of appetite; nausea; peculiar tastes; restlessness; sweating; vomiting; weakness; weight gain or loss
Major Side Effects: Bleeding; convulsions; difficulty in urinating; enlarged or painful breasts (in both sexes); fainting; fever; fluid retention; hair loss; hallucinations; high or low blood pressure; imbalance; impotence; jaundice; mood changes; mouth sores; nervousness; nightmares; numbness in fingers or toes; palpitations; psychosis; ringing in the ears; seizures; skin rash; sleep disorders; sore throat; stroke; tremors; uncoordinated movements
Contraindications: This drug should not be taken by people who are allergic to it, by those who have had a heart attack, or by those who are taking monoamine oxidase inhibitors (ask your pharmacist if you are unsure of the contents of your medications). Consult your doctor immediately if this drug has been prescribed for you and any of these conditions applies.
Warnings: This drug is not recommended for use by children under age 12. • This drug should be used cautiously by pregnant or nursing women and by people who have glaucoma (certain types), heart disease (certain types), high blood pressure, enlarged prostate, epilepsy, urine retention, liver disease, or hyperthyroidism. Be sure your doctor knows if any of these conditions applies to you. • This drug should be used cautiously by patients who are receiving electroshock therapy or those who are about to undergo surgery. • Close medical supervision is required when this drug is taken with guanethidine or Placidyl hypnotic. • This drug may cause changes in blood sugar levels. Diabetics should monitor their blood sugar levels more frequently when first taking this medication. • This drug interacts with alcohol, amphetamine, barbiturates, clonidine, epinephrine, oral anticoagulants, phenylephrine, and depressants; if you are currently taking any drugs of these types, consult your doctor about their use. If you are unsure of the type or contents of your medications, ask your doctor or pharmacist. • This drug may cause drowsiness; avoid tasks that require alertness. • To prevent oversedation, avoid the use of alcohol or other drugs that have sedative properties. • Report any sudden mood changes to your doctor.
Comments: Take this medicine exactly as your doctor prescribes. Do not stop taking it without first checking with your doctor. • While taking this drug, do not take any nonprescription item for weight control, cough, cold, or sinus problems without first checking with your doctor. Be sure your doctor is aware of every medication you use; do not stop or start any other drug without your doctor's approval. • This drug may cause the urine to turn blue-green; this is harmless. • Notify your doctor if you develop signs of jaundice (yellow eyes or skin; dark urine). • The effects of therapy with this drug may not be apparent for two to four weeks. Your doctor may adjust your dosage frequently during the first

few months of therapy to find the best dose for you. • Chew gum or suck on ice chips or a piece of hard candy to reduce mouth dryness. • Avoid long exposure to the sun while taking this drug. • To avoid dizziness or light-headedness when you stand, contract and relax the muscles of your legs for a few moments before rising. Do this by pushing one foot against the floor while raising the other foot slightly, alternating feet so that you are "pumping" your legs in a pedaling motion. • Many people receive as much benefit from taking a single dose of this drug at bedtime as from taking multiple doses throughout the day. Talk to your doctor about this. • This drug is very similar in action to other antidepressants (desipramine, imipramine). If one antidepressant is ineffective or not well tolerated, your doctor may want you to try one of the others.

Amoline bronchodilator (Major Pharmaceuticals), see aminophylline bronchodilator.

amoxicillin antibiotic

Manufacturer: various manufacturers
Ingredient: amoxicillin
Equivalent Products: Amoxil, Beecham Laboratories; Larotid, Beecham Laboratories; Polymox, Bristol Laboratories; Trimox, E. R. Squibb & Sons, Inc.; Utimox, Parke-Davis; Wymox, Wyeth-Ayerst Laboratories
Dosage Forms: Capsule: 250 mg; 500 mg (various colors). Chewable tablet: 125 mg; 250 mg (various colors). Drop (content per ml): 50 mg. Oral suspension (content per 5 ml teaspoon): 125 mg; 250 mg
Use: Treatment of a wide variety of bacterial infections
Minor Side Effects: Diarrhea; gas; loss of appetite; nausea; vomiting
Major Side Effects: Breathing difficulties; fever; joint pain; mouth sores; rash; rectal and vaginal itching; severe diarrhea; sore throat; superinfection
Contraindication: This drug should not be taken by people who are allergic to penicillin-type drugs. Consult your doctor immediately if this drug has been prescribed for you and you have such an allergy.
Warnings: This drug should be used cautiously by pregnant or nursing women and by people who have kidney or liver disease, asthma, severe hay fever, or other significant allergies. Be sure your doctor knows if you have any of these conditions. • Complete blood cell counts and liver and kidney function tests are advisable if you take this drug for a prolonged period of time. • This drug should not be used in conjunction with allopurinol, chloramphenicol, erythromycin, or tetracycline; if you are currently taking any drugs of these types, consult your doctor about their use. If you are unsure of the contents of your medications, ask your doctor or pharmacist. • Severe allergic reactions to this drug (indicated by breathing difficulties and a drop in blood pressure) have been reported with the injectable form but are rare when the drug is taken orally. Notify your doctor if a rash develops. • Prolonged use of this drug may allow organisms that are not susceptible to it to grow wildly. Do not use this drug unless your doctor has specifically told you to do so. Be sure to follow directions carefully and report any unusual reactions to your doctor at once. • In some women, use of certain antibiotics can cause vaginal yeast infections. Contact your doctor if vaginal itching occurs while taking this drug.
Comments: This drug is similar in nature to penicillin and ampicillin. • This drug should be taken as long as prescribed, even if symptoms disappear within that time. For maximum effect, take this drug at even intervals around the clock. • The liquid form of this drug should be stored in the refrigerator. Shake well before using. Discard any unused portion after 14 days. • Diabetics using Clinitest urine test may get a false high sugar reading while taking this drug.

Change to Clinistix, Diastix, Chemstrip UG, or Tes-Tape urine test to avoid this problem. • Amoxicillin can be taken either on an empty stomach or with food or milk (in order to prevent stomach upset).

Amoxil antibiotic (Beecham Laboratories), see amoxicillin antibiotic.

ampicillin antibiotic

Manufacturer: various manufacturers
Ingredient: ampicillin
Equivalent Products: Amcill, Parke-Davis; D-Amp, Dunhall Pharmaceuticals, Inc.; Omnipen, Wyeth-Ayerst Laboratories; Polycillin, Bristol Laboratories; Principen, E. R. Squibb & Sons, Inc.; Totacillin, Beecham Laboratories
Dosage Forms: Capsule: 250 mg; 500 mg (various colors). Oral suspension (content per 5 ml teaspoon): 100 mg; 125 mg; 250 mg; 500 mg
Use: Treatment of a wide variety of bacterial infections
Minor Side Effects: Diarrhea; gas; loss of appetite; nausea; vomiting
Major Side Effects: Abdominal pain; black tongue; breathing difficulties; bruising; cough; fever; mouth irritation; rash; rectal and vaginal itching; severe diarrhea; sore throat; superinfection
Contraindication: This drug should not be taken by people who are allergic to penicillin-type drugs. Consult your doctor immediately if this drug has been prescribed for you and you have such an allergy.
Warnings: This drug should not be used in conjunction with allopurinol, chloramphenicol, erythromycin, or tetracycline; if you are currently taking any drugs of these types, consult your doctor about their use. If you are unsure of the contents of your medications, ask your doctor or pharmacist. • This drug should be used cautiously by pregnant women and by people who have liver or kidney disease, mononucleosis, asthma, severe hay fever, or other significant allergies. Be sure your doctor knows if any of these conditions applies to you. • Complete blood cell counts and liver and kidney function tests are advisable if you take this drug for an extended period of time. • Severe allergic reactions to this drug (indicated by breathing difficulties and a drop in blood pressure) have been reported with the injectable form but are rare when the drug is taken orally. Notify your doctor if a rash develops. • This drug may affect the potency of oral contraceptives. Consult your doctor about using supplementary contraceptive measures while you are taking this drug.
Comments: This drug is similar in nature and action to penicillin and amoxicillin. • This drug should be taken as long as prescribed, even if symptoms disappear within that time. • The liquid form of this drug should be stored in the refrigerator. Shake well before using. Any unused portion should be discarded after 14 days. • Take the drug on an empty stomach (one hour before or two hours after a meal). For maximum effect, take this drug at even intervals around the clock. • Diabetics using Clinitest urine test may get a false high sugar reading while taking this drug. Change to Clinistix, Diastix, Chemstrip UG, or Tes-Tape urine test to avoid this problem.

Anaprox anti-inflammatory (Syntex Laboratories, Inc.), see Naprosyn anti-inflammatory.

Anodynos-DHC analgesic (Forest Pharmaceuticals, Inc.), see Vicodin analgesic.

Antivert antinauseant

Manufacturer: Roerig
Ingredient: meclizine hydrochloride
Equivalent Products: Antrizine, Major Pharmaceuticals; meclizine hydrochloride, various manufacturers; Ru-Vert-M, Reid-Provident Laboratories, Inc.; (see Comments)
Dosage Forms: Chewable tablet: 25 mg (pink). Tablet: 12.5 mg (blue and white); 25 mg (yellow and white); 50 mg (yellow and blue)
Uses: To provide symptomatic relief of dizziness due to ear infections; to prevent or relieve dizziness and nausea due to motion sickness
Minor Side Effects: Blurred vision; drowsiness; dry mouth; headache; insomnia; loss of appetite; nervousness; ringing in the ears; upset stomach
Major Side Effects: Breathing difficulties; fever; painful urination; palpitations; skin rash; sore throat
Contraindications: This drug should be used in pregnant or nursing women only when clearly necessary. If you are pregnant or nursing, discuss the use of this drug with your doctor or pharmacist. • This drug should not be taken by people who are allergic to it. Consult your doctor immediately if this drug has been prescribed for you and you have such an allergy.
Warnings: This drug is not recommended for use by children under 12. • This drug should be used cautiously by people with asthma, glaucoma, stomach ulcer, urinary tract blockage, or prostate trouble. Be sure your doctor knows if you have any of these conditions. • This drug may cause drowsiness; avoid tasks that require alertness. • To prevent oversedation, avoid the use of other sedative drugs or alcohol.
Comments: When used for motion sickness, this drug should be taken one hour before travel, then once every 24 hours during travel. • Although most brands of this drug require a prescription, nonprescription forms are also available. Ask your doctor or pharmacist about them.

Antrizine antinauseant (Major Pharmaceuticals), see Antivert antinauseant.

Anucort steroid-hormone-containing anorectal product (G & W Laboratories, Inc.), see Anusol-HC steroid-hormone-containing anorectal product.

Anugard-HC steroid-hormone-containing anorectal product (Vangard Laboratories), see Anusol-HC steroid-hormone-containing anorectal product.

Anumed HC steroid-hormone-containing anorectal product (Major Pharmaceuticals), see Anusol-HC steroid-hormone-containing anorectal product.

Anusol-HC steroid-hormone-containing anorectal product

Manufacturer: Parke-Davis
Ingredients: benzyl benzoate; bismuth resorcin compound; bismuth subgallate; hydrocortisone acetate; Peruvian balsam; zinc oxide
Equivalent Products: Anucort, G & W Laboratories, Inc.; Anugard-HC, Vangard Laboratories; Anumed HC, Major Pharmaceuticals; hemorrhoidal HC, various manufacturers; Rectacort, Century Pharmaceuticals, Inc.; see Comments

Dosage Forms: Cream: hydrocortisone acetate, 0.5%; bismuth subgallate, 2.25%; bismuth resorcin, 1.75%; benzyl benzoate, 1.2%; zinc oxide, 11%; Peruvian balsam, 1.8%. Suppository: hydrocortisone acetate, 10 mg; bismuth subgallate, 2.25%; bismuth resorcin compound, 1.75%; benzyl benzoate, 1.2%; zinc oxide, 11%; Peruvian balsam, 1.8%

Use: Relief of pain, itching, and discomfort arising from hemorrhoids and irritated anorectal tissues

Minor Side Effect: Burning sensation on application

Major Side Effects: Local inflammation or infection at site of application

Contraindication: This drug should not be used by people who are allergic to any of its ingredients. Consult your doctor immediately if this drug has been prescribed for you and you have such an allergy.

Warnings: This drug should be used with caution by pregnant women. Pregnant women should not use the product unnecessarily, in large amounts, or for prolonged periods. ● If irritation develops, discontinue use of this drug and notify your doctor. ● This drug should be used with caution by children and infants. ● Do not use this drug in the eyes.

Comments: This drug should not be used for more than seven consecutive days, unless your doctor specifically says to do so. If symptoms do not improve after seven days, or if bleeding or seepage occurs while taking this drug, contact your doctor. ● To maintain normal bowel function, drink plenty of fluids, eat a balanced diet, and exercise regularly. Avoid excessive use of laxatives; stool softeners may be helpful. Ask your doctor about them. ● The suppository form of this drug should be stored in a cool, dry place. ● This medicine may stain your clothing; the stain may be removed by washing with laundry detergent. ● There are other steroid-containing anorectal products available—such as Proctocort, Proctofoam-HC, and Corticaine—that have the same action as this drug although their ingredients are somewhat different.

Anxanil antianxiety (Econo Med, Inc.), see Atarax antianxiety.

Aquaphyllin bronchodilator (Ferndale Laboratories, Inc.), see theophylline bronchodilator.

Aquatensen diuretic and antihypertensive (Wallace Laboratories), see Enduron diuretic and antihypertensive.

Armour Thyroid hormone (Rorer Pharmaceuticals), see thyroid hormone.

Asmalix bronchodilator (Century Pharmaceuticals, Inc.), see theophylline bronchodilator.

Aspirin with Codeine analgesic (Halsey Drug Co., Inc.), see Empirin with Codeine analgesic.

Atarax antianxiety

Manufacturer: Roerig
Ingredient: hydroxyzine hydrochloride
Equivalent Products: Anxanil, Econo Med, Inc.; Atozine, Major Pharmaceuticals; Durrax, Dermik Laboratories, Inc.; hydroxyzine hydrochloride, various manufacturers; Vamate (see Comments), Major Pharmaceuticals; Vistaril (see Comments), Pfizer Laboratories Division

Dosage Forms: Syrup (content per 5 ml teaspoon): 10 mg. Tablet: 10 mg (orange); 25 mg (green); 50 mg (yellow); 100 mg (red). See Comments

Uses: Symptomatic relief of anxiety and tension; treatment of itching caused by allergic conditions

Minor Side Effects: Drowsiness; dry mouth

Major Side Effects: Breathing difficulties; chest tightness; convulsions; skin rash; sore throat; tremors

Contraindications: Do not take this drug if you are allergic to it or if you are pregnant. Consult your doctor immediately if the drug has been prescribed for you and either of these conditions applies.

Warnings: This drug should not be used in conjunction with central nervous system depressants, alcohol, or other drugs that have sedative properties; if you are currently taking any drugs of these types, consult your doctor about their use. If you are unsure of the type or contents of your medications, ask your doctor or pharmacist. • This drug may cause drowsiness, especially during the first few days of therapy; avoid tasks that require alertness. • Use of this drug by nursing mothers is not recommended.

Comments: The generic name for Vistaril and Vamate is hydroxyzine pamoate. Both Vistaril and Vamate are available in capsule form (25 mg; 50 mg; 100 mg); Vistaril is also available in suspension form (25 mg per 5 ml teaspoon). Although not generically identical, these products have the same therapeutic effects as Atarax antianxiety and other hydroxyzine hydrochloride products. • Chew gum or suck on ice chips or a piece of hard candy to reduce mouth dryness.

Ativan antianxiety and sedative

Manufacturer: Wyeth-Ayerst Laboratories

Ingredient: lorazepam

Equivalent Products: Alzapam, Major Pharmaceuticals; Loraz, Quantum Pharmics; lorazepam, various manufacturers

Dosage Form: Tablet: 0.5 mg; 1 mg; 2 mg (all are white)

Uses: Relief of anxiety, tension, agitation, irritability, and insomnia

Minor Side Effects: Blurred vision; change in appetite; constipation; depression; diarrhea; dizziness; drowsiness; dry mouth; headache; increased salivation; nausea; rash; unsteadiness; weakness

Major Side Effects: Breathing difficulties; decreased hearing; difficulty in urinating; disorientation; eye function disturbance; fever; hallucinations; jaundice; menstrual irregularities; mouth sores; palpitations; slurred speech; sore throat

Contraindications: This drug should not be used by people who are allergic to it. Consult your doctor immediately if this drug has been prescribed for you and you have such an allergy. • This drug should not be used by people with acute narrow-angle glaucoma or severe mental disorder. Be sure your doctor knows if you have either of these conditions.

Warnings: This drug should be used cautiously by the elderly; children under 12; pregnant or nursing women; and people with impaired liver or kidney function or with certain diseases of the heart, stomach, or lungs. Be sure your doctor knows if any of these conditions applies to you. • This drug may cause drowsiness; avoid tasks that require alertness. • To prevent oversedation, avoid the use of alcohol or other drugs that have sedative properties. • Do not stop taking this drug suddenly without consulting your doctor; if you have been taking this drug for long periods or in high doses, withdrawal symptoms may occur with abrupt cessation. It will be necessary to reduce your dosage gradually. • This drug has the potential for abuse and must be used with caution. Tolerance may develop quickly; do not increase the dose without first consulting

CONSUMER GUIDE®

your doctor. • Persons taking this drug for long periods should have periodic blood and liver function tests. • This drug is safe when used alone. When it is combined with other sedatives, serious adverse reactions may develop. This drug may also interact with cimetidine, phenytoin, levodopa, lithium, and anticoagulants.

Comments: This drug is currently used by many people to relieve nervousness. It is effective for this purpose, but it is important to try to remove the cause of anxiety as well. • Notify your doctor if you develop signs of jaundice (yellow eyes or skin; dark urine). • Chew gum or suck on ice chips or a piece of hard candy to reduce mouth dryness. • Take with food or a full glass of water if stomach upset occurs. • It may take two or three days before this drug's full effects become apparent.

Atozine antianxiety (Major Pharmaceuticals), see Atarax antianxiety.

Augmentin antibiotic

Manufacturer: Beecham Laboratories
Ingredients: amoxicillin, clavulanic acid
Dosage Forms: Chewable Tablet: Augmentin 125: amoxicillin, 125 mg and clavulanic acid, 31.25 mg (yellow); Augmentin 250: amoxicillin, 250 mg and clavulanic acid, 62.5 mg (yellow). Oral suspension (content per 5 ml teaspoon): Augmentin 125: amoxicillin, 125 mg and clavulanic acid, 31.25 mg; Augmentin 250: amoxicillin, 250 mg and clavulanic acid, 62.5 mg. Tablet: Augmentin 250: amoxicillin, 250 mg and clavulanic acid, 125 mg (white); Augmentin 500: amoxicillin, 500 mg and clavulanic acid, 125 mg (white)
Use: Treatment of a wide variety of bacterial infections
Minor Side Effects: Diarrhea; gas; loss of appetite; nausea; vomiting
Major Side Effects: Breathing difficulties; fever; joint pain; mouth sores; rash; rectal or vaginal itching; severe diarrhea; sore throat; superinfection
Contraindication: This drug should not be taken by people who are allergic to penicillin-type drugs. Consult your doctor immediately if this drug has been prescribed for you and you have such an allergy.
Warnings: This drug should be used cautiously by people who have kidney or liver disease, asthma, severe hay fever, or other significant allergies. Be sure your doctor knows if you have any of these conditions. • Complete blood cell counts and liver and kidney function tests are advisable if you take this drug for a prolonged period of time. • This drug should not be used in conjunction with allopurinol, chloramphenicol, erythromycin, or tetracycline; if you are currently taking any drugs of these types, consult your doctor about their use. If you are unsure of the contents of your medications, ask your doctor or pharmacist. • Severe allergic reactions to this drug (indicated by breathing difficulties and a drop in blood pressure) have been reported but are rare when the drug is taken orally. • Prolonged use of this drug may allow organisms that are not susceptible to it to grow wildly. Do not use this drug unless your doctor has specifically told you to do so. Be sure to follow directions carefully and report any unusual reactions to your doctor at once.
Comments: This drug is similar in nature to penicillin, ampicillin, and amoxicillin. • This drug should be taken for at least ten full days, even if symptoms disappear within that time. • The clavulanic acid enables the amoxicillin to be more effective than amoxicillin alone in treating certain bacterial infections. • The liquid form of this drug should be stored in the refrigerator. Shake well before using. Discard the unused portion after ten days. • Diabetics using Clinitest urine tests may get a false high sugar reading while taking this drug.

Change to Clinistix, Diastix, Chemstrip UG, or Tes-Tape urine test to avoid this problem.

Azo-Standard analgesic (Webcon Drug Co.), see Pyridium analgesic.

B-A-C #3 analgesic (Mayrand, Inc.), see Fiorinal with Codeine analgesic.

Bacticort Suspension ophthalmic preparation (Rugby Laboratories), see Cortisporin ophthalmic preparation.

Bactrim and Bactrim DS antibacterials

Manufacturer: Roche Laboratories
Ingredients: sulfamethoxazole; trimethoprim
Equivalent Products: Bethaprim SS and Bethaprim DS, Major Pharmaceuticals; Cotrim and Cotrim DS, Lemmon Company; Septra and Septra DS, Burroughs Wellcome Co.; SMZ-TMP, various manufacturers; sulfamethoxazole and trimethoprim, various manufacturers; Sulfatrim and Sulfatrim DS, various manufacturers; Uroplus DS and Uroplus SS, Shionogi USA
Dosage Forms: Double-strength (DS) tablet: trimethoprim, 160 mg and sulfamethoxazole, 800 mg (white). Liquid (content per 5 ml teaspoon): trimethoprim, 40 mg and sulfamethoxazole, 200 mg. Tablet: trimethoprim, 80 mg and sulfamethoxazole, 400 mg (green)
Uses: Treatment of urinary tract infections, certain respiratory infections, and middle-ear infections; prevention of traveler's diarrhea
Minor Side Effects: Abdominal pain; depression; diarrhea; dizziness; headache; loss of appetite; nausea; sore mouth; sun sensitivity; vomiting
Major Side Effects: Anemia; arthritis; bleeding; blood disorders; breathing difficulties; convulsions; difficulty in urinating; fever; fluid retention; hallucinations; itching; jaundice; kidney disease; rash; ringing in the ears; sore throat; tingling in hands or feet; weakness
Contraindications: This drug should not be taken by people who are allergic to either ingredient, by those with folate deficiency anemia, or by women who are pregnant or nursing. Consult your doctor immediately if any of these conditions applies to you. • This drug should not be used by infants under two months old.
Warnings: This drug should be used cautiously by elderly patients who also take diuretics. • This drug may cause allergic reactions and should, therefore, be used cautiously by people who have asthma, severe hay fever, or other significant allergies. People who have certain vitamin deficiencies or who have liver or kidney disease should also use this drug with caution. Be sure your doctor knows if any of these conditions applies to you. • This drug should not be used to treat strep throat. • This drug can cause blood diseases; notify your doctor immediately if you experience fever, sore throat, or skin discoloration, as these can be early signs of blood disorders. • Complete blood cell counts and liver and kidney function tests should be done if you take this drug for a prolonged period. • This drug should not be used in conjunction with barbiturates, cyclophosphamide, isoniazid, local anesthetics, methenamine hippurate, methenamine mandelate, methotrexate, oral anticoagulants, oral antidiabetics, oxacillin, para-aminobenzoic acid (PABA), penicillins, phenylbutazone, phenytoin, or probenecid; if you are currently taking any drugs of these types, consult your doctor or pharmacist.
Comments: This drug should be taken for as long as prescribed, even if

symptoms disappear within that time. • To be most effective, this drug should be taken at even intervals around the clock. Your doctor or pharmacist can help you set up a dosing schedule. • Take this drug with at least one full glass of water. Drink at least nine or ten glasses of water each day. • This drug may cause you to be especially sensitive to the sun, so avoid exposure to the sun as much as possible and use an effective sunscreen that does not contain PABA. • This drug may interfere with blood and urine laboratory tests. If you are scheduled to take any such tests, remind your doctor that you are taking this drug. • Notify your doctor if you develop signs of jaundice (yellow eyes or skin; dark urine).

Bancap HC analgesic (Forest Pharmaceuticals, Inc.), see Vicodin analgesic.

Banex-LA decongestant and expectorant (LuChem), see Entex LA decongestant and expectorant.

Barbita sedative and hypnotic (Vortech Pharmaceutical, Ltd.), see phenobarbital sedative and hypnotic.

Baridium analgesic (Pfeiffer), see Pyridium analgesic.

Beclovent antiasthmatic (Glaxo, Inc.), see Vanceril antiasthmatic.

Beepen VK antibiotic (Beecham Laboratories), see penicillin potassium phenoxymethyl (penicillin VK) antibiotic.

Belix antihistamine (Halsey Drug Co., Inc.), see Benadryl antihistamine.

belladonna alkaloids with phenobarbital sedative and anticholinergic (various manufacturers), see Donnatal sedative and anticholinergic.

Benadryl antihistamine

Manufacturer: Parke-Davis
Ingredient: diphenhydramine hydrochloride
Equivalent Products: Belix, Halsey Drug Co., Inc.; Benaphen, Major Pharmaceuticals; Diahist, Century Pharmaceuticals, Inc.; Diphen Cough, My-K Labs; diphenhydramine hydrochloride, various manufacturers; Fenylhist, Mallard, Inc.; Genahist, Goldline Laboratories; Nordryl, Vortech Pharmaceutical, Ltd.; Tusstat, Century Pharmaceuticals, Inc.; Valdrene, The Vale Chemical Company; see Comments
Dosage Forms: Capsule: 25 mg; 50 mg (both pink/white). Liquid (content per 5 ml teaspoon): 12.5 mg. Tablet: 25 mg. See Comments
Uses: Treatment of insomnia, motion sickness, Parkinson's disease, and allergy-related itching and swelling; nighttime sleep aid; cough suppressant
Minor Side Effects: Blurred vision; confusion; constipation; diarrhea; difficulty in urinating; dizziness; drowsiness; dry mouth; headache; insomnia; loss of appetite; nasal congestion; nausea; nervousness; restlessness; sweating; vomiting; weakness; wheezing
Major Side Effects: Changes in menstruation; convulsions; decreased sexual

ability; disturbed coordination; fever; low blood pressure; nightmares; palpitations; rash from exposure to sunlight; ringing in ears; severe abdominal pain; shortness of breath; sore throat; tightness in chest; unusual bleeding and bruising

Contraindications: This drug should not be given to infants or taken by nursing mothers. People who are allergic to this drug or similar antihistamines should not use this drug. Consult your doctor immediately if this drug has been prescribed for you and any of these conditions applies to you. • This drug should not be used to treat asthma or other lower respiratory tract symptoms.

Warnings: This drug should be used cautiously by people who have asthma, glaucoma (certain types), ulcers (certain types), enlarged prostate, obstructed bladder, obstructed intestine, thyroid disease, heart disease (certain types), or high blood pressure and by those who are pregnant. Be sure your doctor knows if any of these conditions applies to you. • Elderly people are more likely than others to experience side effects, especially sedation, with this drug and should use it with caution. • This drug should be used cautiously with aminosalicylic acid, oral anticoagulants, and phenytoin. • This drug should not be used in conjunction with central nervous system depressants or monoamine oxidase inhibitors; if you are currently taking any drugs of these types, consult your doctor about their use. If you are unsure of the type or contents of your medications, ask your doctor or pharmacist. • This drug may cause drowsiness; avoid tasks that require alertness. • To prevent oversedation, avoid alcohol or other sedative drugs.

Comments: Chew gum or suck on ice chips or a piece of hard candy to reduce mouth dryness. • Take only the prescribed amount of this drug. An overdose usually sedates an adult but can cause excitation leading to convulsions and death in a child. • While taking this drug, do not take any nonprescription item for weight control, cough, cold, or sinus problems without checking with your doctor or pharmacist. • Valdrene and some generic forms of diphenhydramine hydrochloride are available in 50 mg tablets by prescription. Benadryl is available in topical forms for relief of itching due to minor skin disorders. Benadryl is also available in some strengths and dosage forms without a prescription. In addition, there are a variety of diphenhydramine products available without a prescription. Check with your doctor or pharmacist about using them.

Benaphen antihistamine (Major Pharmaceuticals), see Benadryl antihistamine.

Bentyl antispasmodic

Manufacturer: Lakeside Pharmaceuticals
Ingredient: dicyclomine hydrochloride
Equivalent Products: Byclomine, Major Pharmaceuticals; dicyclomine hydrochloride, various manufacturers; Di-Spaz, Vortech Pharmaceutical, Ltd.
Dosage Forms: Capsule: 10 mg (blue). Liquid (content per 5 ml teaspoon): 10 mg. Tablet: 20 mg (blue).
Uses: Treatment of functional bowel and irritable bowel syndromes
Minor Side Effects: Bloating; blurred vision; confusion; dizziness; drowsiness; dry mouth; increased sensitivity to light; headache; insomnia; interference with milk production; loss of taste; nausea; nervousness; reduced sweating; vomiting; weakness
Major Side Effects: Constipation; difficulty in urinating; fever; impotence; palpitations; rapid heartbeat; rash; sore throat
Contraindications: This drug should not be taken by people who have severe ulcerative colitis, severe hemorrhage, obstructed bladder, obstructed intestine, heart disease (certain types), or myasthenia gravis. This drug should

not be taken by those who are allergic to it. Consult your doctor immediately if this drug has been prescribed for you and you have any of these conditions or such an allergy.

Warnings: This drug should be used cautiously by people who have hiatal hernia, glaucoma, enlarged prostate, high blood pressure, thyroid disease, liver or kidney disease, or heart disease and by women who are pregnant. Be sure your doctor knows if any of these conditions applies to you. • If diarrhea is caused by obstructed intestine, this drug could be harmful. Use of this drug requires careful diagnosis of your condition. • People who have ulcerative colitis should be especially careful about taking this drug and should never increase the dosage unless told to do so by their doctor. • This drug should not be used in conjunction with amantadine, haloperidol, phenothiazines, or antacids; if you are currently taking any drugs of these types, consult your doctor about their use. If you are unsure of the type or contents of your medications, ask your doctor or pharmacist. • This drug always produces certain side effects, which may include dry mouth, blurred vision, reduced sweating, drowsiness, difficulty in urinating, constipation, increased sensitivity to light, and palpitations. • Avoid tasks that require alertness. • Avoid excessive work or exercise in hot weather and drink plenty of fluids. • To prevent oversedation, avoid taking alcohol or other drugs that have sedative properties. • Call your doctor if you notice a rash, flushing, or pain in the eye. • In a few instances, infants less than six weeks old have developed breathing problems after being given this drug. In such a situation, you should call your doctor immediately.

Comments: This drug is best taken one-half to one hour before meals. • Chew gum or suck on ice chips or a piece of hard candy to reduce mouth dryness. • Products combining dicyclomine antispasmodic with phenobarbital are available for persons who are especially nervous or anxious. Despite the phenobarbital content, dicyclomine antispasmodic with phenobarbital has not been shown to have high potential for abuse.

betamethasone valerate topical steroid hormone (various manufacturers), see Valisone topical steroid hormone.

Betapen-VK antibiotic (Bristol Laboratories), see penicillin potassium phenoxymethyl (penicillin VK) antibiotic.

Betatrex topical steroid hormone (Savage Laboratories), see Valisone topical steroid hormone.

Beta-Val topical steroid hormone (Lemmon Company), see Valisone topical steroid hormone.

Bethaprim SS and Bethaprim DS antibacterials (Major Pharmaceuticals), see Bactrim and Bactrim DS antibacterials.

Bexophene analgesic (Mallard, Inc.), see Darvon Compound-65 analgesic.

birth control pills, see oral contraceptives.

Blocadren beta blocker

Manufacturer: Merck Sharp & Dohme
Ingredient: timolol maleate
Dosage Form: Tablet: 5 mg; 10 mg; 20 mg (light blue)
Uses: Treatment of high blood pressure and prevention of heartbeat irregularities following a heart attack
Minor Side Effects: Abdominal pain; blurred vision; bloating; constipation; drowsiness; dry eyes, mouth, or skin; gas or heartburn; headache; insomnia; loss of appetite; nasal congestion; nausea; slowed heart rate; sweating; tiredness; vivid dreams; vomiting
Major Side Effects: Bleeding or bruising; confusion; decreased sexual ability; depression; diarrhea; difficulty in urinating; dizziness; earache; fever; hair loss; hallucinations; mouth sores; night cough; nightmares; numbness and tingling in the fingers and toes; rash; ringing in the ears; shortness of breath; swelling in the hands or feet
Contraindications: This drug should not be used by people who are allergic to timolol maleate or any other beta blocker. This drug should not be taken by people who suffer from certain types of heart disease or lung disease or anyone who has taken any monoamine oxidase inhibitors within the past two weeks. Consult your doctor immediately if this drug has been prescribed for you and any of these conditions applies.
Warnings: This drug should be used with caution by persons with certain respiratory problems, diabetes, certain heart problems, liver and kidney diseases, hypoglycemia, or thyroid disease. Be sure your doctor knows if you have any of these conditions. • This drug should be used cautiously by persons taking other medications, such as theophylline, insulin, salicylates, and other antihypertensive agents. Inform your doctor of all the medications you are taking so that effects can be monitored. • This drug should be used cautiously by pregnant women and by women of childbearing age. • This drug should be used with care during anesthesia and by patients undergoing major surgery. If possible, this drug should be withdrawn 48 hours prior to surgery. • This drug should be used cautiously when reserpine is taken. • Do not abruptly stop taking this drug unless directed to do so by your doctor; usually the dose must be gradually reduced over one to two weeks. • Diabetics taking this drug should watch for signs of altered blood glucose levels.
Comments: Your doctor may want you to take your pulse and monitor your blood pressure every day while you take this medication. Ask your doctor about what your normal values are and what target rates you should be looking for. • Be sure to take your medication doses at the same time each day. • While taking this drug, do not take any nonprescription items for weight control, cough, cold, or sinus problems without first checking with your doctor; such medications may contain ingredients that can increase blood pressure. • Notify your doctor if dizziness, diarrhea, shortness of breath, or slow pulse develops. • There are many different beta blockers available. Your doctor may want you to try different ones in order to find the best one for you. • Timolol maleate is also available as Timoptic, an eye drop used in the management of glaucoma.

Brethine bronchodilator

Manufacturer: Geigy Pharmaceuticals
Ingredient: terbutaline sulfate
Equivalent Product: Bricanyl, Lakeside Pharmaceuticals
Dosage Form: Tablet: 2.5 mg; 5 mg (white)
Uses: Relief of bronchial asthma and bronchospasm associated with bronchitis and emphysema

Minor Side Effects: Anxiety; dizziness; headache; flushing; increased heart rate; insomnia; loss of appetite; muscle cramps; nausea; nervousness; peculiar taste in the mouth; sweating; tension; tremors; vomiting; weakness

Major Side Effects: Breathing difficulties; chest pain; difficulty in urinating; palpitations

Contraindication: This drug should not be taken by people who are allergic to any sympathomimetic amine drug. Consult your doctor immediately if this drug has been prescribed for you and you have an allergy of this type.

Warnings: This drug should be used cautiously by pregnant or nursing women and by people who have diabetes, high blood pressure, thyroid disease, glaucoma, enlarged prostate, Parkinson's disease, heart disease (certain types), or epilepsy. Be sure your doctor knows if any of these conditions applies to you. • This drug is not recommended for use by children under age 12. • This drug should not be used in conjunction with guanethidine, beta blockers, or monoamine oxidase inhibitors; if you are currently taking any drugs of these types, consult your doctor about their use. If you are unsure of the type or contents of your medications, ask your doctor or pharmacist. • While taking this drug, do not take any nonprescription item for weight control, cough, cold, or sinus problems without first checking with your doctor; these items may contain ingredients that can increase blood pressure. Do not take any other drug containing a sympathomimetic amine (a decongestant, for example) without consulting your doctor.

Comments: While taking this drug, drink at least eight glasses of water daily. • Side effects from this drug are usually worse the first week or so of therapy and will lessen in severity after that. • Take this drug as prescribed. Do not increase your dose without consulting your doctor.

Bricanyl bronchodilator (Lakeside Pharmaceuticals), see Brethine bronchodilator.

Bronkodyl bronchodilator (Winthrop-Breon Laboratories), see theophylline bronchodilator.

Bumex diuretic

Manufacturer: Roche Laboratories
Ingredient: bumetanide
Dosage Form: Tablet: 0.5 mg (light green); 1 mg (yellow); 2 mg (peach)
Use: Removal of fluid from body tissues
Minor Side Effects: Abdominal pain; blurred vision; diarrhea; dizziness; fatigue; headache; nausea; weakness
Major Side Effects: Blood disorders; chest pain; dehydration; dry mouth; excessive thirst; hives; impaired coordination; jaundice; loss of appetite; loss of hearing; low blood pressure; muscle cramps; rash; sweating; vomiting
Contraindications: This drug should not be used by persons allergic to it, by persons with anuria (inability to urinate), or by those with severe liver or kidney disease. Consult your doctor immediately if this drug has been prescribed for you and you have any of these conditions.
Warnings: Use of this drug may cause gout, diabetes, hearing loss, and loss of potassium, calcium, water, and salt. Persons taking this drug should have periodic drug tests to monitor for these effects. • Persons hypersensitive to sulfa drugs may also be hypersensitive to this drug. If this drug has been prescribed for you and you are allergic to sulfa drugs, consult your doctor immediately. • This drug should be used with caution by persons with cirrhosis of the liver or other liver problems and by persons with kidney disease. This drug

should be used cautiously by children and by pregnant or nursing women. Be sure your doctor knows if any of these conditions applies to you. • This drug should be used with caution in conjunction with other high blood pressure drugs. If you are taking other such medications, the dosages may require adjustment. • Use of this drug may activate the appearance of systemic lupus erythematosus. • Whenever reactions to this drug are moderate to severe, this drug should be reduced or discontinued. Consult your doctor promptly if such side effects occur. • This drug interacts with aspirin, curare, indomethacin, digitalis, lithium carbonate, steroids, or cephaloridine. If you are currently taking any drugs of these types, consult your doctor about their use. If you are unsure of the type or contents of your medications, ask your doctor or pharmacist.

Comments: This drug causes frequent urination. Expect this effect; it should not alarm you. Try to plan your dosage schedule to avoid taking this drug at night. • This drug has potent activity. If another drug to decrease blood pressure is also prescribed, your doctor may decide to decrease the dose of one of the drugs to avoid an excessive drop in blood pressure. You should learn how to monitor your pulse and blood pressure; discuss this with your doctor. • This drug can cause potassium loss. Signs of such loss include dry mouth, thirst, muscle cramps, weakness, and nausea or vomiting. If you experience any of these side effects, notify your doctor. To help avoid such loss, take this drug with a glass of fresh or frozen orange juice. You may also eat a banana each day. The use of a salt substitute helps prevent potassium loss. Do not change your diet, however, without consulting your doctor. Too much potassium may also be dangerous. • Notify your doctor if you develop signs of jaundice (yellow eyes or skin; dark urine). • To avoid dizziness or light-headedness when you stand, contract and relax the muscles of your legs for a few minutes before rising. Do this by pushing one foot against the floor while raising the other foot slightly, alternating feet so that you are "pumping" your legs in a pedaling motion. • Persons taking this drug and digitalis should watch carefully for symptoms of increased digitalis toxicity (e.g., nausea, blurred vision, palpitations), and notify their doctor immediately if symptoms occur. • If you have high blood pressure, do not take any nonprescription item for weight control, cough, cold, or sinus problems without first checking with your doctor. Such medications may contain ingredients which can increase blood pressure. • When taking this drug (or other drugs for high blood pressure), limit the use of alcohol to avoid dizziness or light-headedness. • Take this drug exactly as directed. It is usually taken in the morning with food. Do not take extra doses or skip a dose without first consulting your doctor.

butalbital compound analgesic (various manufacturers), see Fiorinal analgesic.

Byclomine antispasmodic (Major Pharmaceuticals), see Bentyl antispasmodic.

Calan antianginal and antihypertensive (Searle & Co.), see Isoptin antianginal and antihypertensive.

Capital with Codeine analgesic (Carnrick Laboratories, Inc.), see acetaminophen with codeine analgesic.

Capoten antihypertensive

Manufacturer: E.R. Squibb & Sons, Inc.
Ingredient: captopril

Dosage Form: Tablet: 12.5 mg; 25 mg; 50 mg; 100 mg (white)

Uses: Treatment of high blood pressure; treatment of heart failure

Minor Side Effects: Cough; diarrhea; dizziness; fatigue; frequent urination; gastrointestinal upset; headache; impairment or loss of taste perception; insomnia; light-headedness; nausea; swelling of face, hands, or feet

Major Side Effects: Blood disorders; breathing difficulties; chest pain; chills; fainting; fast or irregular heartbeat; fever; itching; skin rash; sore throat

Contraindication: This drug should not be taken by people who are allergic to it. Consult your doctor if this drug has been prescribed for you and you have such an allergy.

Warnings: This drug should be used cautiously by the elderly; by pregnant or nursing women; and by people with kidney diseases or blood disorders. Be sure your doctor knows if any of these conditions applies to you. • This drug should be used with caution with other medicines. Inform your doctor if you are taking any cancer medicines, diuretics, antihypertensive drugs, steroids, indomethacin, or potassium supplements. The effectiveness of Capoten may be reduced by aspirin and by indomethacin. Check with your doctor before taking any product containing either of these drugs. • Because this medicine may initially cause dizziness or fainting, your doctor may start you on a low dose and gradually increase it. • Do not use salt substitutes or low-salt milk that contains potassium without first checking with your doctor. • Periodic kidney function tests and blood tests are recommended if this drug is prescribed for a long time. • While taking this drug, do not take any nonprescription item for weight control, cough, cold, or sinus problems without first checking with your doctor; these items may contain ingredients that can increase blood pressure.

Comments: For maximum effect, take this drug on an empty stomach one hour before meals. Take this drug exactly as directed. Do not take extra doses or skip doses without consulting your physician. • While taking this drug, you should limit your consumption of alcoholic beverages in order to minimize dizziness and light-headedness. Sudden changes in posture may cause dizziness or light-headedness. To relieve this, contract and relax the muscles of your legs for a few moments before rising. Do this by pushing one foot against the floor while raising the other foot slightly, alternating feet so that your legs are "pumping" in a pedaling motion. • Notify your physician if you develop mouth sores, sore throat, fever, chest pains, or swelling of hands or feet.

Carafate antiulcer

Manufacturer: Marion Laboratories, Inc.

Ingredient: sucralfate

Dosage Form: Tablet: 1 g (pink)

Use: Short-term treatment of ulcers

Minor Side Effects: Back pain; constipation; diarrhea; dizziness; drowsiness; dry mouth; indigestion; itching; nausea; rash; stomach upset

Major Side Effects: None

Contraindication: This drug should not be used by people who are allergic to it. Consult your doctor immediately if this drug has been prescribed for you and you have such an allergy.

Warnings: This drug should be used with caution by pregnant women and nursing mothers. • If you are also taking tetracycline, phenytoin, or cimetidine, it is best to separate dosing of these drugs and Carafate by two hours. Consult your doctor if these drugs have been prescribed for you.

Comments: This drug has only been shown to be effective for short time periods (up to eight weeks). • Take this drug on an empty stomach at least one hour before or two hours after a meal and at bedtime. • Do not take antacids within 30 minutes before or after taking this drug. • Continue taking this medication for the full time prescribed by your doctor, even if your symptoms disappear. • Sucralfate forms a protective layer at the ulcer site. It is virtually not absorbed into the body, so side effects are minimal.

carbamazepine anticonvulsant (Rugby Laboratories), see Tegretol anticonvulsant.

Cardizem antianginal

Manufacturer: Marion Laboratories, Inc.
Ingredient: diltiazem
Dosage Form: Tablet: 30 mg (green); 60 mg (yellow); 90 mg (green); 120 mg (yellow)
Use: Treatment of various types of angina (chest pain)
Minor Side Effects: Constipation; diarrhea; dizziness; drowsiness; fatigue; flushing; gastric upset; headache; increased frequency of urination; indigestion; light-headedness; nausea; nervousness; weakness
Major Side Effects: Confusion; depression; fainting; hallucinations; low blood pressure; rapid or pounding heartbeat; skin rash; swelling of the feet, ankles, or lower legs; tingling of hands or feet
Contraindications: This drug should not be used by people who are allergic to it or by people with very low blood pressure. Consult your doctor immediately if this drug has been prescribed for you and either of these conditions applies.
Warnings: This drug should be used cautiously by pregnant or nursing women and by people with low blood pressure, certain heart diseases, kidney disease, or liver disease. Be sure your doctor knows if any of these conditions applies to you. • This drug may interact with beta blockers, calcium supplements, antihypertensive medications, and digoxin. If you are taking any of these medicines, consult your doctor about their use. • This drug may make you dizzy, especially during the first few days of use. Avoid activities that require alertness and avoid alcohol, which may exaggerate this effect.
Comments: Your physician may want to see you regularly when you begin taking this drug in order to check your response to the therapy. You should learn how to monitor your pulse and blood pressure; discuss this with your doctor. • This drug must be taken as directed. It is important that you continue to take Cardizem to prevent chest pain. This drug is not effective in treating an attack of angina already in progress. • Contact your doctor if this drug causes severe or persistent dizziness, constipation, nausea, swelling of hands and feet, shortness of breath, or irregular heartbeat.

Carfin anticoagulant (Major Pharmaceuticals), see Coumadin anticoagulant.

Carmol HC topical steroid (Syntex Laboratories, Inc.), see hydrocortisone topical steroid.

Catapres antihypertensive

Manufacturer: Boehringer Ingelheim
Ingredient: clonidine hydrochloride
Equivalent Product: clonidine HCl, various manufacturers
Dosage Forms: Tablet: 0.1 mg (tan); 0.2 mg (orange); 0.3 mg (peach). Transdermal Patch (see Comments)
Use: Treatment of high blood pressure
Minor Side Effects: Anxiety; constipation; decreased sexual desire; depres-

sion; dizziness; drowsiness; dry eyes; dry mouth; fatigue; headache; increased sensitivity to alcohol; insomnia; itching; jaw pain; loss of appetite; nasal congestion; nausea; nervousness; nightmares; vomiting

Major Side Effects: Breathing difficulties; chest pain; cold feeling in fingertips or toes; enlarged breasts (in both sexes); hair loss; heart failure; hives; impotence; jaundice; pain; rash; rise in blood sugar; urine retention; weight gain

Contraindications: This drug should not be used by people who are allergic to it. The transdermal patch should not be used by people allergic to the adhesive layer.

Warnings: This drug is not recommended for use by women who are pregnant or who may become pregnant. • This drug should be used cautiously by children. • This drug should be used with caution by persons with severe heart disease, depression, or chronic kidney failure and by those who have had a stroke or heart attack. Be sure your doctor knows if any of these conditions applies to you. • This drug should not be used with alcohol, barbiturates, or other sedatives. If you are currently taking any drugs of these types, consult your doctor about their use. If you are unsure of the type or content of the medications you are taking, ask your doctor or pharmacist. • Tolerance to this drug develops occasionally; consult your doctor if you feel the drug is becoming less effective. Do not stop using this drug without consulting your doctor first. Your doctor will advise you on how to discontinue the drug gradually. • You should receive periodic eye examinations while taking this drug. • This drug can cause drowsiness; avoid tasks that require alertness.

Comments: Your physician may want to see you regularly when you first begin taking this drug in order to check your response. Dosage adjustments may be made frequently. You should learn how to monitor your pulse and blood pressure; discuss this with your doctor. • Mild side effects from this drug (e.g., nasal congestion) are most noticeable during the first two weeks of therapy and become less bothersome after this period. • Notify your doctor if you develop signs of jaundice (yellow eyes or skin; dark urine) while taking this drug. • While taking this drug, do not take any nonprescription item for weight control, cough, cold, or sinus problems without first checking with your doctor; such products often contain ingredients that may increase blood pressure. • To avoid dizziness or light-headedness when you stand, contract and relax the muscles of your legs for a few moments before rising. Do this by pushing one foot against the floor while raising the other foot slightly, alternating feet so that you are "pumping" your legs in a pedaling motion. • Chew gum or suck on ice chips or a piece of hard candy to reduce mouth dryness. • Take this drug exactly as directed. Do not take extra doses or skip a dose without first consulting your doctor. • The transdermal patches (called Catapres-TTS) are designed to continually release the medication over a seven-day period. The patch should be applied to a hairless area (shaving may be necessary) on the upper arm or chest. Do not apply a patch to the lower arm or to the legs. Change the site of application with each new patch. Avoid placing the patch on irritated or damaged skin. It is safe to bathe and shower with a patch in place. If it loosens, apply a new one. Store the patches in a cool, dry place. Do not refrigerate. Patient instructions for application are available. Ask your pharmacist for them if they are not provided with your prescription. For maximum benefit, read and follow the instructions carefully. If you are currently taking clonidine tablets, discuss the use of transdermal patches with your doctor.

Ceclor antibiotic

Manufacturer: Eli Lilly & Co.
Ingredient: cefaclor

Dosage Forms: Capsule: 250 mg (white/purple); 500 mg (gray/purple). Liquid (content per 5 ml teaspoon): 125 mg; 250 mg

Use: Treatment of a wide variety of bacterial infections

Minor Side Effects: Diarrhea; fatigue; heartburn; loss of appetite; mouth sores; nausea; rectal or vaginal itching; vomiting

Major Side Effects: Blood disorders; breathing difficulties; jaundice; kidney disease; rash; severe diarrhea; superinfection; tingling in hands and feet

Contraindications: This drug should not be used by people who are allergic to it or to other antibiotics similar to it. Consult your doctor immediately if this drug has been prescribed for you and you have such an allergy.

Warnings: This drug should be used cautiously by people who are allergic to penicillin or cephalosporin antibiotics or who have other allergies; by women who are pregnant or nursing; and by people with kidney disease. Be sure your doctor knows if any of these conditions applies to you. • This drug should be used cautiously in newborns. • Prolonged use of this drug may allow organisms that are not susceptible to it to grow wildly. Do not use this drug unless your doctor has specifically told you to do so. Be sure to follow directions carefully and report any unusual reactions to your doctor at once. • This drug should be used cautiously in conjunction with diuretics, oral anticoagulants, and probenecid. • This drug may interfere with some blood tests. Be sure your doctor knows you are taking it. • Diabetics using Clinitest urine test may get a false high sugar reading. Change to Clinistix urine test or Tes-Tape urine test to avoid this problem.

Comments: It is generally believed that about ten percent of all people who are allergic to penicillin will be allergic to an antibiotic like this as well. • This drug is usually prescribed after unsuccessful treatment with another antibiotic like penicillin or Bactrim. Ceclor is more potent and more expensive, so it is generally reserved for second-line use. • Notify your doctor if you develop signs of jaundice (yellow eyes or skin; dark urine) while taking this drug. • Take this drug with food or milk if stomach upset occurs. • The liquid form of this drug should be stored in the refrigerator. Any unused portion should be discarded after 14 days. Shake well before using. Finish all the medicine — even if you feel better — to ensure that the infection is eradicated. For maximum effect, take this drug at evenly spaced intervals around the clock. Ask your doctor or pharmacist to help you establish a dosing schedule.

Cena-K potassium chloride replacement (Century Pharmaceuticals, Inc.), see potassium chloride replacement.

Centrax antianxiety

Manufacturer: Parke-Davis

Ingredient: prazepam

Dosage Forms: Capsule: 5 mg (celery); 10 mg (aqua); 20 mg (yellow). Tablet: 10 mg (blue)

Use: Treatment of anxiety and its symptoms

Minor Side Effects: Confusion; constipation; decrease or increase in sex drive; depression; diarrhea; dizziness; drowsiness; dry mouth; excess saliva; fatigue; headache; heartburn; loss of appetite; nausea; sweating; vomiting

Major Side Effects: Blurred vision; breathing difficulties; difficulty in urinating; double vision; excitement; fever; hallucinations; jaundice; low blood pressure; menstrual irregularities; mouth sores; rapid, pounding heartbeat; rash; slurred speech; sore throat; stimulation; tremors; uncoordinated movements

Contraindications: This drug should not be given to children under six months of age. This drug should not be taken by persons with certain types of glaucoma or severe mental disorder, by pregnant or nursing women, or by

CONSUMER GUIDE®

people who are allergic to it. Consult your doctor immediately if any of these conditions applies to you.

Warnings: This drug should be used cautiously by the elderly or debilitated and by people with epilepsy, respiratory problems, myasthenia gravis, porphyria, a history of drug abuse, or impaired liver or kidney function. Be sure your doctor knows if any of these conditions applies to you. • This drug may cause drowsiness, especially during the first few days of therapy; avoid tasks that require alertness. • This drug should not be taken simultaneously with alcohol or other central nervous system depressants that exaggerate its effects; serious adverse reactions may develop. • This drug should be used cautiously with phenytoin, cimetidine, and oral anticoagulants. • Do not stop taking this drug without informing your doctor. If you have been taking the drug regularly and wish to discontinue use, you must decrease the dose gradually, according to your doctor's instructions. • This drug has the potential for abuse and must be used with caution. Tolerance may develop quickly; do not increase the dose without first consulting your doctor. • Persons taking this drug should have periodic blood counts and liver function tests.

Comments: This drug currently is used by many people to relieve nervousness. It is effective for this purpose, but it is important to try to remove the cause of the anxiety as well. • Notify your doctor if you develop signs of jaundice (yellow eyes or skin; dark urine). • Chew gum or suck on ice chips or a piece of hard candy to reduce mouth dryness. • To lessen stomach upset, take with food or a full glass of water. • The full effects of this drug may not be apparent until it has been taken for two to three days. • Drowsiness is common during the first few days of therapy and should subside with continued use. Because this drug causes drowsiness, it may be best to take Centrax at bedtime. Discuss this with your doctor.

cephalexin antibiotic (various manufacturers), see Keflex antibiotic.

chlordiazepoxide hydrochloride antianxiety (various manufacturers), see Librium antianxiety.

Chlorpazine phenothiazine (Major Pharmaceuticals), see Compazine phenothiazine.

Chlorpropamide oral antidiabetic (various manufacturers), see Diabinese oral antidiabetic.

chlorthalidone diuretic and antihypertensive (various manufacturers), see Hygroton diuretic and antihypertensive.

Cin-Quin antiarrhythmic (Reid-Rowell), see quinidine sulfate antiarrhythmic.

Clindex antianxiety (Rugby Laboratories), see Librax antianxiety.

Clinoril anti-inflammatory

Manufacturer: Merck Sharp & Dohme
Ingredient: sulindac
Dosage Form: Tablet: 150 mg; 200 mg (both yellow)

Uses: Reduction of pain, redness, and swelling due to acute or chronic arthritis, painful shoulder, or acute gouty arthritis

Minor Side Effects: Abdominal pain; constipation; cramps; diarrhea; dry mouth; gas; headache; heartburn; indigestion; itching; loss of appetite; nausea; nervousness; nosebleed; sore mouth; vomiting

Major Side Effects: Black stools; chest tightness; chills; depression; dizziness; edema; fever; gastrointestinal bleeding; headache; hearing loss; high blood pressure; jaundice; kidney disease; menstrual irregularities; numbness or tingling in fingers or toes; palpitations; peptic ulcer; psychosis; rectal bleeding; ringing in the ears; shortness of breath; skin rash; sore throat; swelling of the feet; visual disturbance; weight gain; wheezing

Contraindications: This drug should not be taken by people who are allergic to it or to aspirin or other nonsteroidal anti-inflammatory agents. Consult your doctor immediately if this drug has been prescribed for you and you have such an allergy.

Warnings: This drug should be used with caution by persons with asthma, peptic ulcer, certain blood diseases, gastrointestinal bleeding, high blood pressure, fluid retention, history of gastrointestinal disease, blood clotting disorders, liver or kidney disease, or certain types of heart disease. Be sure your doctor knows if any of these conditions applies to you. • This drug should not be used by pregnant women, nursing mothers, or children. • Persons using this drug who experience eye problems should immediately bring these symptoms to their doctor's attention so that eye tests can be initiated. • This drug interacts with aspirin, beta blockers, diuretics, phenytoin, and probenecid. People taking anticoagulants and antidiabetics should be monitored carefully. If you are currently taking any drugs of these types, consult your doctor about their use. If you are unsure about the type or contents of your medications, ask your doctor or pharmacist. • Do not stop taking this drug without informing your doctor. • This drug may cause dizziness or blurred vision and therefore may impair your ability to perform potentially hazardous tasks, such as driving or operating machinery.

Comments: This drug is a potent pain reliever and is not intended for general aches and pains. • Regular medical checkups, including blood tests and eye examinations, are required of persons taking this drug. • This drug must be taken with food or milk. Never take this drug on an empty stomach or with aspirin, and never take more than directed. • In numerous tests, this drug has been shown to be as effective as aspirin in the treatment of arthritis, but aspirin is still the drug of choice for the disease. Because of the high cost of this drug, consult your doctor about prescribing proper doses of aspirin instead. • Do not drink alcohol while taking this drug without first consulting your doctor. • You should note improvement in your condition soon after you start using this drug; however, full benefit may not be obtained for as long as a month. It is important not to stop taking this drug even though symptoms have diminished or disappeared. • This drug is not a substitute for rest, physical therapy, or other measures recommended by your doctor. • This drug is similar in action to other anti-inflammatory agents, such as Motrin and Indocin. If this drug is not well tolerated, your doctor may have you try the other ones to see which one works best for you. • Notify your doctor if you develop signs of jaundice (yellow eyes or skin; dark urine).

Clinoxide antianxiety (Geneva Generics, Inc.), see Librax antianxiety.

Clipoxide antianxiety (Henry Schein, Inc.), see Librax antianxiety.

clonidine HCl antihypertensive (various manufacturers), see Catapres antihypertensive.

Clopra gastrointestinal stimulant (Quantum Pharmics), see Reglan gastrointestinal stimulant.

Codap analgesic (Reid-Rowell), see acetaminophen with codeine analgesic.

Codoxy analgesic (Halsey Drug Co., Inc.), see Percodan analgesic.

Cogentin antiparkinson drug

Manufacturer: Merck Sharp & Dohme
Ingredient: benztropine mesylate
Dosage Form: Tablet: 0.5 mg; 1 mg; 2 mg (all white)
Uses: Treatment of symptoms of Parkinson's disease or control of side effects of phenothiazines
Minor Side Effects: Bloating; blurred vision; constipation; depression; dizziness; drowsiness; dry mouth; headache; increased sensitivity of eyes to light; mild nausea; nervousness; reduced sweating; weakness
Major Side Effects: Difficulty in urinating; hallucinations; involuntary muscle movements; numbness of the fingers; palpitations. Some people with arteriosclerosis or with a history of abnormal reactions to other drugs may exhibit symptoms of mental confusion, agitation, disturbed behavior, or nausea and vomiting. Psychiatric disturbances can result from indiscriminate use leading to overdosage; narrow-angle glaucoma has also been reported.
Contraindications: This drug should not be taken by people who are allergic to it or by people with narrow-angle glaucoma, intestinal obstructions, stomach ulcers, an enlarged prostate gland, urinary tract blockage, myasthenia gravis, or achalasia. Consult your doctor if this drug has been prescribed for you and any of these conditions applies. • Children under the age of three should not use this drug.
Warnings: People treated with this drug should have close monitoring of intraocular pressures at regular intervals. • Careful and constant observation of people using this drug long-term should be undertaken to avoid allergic and certain other reactions. • This drug should be used with caution by people with heart, liver, or kidney disorders and by those who suffer from high blood pressure, thyroid disease, or alcoholism. People with any of these conditions should be under close medical observation. • This drug should be used with caution by people with glaucoma or obstructive diseases of the intestine or bowel, by pregnant women, and by elderly males with possible prostate gland problems. If any of these conditions applies to you, be sure to inform your doctor. • Persons over 60 years of age require strict dosage regulation; they frequently develop increased sensitivity to this drug. • This drug may cause dizziness or drowsiness; avoid tasks that require alertness, such as driving a vehicle or operating potentially dangerous machinery.
Comments: This drug is frequently prescribed along with phenothiazine drugs such as Thorazine and Stelazine to reduce the tremors caused by phenothiazines. You should talk with your doctor about waiting before taking this drug to see if you really need it. Many people can take phenothiazine drugs successfully and may not need this drug. • Do not stop taking this drug without first consulting your physician. • Chew gum or suck on ice chips or a piece of hard candy to reduce mouth dryness. • Because this drug reduces sweating, avoid excessive work or exercise in hot weather and drink plenty of fluids. • Certain other drugs, such as Artane (Lederle Laboratories) antiparkinson drug, have actions similar to those of this drug. • If this drug makes it difficult for you to urinate, try to do so just before each dose.

Co-Gesic analgesic (Central Pharmaceuticals, Inc.), see Vicodin analgesic.

Compazine phenothiazine

Manufacturer: Smith Kline & French Laboratories
Ingredient: prochlorperazine
Equivalent Products: Chlorpazine, Major Pharmaceuticals; prochlorperazine, various manufacturers
Dosage Forms: Suppository: 2.5 mg; 5 mg; 25 mg. Syrup (per 5 ml teaspoon): 5 mg. Tablet: 5 mg; 10 mg; 25 mg (all yellow). Time-release capsule: 10 mg; 15 mg; 30 mg (all are black/clear with yellow and white beads)
Uses: Control of severe nausea and vomiting; relief of certain kinds of anxiety, tension, agitation, psychiatric disorders
Minor Side Effects: Blurred vision; constipation; diarrhea; dizziness; drooling; drowsiness; dry mouth; fatigue; headache; impotence; insomnia; jitteriness; loss of appetite; milk production; nasal congestion; nausea; photosensitivity; reduced sweating; restlessness; tremors; weakness
Major Side Effects: Asthma; arthritis; blood disorders; breast enlargement (in both sexes); convulsions; difficulty in urinating; eye changes; fever; fluid retention; heart attack; involuntary movements of the mouth, face, neck, and tongue; liver damage; low blood pressure; menstrual irregularities; mouth sores; palpitations; rash; skin darkening; sore throat
Contraindications: This drug should not be taken by people who are suffering from drug-induced depression or by those who have blood diseases, severe high or low blood pressure, Parkinson's disease, or liver disease. Consult your doctor immediately if this drug has been prescribed for you and you have such a condition. • This drug should not be given to people who are comatose or to children undergoing surgery.
Warnings: This drug should be used cautiously by people with glaucoma; heart, lung, brain, or kidney disease; diabetes; epilepsy; breast cancer; ulcers; or an enlarged prostate gland; by pregnant women; and by people who have previously had an allergic reaction to any phenothiazine. Be sure your doctor knows if any of these conditions applies to you. • This drug may cause drowsiness; avoid tasks that require alertness. To prevent oversedation, avoid the use of alcohol or other drugs that have sedative properties. • This drug interacts with oral antacids and anticholinergics; if you are currently taking any drugs of these types, consult your doctor about their use. If you are unsure of the type or contents of your medications, ask your doctor or pharmacist. • When taking this drug, do not take any nonprescription item for weight control, cough, cold, or sinus problems without first checking with your doctor. • This drug may cause motor restlessness, uncoordinated movements, and muscle spasms. If you notice any of these effects, contact your doctor immediately — the drug may need to be stopped or the dosage may need to be adjusted. • This drug may cause urine to turn pink or red-brown; this is harmless. • Children with acute illnesses should take this drug only under close supervision. Their dosage may need adjustment. • If you take this drug for a prolonged time, it may be desirable for you to stop taking it for a while in order to see if you still need it. Do not stop taking the drug, however, without talking to your doctor first. You may have to reduce your dosage gradually.
Comments: The effects of this drug may not be apparent for at least two weeks. • Chew gum or suck on ice chips or a piece of hard candy to reduce mouth dryness. • To avoid dizziness or light-headedness when you stand, contract and relax the muscles of your legs for a few moments before rising. Do this by pushing one foot against the floor while raising the other foot slightly, alternating feet so that you are "pumping" your legs in a pedaling motion. •

Because this drug reduces sweating, avoid excessive work or exercise in hot weather and drink plenty of fluids. • The capsule form of this drug has sustained action. Never take it more frequently than your doctor prescribes; a serious overdose may result. The capsules are to be swallowed whole. Do not crush or chew them. • If you notice a sore throat, darkening vision, or fine tremors of your tongue, call your doctor. • Some side effects caused by this drug can be controlled by taking an antiparkinson drug. Discuss this with your doctor. • This drug may interfere with certain blood and urine laboratory tests. If you are scheduled for any such tests, remind your doctor that you are taking this medication.

Condrin-LA antihistamine and decongestant (Mallard, Inc.), see Ornade Spansules antihistamine and decongestant.

conjugated estrogen hormone (various manufacturers), see Premarin estrogen hormone.

Constant-T bronchodilator (Geigy Pharmaceuticals), see theophylline bronchodilator.

Contac 12 Hour antihistamine and decongestant (SmithKline Consumer Products), see Ornade Spansules antihistamine and decongestant.

contraceptives (oral), see oral contraceptives.

Corgard beta blocker

Manufacturer: Princeton Pharmaceutical Products
Ingredient: nadolol
Dosage Form: Tablet: 20 mg; 40 mg; 80 mg; 120 mg; 160 mg (all are blue)
Uses: Treatment of chest pain and high blood pressure
Minor Side Effects: Abdominal pain; bloating; blurred vision; constipation; drowsiness; dry eyes, mouth, or skin; gas or heartburn; headache; insomnia; loss of appetite; nasal congestion; nausea; slowed heart rate; sweating; vivid dreams; vomiting
Major Side Effects: Bleeding or bruising; confusion; decreased sexual ability; depression; diarrhea; difficulty in urinating; dizziness; earache; fever; hair loss; hallucinations; mouth sores; night cough; nightmares; numbness and tingling in the fingers and toes; rash; ringing in the ears; shortness of breath; swelling in the hands or feet
Contraindications: This drug should not be used by people who are allergic to nadolol or any other beta blocker. This drug should not be taken by people who suffer from certain types of heart disease or lung disease or by anyone who has taken any monoamine oxidase inhibitors within the past two weeks. Consult your doctor immediately if this drug has been prescribed for you and any of these conditions applies.
Warnings: This drug should be used with caution by persons with certain respiratory problems, diabetes, certain heart problems, liver disease, kidney disease, hypoglycemia, or thyroid disease. Be sure your doctor knows if you have any of these conditions. • Diabetics should watch for signs of altered blood glucose levels. • This drug should be used cautiously by pregnant women and by women of childbearing age. • This drug should be used with care during anesthesia and by patients undergoing major surgery. If possible,

this drug should be withdrawn 48 hours prior to surgery. • This drug should be used cautiously when reserpine is taken. • This drug may interact with cimetidine, chlorpromazine, oral contraceptives, salicylates, phenytoin, and theophyllines. If you are currently taking any of these types of drugs, consult your doctor about their use. If you are unsure about the type or contents of your medications, ask your doctor or pharmacist. • Do not abruptly stop taking this medication unless directed to do so by your doctor. Chest pain—even heart attacks—can occur when this drug is suddenly stopped. Your doctor will gradually reduce the dosage or substitute another medication.

Comments: Your doctor may want you to take your pulse and monitor your blood pressure every day while you take this medication. Discuss with your doctor what your normal pulse and blood pressure values are and what they should be. • Be sure to take this medication at the same time each day. • While taking this drug, do not take any nonprescription items for weight control, cough, cold, or sinus problems without first checking with your doctor; such items may contain ingredients that may increase blood pressure. • Notify your doctor if you develop dizziness, diarrhea, or a slow pulse or if you have breathing difficulties while on this medication. • This drug may make you more sensitive to the cold. Dress warmly. • There are many different beta blockers available. Your doctor may have you try different ones to find the one that's best for you.

Cortaid topical steroid (The Upjohn Company), see hydrocortisone topical steroid.

Cortatrigen Modified otic preparation (Goldline Laboratories), see Cortisporin Otic preparation.

Cort-Dome topical steroid (Miles Pharmaceutical), see hydrocortisone topical steroid.

Cortef Acetate topical steroid (The Upjohn Company), see hydrocortisone topical steroid.

Cortef oral steroid hormone (The Upjohn Company), see hydrocortisone oral steroid hormone.

cortisol oral steroid hormone (various manufacturers), see hydrocortisone oral steroid hormone.

Cortisporin ophthalmic preparation

Manufacturer: Burroughs Wellcome Co.
Ingredients: polymyxin B sulfate; neomycin sulfate; hydrocortisone; thimerosal (drops only); bacitracin (ointment only)
Equivalent Products: Bacticort Suspension, Rugby Laboratories; triple antibiotic, various manufacturers; Triple-Gen, Goldline Laboratories
Dosage Forms: Drop (content per ml): polymyxin B sulfate, 10,000 units; neomycin sulfate, 0.35%; hydrocortisone, 1%; thimerosal, 0.001%. Ointment (content per gram): polymyxin B sulfate, 10,000 units; neomycin sulfate, 0.35%; hydrocortisone, 1%; bacitracin, 400 units
Use: Short-term treatment of bacterial infections of the eye
Minor Side Effects: Blurred vision; burning; eye redness; stinging

Major Side Effects: Disturbed or reduced vision; eye pain; headache; severe irritation

Contraindications: This product should not be used for fungal or viral infections of the eye or for eye infections with pus. Nor should this product be used for conditions involving the back part of the eye. This drug should not be used by people who are allergic to any of its ingredients or by those with tuberculosis. Consult your doctor immediately if this drug has been prescribed for you and any of these conditions applies.

Warnings: Frequent eye examinations are advisable while this drug is being used, particularly if it is necessary to use the drug for an extended period of time. • This drug should be used cautiously by people with inner ear disease, kidney disease, or myasthenia gravis. • Prolonged use of this drug may result in secondary infection, cataracts, and eye damage. Contact your doctor immediately if you notice any visual disturbances (dimming or blurring of vision, reduced night vision, halos around lights), eye pain, or headache.

Comments: As with all eye medications, this drug may cause minor, temporary clouding or blurring of vision when first applied. • When you have used this product for the prescribed amount of time, discard any unused portion. • Consult your doctor if symptoms reappear. • The suspension should be shaken well before using. • Be careful about the contamination of medications used for the eyes. Do not touch the dropper or ointment tube to the eye surface. Wash your hands before administering eye medications. Do not wash or wipe the dropper before replacing it in the bottle. Close the bottle tightly to keep out moisture. • See the chapter on Administering Medication Correctly for instructions on using eye medications.

Cortisporin Otic preparation

Manufacturer: Burroughs Wellcome Co.

Ingredients: hydrocortisone; neomycin sulfate; polymyxin B sulfate

Equivalent Products: AK-Spore H.C. Otic, Akorn, Inc.; Cortatrigen Modified, Goldline Laboratories; Drotic, B.F. Ascher & Company, Inc.; Ortega Otic M, Ortega Pharmaceutical Company; Otocort, Lemmon Company; Otomycin-Hpn Otic, Misemer Pharmaceuticals, Inc.; Otoreid-HC, Reid-Rowell

Dosage Forms: Solution (per ml): hydrocortisone, 1%; neomycin sulfate, 5 mg; polymyxin B sulfate, 10,000 units. Suspension (per ml): hydrocortisone, 1%; neomycin sulfate, 5 mg; polymyxin B sulfate, 10,000 units

Use: Treatment of superficial bacterial infections of the outer ear

Minor Side Effects: Burning sensation; itching; rash

Major Side Effects: None

Contraindications: This drug should not be used to treat viral or fungal infections. This drug should not be taken by people who are allergic to it. Consult your doctor immediately if you have such a condition or allergy.

Warnings: Do not use this drug for more than ten days, unless your doctor directs you to do so. • This drug should be used cautiously if there is a possibility that the patient has a punctured eardrum. • This drug should be used cautiously by persons with myasthenia gravis or kidney disease. • Notify your doctor if your skin becomes red and swollen, scaly, or itchy; allergic reactions to neomycin are common.

Comments: To administer ear drops, tilt your head to one side with the affected ear turned upward. Grasp the earlobe and pull it upward and back to straighten the ear canal. (If administering ear drops to a child, gently pull the earlobe downward and back.) Fill the dropper and place the prescribed number of drops in the ear. Be careful not to touch the dropper to the ear canal, as the dropper can easily become contaminated this way. Keep the ear tilted upward for five to ten seconds, then gently insert a small piece of cotton into the ear to prevent the drops from escaping. • Do not wash or wipe the dropper after use. Close the bottle tightly to keep out moisture. • Discard any remaining medicine after treatment has been completed so that you will not be tempted to use the medication for a subsequent ear problem without consulting a doctor. • If you wish to warm the drops before administration, roll the bottle back and forth between your hands. Do not place the bottle in boiling water.

Cortizone-5 topical steroid (Thompson Medical), see hydrocortisone topical steroid.

Cortril topical steroid (Pfipharmecs Division), see hydrocortisone topical steroid.

Cotrim and Cotrim DS antibacterials (Lemmon Company), see Bactrim and Bactrim DS antibacterials.

Coumadin anticoagulant

Manufacturer: Du Pont Pharmaceuticals, Inc.
Ingredient: warfarin sodium
Equivalent Products: Carfin, Major Pharmaceuticals; Panwarfin, Abbott Laboratories; Sofarin, Lemmon Company; warfarin sodium, various manufacturers
Dosage Form: Tablet: 2 mg (lavender); 2.5 mg (orange); 5 mg (peach); 7.5 mg (yellow); 10 mg (white)
Use: Prevention of blood clot formation in conditions such as heart disease
Minor Side Effects: Blurred vision; cramps; decreased appetite; diarrhea; heavy bleeding from cuts; nausea
Major Side Effects: Black stools; coughing up blood; fever; hemorrhage; jaundice; loss of hair; mouth sores; nausea; rash; red urine; severe headache
Contraindications: This drug should not be taken if any condition or circumstance exists in which bleeding is likely to be worsened by taking the drug (such as ulcers or certain surgeries). Be sure that you have given your doctor a complete medical history. • This drug should not be taken by people who are allergic to it or by pregnant women. Consult your doctor immediately if this drug has been prescribed for you and either of these conditions applies.
Warnings: This drug should be used cautiously by people who have any condition where bleeding is an added risk, including those suffering malnutrition, and by people who have liver disease, kidney disease, intestinal infection, wounds or injuries, high blood pressure, blood disease (certain types), diabetes, menstrual difficulties, indwelling catheters, or congestive heart failure. The drug should be used cautiously by nursing mothers. Be sure your doctor knows if any of these conditions applies to you. • This drug interacts with alcohol, allopurinol, aminosalicylic acid, anabolic steroids, antibiotics, antidepressants, antipyrine, Bactrim/Septra, barbiturates, bromelains, chloral hydrate, chloramphenicol, chlordiazepoxide, chlorpropamide, cholestyramine, chymotrypsin, cimetidine, cinchophen, clofibrate, dextran, dextrothyroxine, diazoxide, diuretics, disulfiram, ethacrynic acid, ethchlorvynol, glucagon, glutethimide, griseofulvin, haloperidol, indomethacin, mefenamic acid, meprobamate, methyldopa, methylphenidate, metronidazole, monoamine oxidase inhibitors, nalidixic acid, neomycin, oral antidiabetics, oral contraceptives, oxyphenbutazone, paraldehyde, phenylbutazone, phenytoin, primidone, quinidine, quinine, rifampin, salicylates, steroids, sulfinpyrazone, sulfonamides, sulindac, thyroid drugs, tolbutamide, triclofos sodium, and vitamin C. If you are currently taking any

drugs of these types, consult your doctor about their use. If you are unsure of the type or contents of your medications, ask your doctor or pharmacist.

Comments: Do not start or stop taking any other medication, including aspirin, without checking with your doctor. • Although there are many equivalent products, you should not change brands. If you must switch brands, discuss the impact with your doctor or pharmacist. • Regular blood coagulation tests are essential while you are taking this drug. Many factors — including diet, environment, exercise, and other medications — may affect your response to this drug, so blood tests will need to be repeated often. • Avoid eating large amounts of leafy green vegetables and avoid drastic dietary changes while taking this drug. • If clots fail to form over cuts and bruises or if purple or brown spots appear under bruised skin, call your doctor immediately. • Do not increase your dose or take this drug more frequently than your doctor prescribes. • While taking this drug, avoid drinking alcoholic beverages. • A change in urine color may or may not be serious; if you notice a change, contact your doctor. • Notify your doctor if you develop yellow eyes or skin. • Be sure all of your health care professionals know you are taking this drug. It is advisable to wear a medical alert bracelet and to carry a medical information card that states that you are taking this drug. • It is important that you take this drug as prescribed and that you take it at the same time each day. Never take more than the prescribed dose. Your doctor or pharmacist may have a special calendar or chart you can use to keep track of your doses.

Curretab progesterone hormone (Reid-Provident Laboratories, Inc.), see Provera progesterone hormone.

Cyclopar antibiotic (Parke-Davis), see tetracycline hydrochloride antibiotic.

Dalmane sedative and hypnotic

Manufacturer: Roche Products Inc.
Ingredient: flurazepam hydrochloride
Equivalent Products: Durapam, Major Pharmaceuticals; flurazepam, various manufacturers
Dosage Form: Capsule: 15 mg (orange/ivory); 30 mg (red/ivory)
Use: Relief of insomnia
Minor Side Effects: Bitter taste in mouth; constipation; depression; diarrhea; dizziness; drowsiness; dry mouth; fatigue; flushing; headache; heartburn; loss of appetite; nausea; nervousness; sweating; vomiting
Major Side Effects: Blurred vision; chest pain; difficulty in urinating; double vision; fainting; falling; jaundice; joint pain; low blood pressure; mouth sores; nightmares; palpitations; rash; shortness of breath; slurred speech; sore throat; stimulation; uncoordinated movements
Contraindications: This drug should not be taken by people who are allergic to it or by pregnant women. Consult your doctor immediately if this drug has been prescribed for you and either of these conditions applies.
Warnings: This drug should be used cautiously by people with impaired liver or kidney function, lung disease, or myasthenia gravis; by the elderly or debilitated; and by people who are severely depressed. Be sure your doctor knows if any of these conditions applies to you. • This drug is not recommended for use by people under the age of 15. • This drug causes drowsiness; avoid tasks that require alertness. • Periodic blood counts and liver function tests should be performed if this drug is used over a long period. • To prevent oversedation and avoid serious adverse reactions, this drug should not be taken with alcohol or

other sedative drugs or central nervous system depressants. This drug may interact with cimetidine, oral anticoagulants, disulfiram, isoniazid, and rifampin. If you are currently taking any drugs of these types, consult your doctor about their use. If you are unsure of the type or contents of your medications, ask your doctor or pharmacist. • This drug has the potential for abuse and must be used with caution. Tolerance may develop quickly; do not increase the dose of the drug without first consulting your doctor. • If this drug has been used consistently for a prolonged period of time, it should not be stopped suddenly. The dosage should be reduced gradually. Consult your doctor.

Comments: This drug is widely used for inducing sleep. It is effective, but eliminating the cause of the insomnia is also important. • This drug should be taken 30 to 60 minutes before retiring. • Take this medication with food or a full glass of water if stomach upset occurs. Do not take it with a dose of antacids since they may retard absorption of the drug. • Notify your doctor if you develop signs of jaundice (yellow skin or eyes; dark urine). • Chew gum or suck on ice chips or a piece of hard candy to reduce mouth dryness. • This medication may cause you to feel lethargic and drowsy in the morning. Taking the drug in the early evening may help relieve the "hangover feeling." If drowsiness is a continual problem, you may want to discuss alternative sleep-aid products with your doctor or pharmacist. • Restoril and Halcion are also sedative and hypnotic agents that act similarly to Dalmane but are not as long lasting. The short-acting agents are preferred for use in the elderly.

Damacet-P analgesic (Mason Pharmaceuticals), see Vicodin analgesic.

D-Amp antibiotic (Dunhall Pharmaceuticals, Inc.), see ampicillin antibiotic.

Darvocet-N analgesic

Manufacturer: Eli Lilly & Co.
Ingredients: propoxyphene napsylate; acetaminophen
Equivalent Products: Doxapap-N, Major Pharmaceuticals; Propacet 100, Lemmon Company; propoxyphene napsylate and acetaminophen analgesic, various manufacturers
Dosage Form: Tablet: Darvocet-N 50: propoxyphene napsylate, 50 mg and acetaminophen, 325 mg (orange); Darvocet-N 100: propoxyphene napsylate, 100 mg and acetaminophen, 650 mg (orange)
Use: Relief of mild to moderate pain
Minor Side Effects: Abdominal pain; blurred vision; constipation; dizziness; drowsiness; euphoria; fatigue; headache; light-headedness; loss of appetite; nausea; restlessness; sedation; vomiting; weakness
Major Side Effects: Breathing difficulties; diarrhea; hives; liver dysfunction; palpitations; rash; ringing in the ears; seizures; sore throat; stomach cramps
Contraindication: This drug should not be used by persons allergic to either of its ingredients. Consult your doctor immediately if this drug has been prescribed for you and you have such an allergy.
Warnings: This drug should be used cautiously by people with blood disorders or heart, lung, liver, or kidney disease; it should be used cautiously by pregnant or nursing women. Be sure your doctor knows if any of these conditions applies to you. • This drug is not recommended for use by children under 12. • This drug has the potential for abuse and must be used with caution. Tolerance may develop quickly; do not increase your dose without consulting your doctor. • This drug can cause drowsiness; avoid tasks that require alertness. •

To prevent oversedation, avoid alcohol and other drugs that have sedative properties. • This drug should be used with extreme caution by patients taking tranquilizers or antidepressant drugs. If you are currently taking any drugs of these types, consult your doctor about their use. If you are unsure of the type or contents of your medications, ask your doctor or pharmacist.

Comments: Aspirin or acetaminophen should be tried before therapy with this drug is undertaken. If aspirin or acetaminophen does not relieve pain, this drug may be effective. • Since the napsylate form of this drug is converted to hydrochloride once it is in the stomach, you may want to ask your doctor to prescribe a generic brand of propoxyphene hydrochloride instead of the napsylate form; it may be less expensive. • Side effects from this drug may be somewhat relieved by lying down. • If stomach upset occurs, take this medication with food. • This drug may interfere with certain urine laboratory tests. Tell your doctor you are taking this drug before undergoing any urine tests.

Darvon Compound-65
analgesic

Manufacturer: Eli Lilly & Co.

Ingredients: aspirin; caffeine; propoxyphene hydrochloride

Equivalent Products: Bexophene, Mallard, Inc.; Doxaphene Compound, Major Pharmaceuticals; propoxyphene hydrochloride compound, various manufacturers

Dosage Form: Capsule: aspirin, 389 mg; caffeine, 32.4 mg; propoxyphene hydrochloride, 65 mg (crimson/light gray)

Use: Relief of mild to moderate pain

Minor Side Effects: Abdominal pain; anxiety; blurred vision; constipation; dizziness; drowsiness; euphoria; headache; indigestion; light-headedness; nausea; restlessness; ringing in the ears; sedation; vomiting; weakness

Major Side Effects: Chest tightness; kidney disease; liver dysfunction; rash; seizures; shortness of breath; sore throat

Contraindications: This drug should not be used by people allergic to any of its ingredients. It may cause allergic reactions and should not, therefore, be taken by people who have asthma, severe hay fever, or other significant allergies. Be sure your doctor knows if any of these conditions applies to you.

Warnings: This drug should be used cautiously by pregnant or nursing women; by children under 12; and by persons with diabetes, ulcers, liver disease, or kidney disease. Be sure your doctor knows if any of these conditions applies to you. • Persons who take this drug in high doses over long periods may develop kidney disease. Follow your doctor's dosage instructions carefully. • This drug may cause drowsiness; avoid tasks that require alertness. • To prevent oversedation, avoid the use of alcohol or other central nervous system depressants or drugs that have sedative qualities. • This drug should not be used in conjunction with alcohol, methotrexate, oral anticoagulants, orphenadrine, probenecid, or sulfinpyrazone. If you are currently taking any drugs of these types, consult your doctor about their use. If you are unsure of the type or contents of your medications, ask your doctor or pharmacist. • This drug has the potential for abuse and must be used with caution. Tolerance may develop quickly; do not increase the dose of this drug without first consulting your doctor. • If your ears feel unusual, if you hear buzzing or ringing, or if your stomach hurts, your dosage may need adjustment. Call your doctor.

Comments: An aspirin or acetaminophen product should be tried before this drug. If aspirin or acetaminophen does not relieve the pain, this drug may be effective. Eli Lilly & Co. also makes a Darvon compound with the same ingredients that contains only 32 mg of the propoxyphene. • Side effects from this drug may be somewhat relieved by lying down. • If stomach upset occurs, take this medication with food.

Decongestabs decongestant and antihistamine (various manufacturers), see Naldecon decongestant and antihistamine.

Dehist antihistamine and decongestant (Forest Pharmaceuticals, Inc.), see Ornade Spansules antihistamine and decongestant.

Delacort topical steroid (Mericon), see hydrocortisone topical steroid.

Deltasone steroid hormone (The Upjohn Company), see prednisone steroid hormone.

Deponit transdermal antianginal (Wyeth-Ayerst Laboratories), see nitroglycerin transdermal antianginal.

Dermacort topical steroid (Reid-Rowell), see hydrocortisone topical steroid.

DermiCort topical steroid (Republic Drug), see hydrocortisone topical steroid.

Dermolate topical steroid (Schering Corp.), see hydrocortisone topical steroid.

Dermtex HC topical steroid (Pfeiffer), see hydrocortisone topical steroid.

Desyrel antidepressant

Manufacturer: Mead Johnson Pharmaceuticals
Ingredient: trazodone
Equivalent Products: trazodone HCl, various manufacturers; Trialodine, Quantum Pharmics
Dosage Form: Tablet: 50 mg (orange); 100 mg (white); 150 mg (orange); 300 mg (yellow)
Use: Relief of depression
Minor Side Effects: Bad taste in mouth; blurred vision; constipation; diarrhea; dizziness; drowsiness; dry mouth; headache; insomnia; light-headedness; loss of appetite; nasal congestion; sweating; weight loss or gain
Major Side Effects: Chest pain; decreased sexual desire; disorientation; fluid retention; memory loss; menstrual changes; nightmares; numbness; prolonged or inappropriate erections; rapid heartbeat; seizures; shortness of breath; skin rash; tingling in fingers or toes; tremors; uncoordinated movements
Contraindications: This drug should not be taken by people who are allergic to it, by those with a history of alcoholism, or by those who have recently had a heart attack. Consult your doctor immediately if this drug has been prescribed for you and any of these conditions applies.
Warnings: This drug is not recommended for use by children under age 18.
• Male patients who experience prolonged or inappropriate erections should consult their doctor immediately. • This drug should be used cautiously by people who have certain types of heart disease, liver disease, or kidney disease and by pregnant or nursing women. Be sure your doctor knows if any of these conditions applies to you. • This drug interacts with digoxin, phenytoin, cloni-

dine, and barbiturates. If you are also taking antihypertensive drugs, you may require a decreased dose. If you are taking any drugs of these types, consult your doctor about their use. If you are unsure of the type or contents of your medications, ask your doctor or pharmacist. • This drug should be used with caution by people who are receiving electroshock therapy and by those about to undergo surgery. • This drug may cause dry mouth, irregular heartbeat, nausea, vomiting, or shortness of breath. Consult your doctor if these symptoms become bothersome or if they last for more than a few days. • This drug may cause drowsiness; avoid tasks that require alertness. To prevent oversedation, avoid the use of alcohol or other sedative agents.

Comments: Take this medicine exactly as your physician prescribes. Do not stop taking it without first checking with your doctor. It may be two to four weeks before the full effect of this drug becomes apparent. Your dose may be adjusted frequently at first until the best response is obtained. • While taking this drug, do not take any nonprescription item for weight control, cough, cold, or sinus problems without first checking with your doctor or pharmacist. • To minimize dizziness and light-headedness, take this medicine with food. To avoid dizziness or light-headedness when you stand, contract and relax the muscles of your legs for a few minutes before rising. Do this by pushing one foot against the floor while raising the other foot slightly, alternating feet so that you are "pumping" your legs in a pedaling motion. • Chew gum or suck on ice chips or hard candy to reduce mouth dryness.

DiaBeta oral antidiabetic (Hoechst-Roussel Pharmaceutical, Inc.), see Micronase oral antidiabetic.

Diabinese oral antidiabetic

Manufacturer: Pfizer Laboratories Division
Ingredient: chlorpropamide
Equivalent Product: chlorpropamide, various manufacturers
Dosage Form: Tablet: 100 mg; 250 mg (both blue)
Use: Treatment of diabetes mellitus not controlled by diet and exercise alone
Minor Side Effects: Cramps; diarrhea; dizziness; fatigue; headache; heartburn; increased sensitivity to sunlight; loss of appetite; nausea; stomach upset; vomiting; weakness
Major Side Effects: Anemia; breathing difficulties; fluid retention; jaundice; low blood sugar; numbness or tingling of fingers and toes; rash; ringing in the ears; sore throat
Contraindications: This drug should not be used by people with juvenile or insulin-dependent diabetes (see Comments); severe or unstable "brittle" diabetes; diabetes complicated by ketosis and acidosis, major surgery, severe infection, or severe trauma; by people with severe liver, thyroid, or kidney disease; or by people with an allergy to sulfonylureas. Be sure your doctor knows if any of these conditions applies to you.
Warnings: This drug should be used cautiously during pregnancy. If you are pregnant, or if you become pregnant while taking this drug, talk to your doctor about its use. • This drug should be used cautiously by people with Addison's disease. If you have this disease, be sure your doctor knows. • If you have any signs of liver damage, such as jaundice (marked by dark urine or yellow eyes or skin), itching, rash, low-grade fever, sore throat, or diarrhea, call your doctor. • This drug should be used cautiously in conjunction with alcohol, antibacterial sulfonamides, anticonvulsants, barbiturates, chloramphenicol, dicumarol, guanethidine, monoamine oxidase inhibitors, oral anticoagulants, oral contraceptives, phenylbutazone, probenecid, rifampin, salicylates, and steroids. If you

are currently taking any drugs of these types, consult your doctor about their use. If you are unsure of the type or contents of your medications, ask your doctor or pharmacist. • Use of this drug in combination with certain other drugs may bring about hypoglycemia. When starting this drug, your urine should be tested for sugar and acetone at least three times daily; your doctor should review the results at least once a week. Your doctor may also want you to have frequent laboratory tests of liver function. • Call your doctor if you develop an infection, fever, sore throat, rash, excessive thirst, dark urine, or light-colored stools while taking this drug. • It may be necessary for you to use insulin while taking this drug, particularly during the transition period from insulin to this oral antidiabetic, or when under severe stress or trauma.

Comments: Oral antidiabetic drugs such as this are not effective in the treatment of diabetes in children under age 12. • Studies have shown that a balanced diet and exercise program is extremely important in controlling diabetes. Persons taking antidiabetic drugs must still maintain their diet and exercise program and practice good personal hygiene. • During the first few weeks of therapy with this drug, visit your doctor frequently. • While taking this drug, check your urine/blood for sugar and ketones at least three times a day. • You will have to be switched to insulin therapy if complications (e.g., ketoacidosis, severe trauma, severe infection, diarrhea, nausea, or vomiting) or the need for major surgery develops. • This drug should be taken at the same time each day. Do not stop taking this drug unless told to do so by your doctor. • Persons taking this drug should know how to recognize the signs of low blood sugar, which include chills; cold sweat; cool, pale skin; drowsiness; headache; rapid pulse; tremors; and weakness. If any of these symptoms develops, eat or drink something containing sugar and call your doctor. • If this drug causes stomach upset, it may be taken with food. • Do not use alcohol while taking this drug. Avoid the use of any other drugs, including nonprescription cold remedies and aspirin, unless your doctor tells you to take them. • You may sunburn easily while taking this product. Avoid exposure to the sun as much as possible. • Be careful to watch for swollen feet or hands or a rapid weight gain, each of which could be indicative of fluid retention. • It is advised that you carry a medical alert card or wear a medical alert bracelet indicating that you are taking this medication. • There are other drugs similar to this one that vary slightly in activity (see Glucotrol, Micronase, Orinase, Tolinase). Certain persons who do not benefit from one type of oral antidiabetic agent may benefit from another.

Diahist antihistamine (Century Pharmaceuticals, Inc.), see Benadryl antihistamine.

Diaqua diuretic and antihypertensive (W. E. Hauck, Inc.), see hydrochlorothiazide diuretic and antihypertensive.

diazepam antianxiety (various manufacturers), see Valium antianxiety.

Di-Azo analgesic (Kay Pharmacal Co., Inc.), see Pyridium analgesic.

dicyclomine hydrochloride antispasmodic (various manufacturers), see Bentyl antispasmodic.

digoxin heart drug (various manufacturers), see Lanoxin heart drug.

Dilantin anticonvulsant

Manufacturer: Parke-Davis

Ingredient: phenytoin sodium

Equivalent Products: Diphenylan Sodium, The Lannett Company, Inc.; phenytoin sodium, various manufacturers (see Comments)

Dosage Forms: Capsule: 30 mg (white with pink stripe); 100 mg (white with orange stripe). Chewable tablet: 50 mg (yellow). Liquid (content per 5 ml teaspoon): 30 mg; 125 mg

Use: Control of seizure disorders

Minor Side Effects: Bleeding, tender gums; blurred vision; constipation; drowsiness; headache; insomnia; muscle twitching; nausea; vomiting

Major Side Effects: Arthritis; blood disorders; change in facial features; chest pain; confusion; dizziness; gland swelling; gum enlargement; hairiness; liver damage; nervousness; numbness; rash; slurred speech; sore throat; uncoordinated movements

Contraindication: This drug should not be taken by people who are allergic to it. Consult your doctor immediately if this drug has been prescribed for you and you have such an allergy.

Warnings: This drug should be used cautiously by the elderly, by people who have impaired liver function, and by pregnant women. Be sure your doctor knows if any of these conditions applies to you. • Diabetics who need to take this drug should check their urine sugar more frequently than usual, as this medication may raise blood sugar levels. • This drug should not be used to treat seizures if they are due to hypoglycemia. Careful diagnosis is essential before this drug is prescribed. • While taking this drug, you should see your doctor regularly for blood tests to monitor effectiveness. Talk to your doctor about these blood-level tests and gain an understanding of what they mean. You should be aware of the test results. • Because the metabolism of this drug may be significantly altered by the use of other drugs, great care must be taken when this drug is used concurrently with other drugs. Be sure that your doctor is aware of every medication that you take. Do not start or stop taking any other medication without first consulting your doctor. This drug interacts with barbiturates, carbamazepine, chloramphenicol, cimetidine, disulfiram, doxycycline, isoniazid, oral anticoagulants, oral antidiabetics, oral contraceptives, phenylbutazone, quinidine, steroids, sulfaphenazole, and tricyclic antidepressants; if you are currently taking any drugs of these types, consult your doctor about their use. If you are unsure of the type or contents of your medications, ask your doctor or pharmacist. • The results of certain lab tests may be altered if you are taking this drug. If you need any lab tests, remind your doctor that you are taking this drug. • Depending on the type of seizure being treated, this drug may be used in combination with other anticonvulsants. • Do not abruptly stop taking this drug or change your dosage without your doctor's advice; you may start to convulse.

Comments: Although several generic versions of this drug are available, you should not switch from one to another without your doctor's complete approval and careful assessment. • Some phenytoin products are taken once a day (for example, Phenytoin Sodium, Bolar Laboratories, and Dilantin Kapseals, Parke-Davis). Other products are generally taken in three daily doses. • Take this drug with food to minimize stomach upset. • Do not use this drug to treat headaches unless your doctor specifically recommends it. • Therapy with this drug may cause your gums to enlarge enough to cover the teeth. Gum enlargement can be minimized, at least partially, by good dental care — frequent brushing and massaging the gums with the rubber tip of a good toothbrush. Inform your dentist if you are taking this drug. • This drug may cause drowsiness, especially during the first few weeks of therapy; avoid tasks that require alertness. • To prevent oversedation, avoid the use of alcohol or other drugs that have sedative properties. • It is recommended you carry a medical alert card or wear a medical alert bracelet indicating that you are taking phenytoin. • It is important to take all doses of this medicine on time. • Notify your doctor if any of the following symptoms develop: fever; impaired coordination; mouth and gum sores; persistent headache; prolonged weakness; rash; slurred speech; sore throat; or unusual bleeding or bruising. • The liquid form of this drug must be shaken thoroughly before use. • If you take phenobarbital in addition to this drug, you may be able to take them together in a single product, Dilantin with Phenobarbital anticonvulsant. Consult your doctor.

Dilantin with Phenobarbital anticonvulsant (Parke-Davis), see Dilantin anticonvulsant (comments).

Dilatrate-SR antianginal (Reed & Carnrick), see Isordil antianginal.

Diphenatol antidiarrheal (Rugby Laboratories), see Lomotil antidiarrheal.

Diphen Cough antihistamine (My-K Labs), see Benadryl antihistamine.

diphenhydramine hydrochloride antihistamine (various manufacturers), see Benadryl antihistamine.

diphenoxylate hydrochloride with atropine sulfate antidiarrheal (various manufacturers), see Lomotil antidiarrheal.

Diphenylan Sodium anticonvulsant (The Lannett Company, Inc.), see Dilantin anticonvulsant.

dipyridamole antianginal and anticoagulant (various manufacturers), see Persantine antianginal and anticoagulant.

disopyramide phosphate antiarrhythmic (various manufacturers), see Norpace antiarrhythmic.

Di-Spaz antispasmodic (Vortech Pharmaceutical, Ltd.), see Bentyl antispasmodic.

Diulo diuretic and antihypertensive (Searle & Co.), see Zaroxolyn diuretic and antihypertensive.

Dolacet analgesic (W. E. Hauck, Inc.), see Vicodin analgesic.

Dolobid anti-inflammatory analgesic

Manufacturer: Merck Sharp & Dohme
Ingredient: diflunisal
Dosage Form: Tablet: 250 mg (peach); 500 mg (orange)
Uses: Symptomatic treatment of mild to moderate pain; treatment of osteoarthritis and rheumatoid arthritis

Minor Side Effects: Bloating: confusion; constipation; diarrhea; dizziness; drowsiness; gas; headache; heartburn; insomnia; loss of appetite; nausea; vomiting

Major Side Effects: Anemia; asthma; blood disorders; blood in stools, urine, or mouth; blurred vision; breathing difficulties; depression; fatigue; fluid retention; high blood pressure; itching; jaundice; loss of hair; loss of hearing; numbness or tingling in fingers or toes; rash; ringing in the ears; severe abdominal pain; sore throat; ulcer; weight gain

Contraindications: This drug should not be used by people who are allergic to it or to aspirin or other nonsteroidal anti-inflammatory drugs. Consult your doctor immediately if this drug has been prescribed for you and you have such an allergy. • This drug should not be used by pregnant or nursing women. If this drug has been prescribed for you and either of these conditions applies, consult your doctor immediately.

Warnings: This drug should be used cautiously by elderly people; children under 14; people with a history of gastrointestinal disorders; and people with mental illness, epilepsy, Parkinson's disease, infections, bleeding disorders, kidney or liver disease, high blood pressure, or heart failure. Be sure your doctor knows if any of these conditions applies to you. • Nursing women who must use this drug should stop nursing. • The severity of the side effects caused by this drug depends upon the dosage taken. Use the least amount possible and watch carefully for side effects. • This drug may cause ulcers. Call your doctor if you experience stomach pain or if your stools are black and tarry. • If you notice changes in your vision or if you experience headaches while taking this drug, call your doctor. • This drug may cause drowsiness; avoid tasks that require alertness. • Side effects are more likely to occur in the elderly. • This drug interacts with aspirin, acetaminophen, other anti-inflammatories, probenecid, lithium, phenytoin, anticoagulants, steroids, sulfa drugs, diabetes drugs, and diuretics. If you are currently taking any drugs of these types, talk to your doctor about their use. Do not take aspirin or acetaminophen with this drug unless told to do so by your doctor. If you are not sure about the type or contents of your medications, talk to your doctor or pharmacist.

Comments: This drug is not intended for general aches and pains. • Regular medical checkups, including blood tests, are required of persons taking this drug. • Notify your doctor if you develop signs of jaundice (yellow eyes or skin; dark urine). • This drug may be taken with food or milk immediately after meals, or with antacids (other than sodium bicarbonate). Never take this drug on an empty stomach or with aspirin or alcohol. Do not crush or chew the tablets; swallow them whole. • If you are taking an anticoagulant (blood thinner), remind your doctor. • This drug may cause discoloration of the urine or feces. If you notice a change in color, call your doctor. • It may take a month before you feel the full effect of this drug. If you are taking diflunisal to relieve osteoarthritis, you must take it regularly, as directed by your doctor.

Donnamor sedative and anticholinergic (H. L. Moore, Inc.), see Donnatal sedative and anticholinergic.

Donnapine sedative and anticholinergic (Major Pharmaceuticals), see Donnatal sedative and anticholinergic.

Donna-Sed sedative and anticholinergic (Vortech Pharmaceutical, Ltd.), see Donnatal sedative and anticholinergic.

Donnatal sedative and anticholinergic

Manufacturer: A. H. Robins Company

Ingredients: atropine sulfate; scopolamine hydrobromide; hyoscyamine sulfate; phenobarbital

Equivalent Products: belladonna alkaloids with phenobarbital, various manufacturers; Donnamor, H. L. Moore, Inc.; Donnapine, Major Pharmaceuticals; Donna-Sed, Vortech Pharmaceutical, Ltd.; Hyosophen, Rugby Laboratories; Malatal, Mallard, Inc.; Relaxadon, Geneva Generics, Inc.; Spaslin, Blaine Co., Inc.; Spasmolin, various manufacturers; Spasmophen, The Lannett Company, Inc.; Spasquid, Geneva Generics, Inc.; Susano, Halsey Drug Co., Inc.

Dosage Forms: Capsule (green/white); Liquid (content per 5 ml teaspoon); Tablet (white): atropine sulfate, 0.0194 mg; scopolamine hydrobromide, 0.0065 mg; hyoscyamine sulfate, 0.1037 mg; phenobarbital, 16.2 mg. Sustained-action tablet: atropine sulfate, 0.0582 mg; scopolamine hydrobromide, 0.0195 mg; hyoscyamine sulfate, 0.3111 mg; phenobarbital, 48.6 mg (green)

Uses: Treatment of bed-wetting, motion sickness, premenstrual tension, stomach and intestinal disorders, urinary frequency

Minor Side Effects: Blurred vision; confusion; constipation; decreased sexual desire; dizziness; drowsiness; drying up of breast milk; dry mouth; headache; insomnia; loss of taste; muscle pain; nausea; nervousness; rapid heart rate; reduced sweating; sensitivity of eyes to sunlight; vomiting; weakness

Major Side Effects: Breathing difficulties; difficulty in urinating; hallucinations; hot and dry skin; impotence; jaundice; palpitations; rash; slurred speech; sore throat

Contraindications: This drug should not be taken by people who have glaucoma, enlarged prostate, obstructed bladder, obstructed intestine, acute hemorrhage, severe ulcerative colitis, liver disease, myasthenia gravis, hiatal hernia, or porphyria or by those who are allergic to any of the ingredients in this drug. Consult your doctor immediately if the drug has been prescribed for you and you have any of these conditions or such an allergy.

Warnings: This drug should be used cautiously in conjunction with amantadine, haloperidol, antacids, phenothiazines, alcohol, griseofulvin, tranquilizers, oral anticoagulants, steroids, sulfonamides, tetracycline, tricyclic antidepressants, quinidine, digitalis, rifampin, oral contraceptives, chloramphenicol, and phenytoin; if you are currently taking any drugs of these types, consult your doctor about their use. If you are unsure of the type or contents of your medications, ask your doctor or pharmacist. • Do not use this drug to treat diarrhea caused by an obstructed intestine. • Despite its phenobarbital content, this drug has not been shown to have high potential for abuse. Nonetheless, be sure to follow dosage instructions carefully. • This drug should be used with caution by people with kidney, thyroid, or heart disease; by those with high blood pressure; and by pregnant or nursing women. Be sure your doctor knows if any of these conditions applies to you. • This drug may cause drowsiness; avoid tasks that require alertness. To prevent oversedation, avoid taking alcohol or other drugs that have sedative properties.

Comments: This drug is best taken one-half to one hour before meals. • This drug does not cure ulcers but may help them improve. • If this drug makes it difficult for you to urinate, try to do so just before taking each dose. • Notify your doctor if you develop signs of jaundice (yellow eyes or skin; dark urine). • Chew gum or suck on ice chips or hard candy to relieve mouth dryness. • Because this drug may reduce sweating, avoid excessive work or exercise in hot weather and drink plenty of fluids. • The elderly may be more sensitive to this drug's side effects. • If side effects persist or become bothersome, call your doctor.

Doxapap-N analgesic (Major Pharmaceuticals), see Darvocet-N analgesic.

Doxaphene Compound analgesic (Major Pharmaceuticals), see Darvon Compound-65 analgesic.

Doxepin HC antidepressant and antianxiety (various manufacturers), see Sinequan antidepressant and antianxiety.

Drize antihistamine and decongestant (B. F. Ascher & Company, Inc.), see Ornade Spansules antihistamine and decongestant.

Drotic otic preparation (B.F. Ascher & Company, Inc.), see Cortisporin Otic preparation.

Duradyne DHC analgesic (Forest Pharmaceuticals, Inc.), see Vicodin analgesic.

Durapam sedative and hypnotic (Major Pharmaceuticals), see Dalmane sedative and hypnotic.

Dura-Vent decongestant and expectorant (Dura Pharmaceuticals, Inc), see Entex LA decongestant and expectorant.

Duricef antibiotic

Manufacturer: Mead Johnson Pharmaceuticals
Ingredient: cefadroxil
Equivalent Product: Ultracef, Bristol Laboratories
Dosage Forms: Capsule: 500 mg (white/burgundy). Liquid (content per 5 ml teaspoon): 125 mg; 250 mg; 500 mg. Tablet: 1 g (white)
Use: Treatment of bacterial infections
Minor Side Effects: Diarrhea; dizziness; headache; heartburn; nausea; vomiting
Major Side Effects: Breathing difficulties; hypersensitivity reactions such as rash, itching, muscle aches, and fever; severe diarrhea; vaginal itching; superinfection
Contraindications: This drug should not be used by persons who are allergic to it, to other cephalosporin antibiotics, or to penicillin antibiotics (see Comments). Consult your doctor if this drug has been prescribed for you and you have such an allergy.
Warnings: This drug should be used cautiously by persons with kidney disease or a history of colitis and by pregnant or nursing women. Make sure your doctor knows if any of these conditions applies to you. • Contact your doctor if you develop diarrhea while taking this medication, especially if it is severe or contains blood. • Diabetics using Clinitest urine test may get a false high sugar reading while taking this drug. Change to Clinistix, Diastix, Chemstrip UG, or Tes-Tape while taking this drug to avoid this problem.
Comments: It is generally believed that ten percent of all people allergic to penicillin drugs may be allergic to a cephalosporin-type antibiotic such as Duricef. Talk to your doctor or pharmacist about alternative medicines if you have such an allergy. • If stomach upset occurs, take this drug with food or milk. • Finish all of this medication, even if your symptoms disappear after a

few days. The drug is usually taken for a full ten days. Stopping treatment early may lead to reinfection. For best results, take the antibiotic at evenly spaced intervals around the clock. Ask your doctor or pharmacist to help you determine a dosage schedule. • The liquid form must be stored in the refrigerator and shaken well before using. Discard any unused portion after 14 days.

Durrax antianxiety (Dermik Laboratories, Inc.), see Atarax antianxiety

Dyazide diuretic and antihypertensive

Manufacturer: Smith Kline & French Laboratories
Ingredients: hydrochlorothiazide; triamterene
Equivalent Product: triamterene with hydrochlorothiazide, various manufacturers
Dosage Form: Capsule: hydrochlorothiazide, 25 mg and triamterene, 50 mg (maroon/white)
Uses: Treatment of high blood pressure; removal of fluid from the tissues
Minor Side Effects: Constipation; diarrhea; dizziness; drowsiness; dry mouth; fatigue; headache; itching; loss of appetite; nausea; restlessness; sun sensitivity; upset stomach; vomiting; weakness
Major Side Effects: Asthma; bruising; elevated blood sugar; elevated uric acid; jaundice; kidney stones; mood changes; muscle cramps or spasms; palpitations; rash; sore throat; tingling in fingers or toes; weak pulse
Contraindications: This drug should not be used by persons with severe liver or kidney disease, hyperkalemia (high blood levels of potassium), or anuria (inability to urinate). Be sure your doctor knows if you have any of these conditions. • This drug should not be used routinely during pregnancy in otherwise healthy women, since mother and fetus are being exposed unnecessarily to possible hazards. • This drug should not be used by persons allergic to it or to sulfa drugs. Consult your doctor immediately if this drug has been prescribed for you and you have such an allergy.
Warnings: Unlike many diuretic drugs, this drug usually does not cause the loss of potassium. Do not take potassium supplements while taking this drug unless directed to do so by your doctor. • This drug should be used cautiously by pregnant women; children; and people with diabetes, allergy, asthma, liver disease, anemia, blood diseases, high calcium levels, or gout. Nursing mothers who must take this drug should stop nursing. Be sure your doctor knows if any of these conditions applies to you. • This drug may affect the results of thyroid function tests. Be sure your doctor knows you are taking this drug if you must have such tests. • Regular blood tests should be performed if you must take this drug for a long time. You should also be tested for kidney function. • If you develop a sore throat, bleeding, bruising, dry mouth, weakness, or muscle cramps, call your doctor. • Persons who take this drug with digitalis should watch for signs of increased toxicity (e.g., nausea, blurred vision, palpitations). Call your doctor if such symptoms develop. • If you must undergo surgery, remind your doctor that you are taking this drug. • This drug interacts with curare, digitalis, lithium carbonate, oral antidiabetics, potassium salts, steroids, and spironolactone. If you are currently taking any drugs of these types, consult your doctor about their use. If you are unsure of the type or contents of your medications, ask your doctor or pharmacist.
Comments: This drug causes frequent urination. Expect this effect; it should not alarm you. This drug may cause the urine to turn blue; this is harmless. • Take this drug with food or milk. • Take this drug exactly as directed. Do not skip a dose or take extra doses without first consulting your doctor. • While taking this drug (as with many drugs that lower blood pressure), you should limit

your consumption of alcoholic beverages in order to prevent dizziness or light-headedness. • To avoid dizziness or light-headedness when you stand, contract and relax the muscles of your legs for a few moments before rising. Do this by pushing one foot against the floor while raising the other foot slightly, alternating feet so that you are "pumping" your legs in a pedaling motion. • If you are allergic to a sulfa drug, you may likewise be allergic to this drug. Be sure to inform your doctor if you have a sulfa-drug allergy. • When taking this drug, do not take any nonprescription item for weight control, cough, cold, or sinus problems without first checking with your doctor; such items may contain ingredients that can increase blood pressure. • Notify your doctor if you develop signs of jaundice (yellow eyes or skin; dark urine). • A doctor should probably not prescribe this drug or other fixed dose products as the first choice in the treatment of high blood pressure. The patient should receive each of the individual ingredients singly, and if the response is adequate to the fixed doses contained in Dyazide, it can be substituted. The advantage of a combination product such as this drug is increased convenience to the patient. • This drug has the same ingredients as Maxzide, but the strengths are different.

E.E.S. antibiotic (Abbott Laboratories), see erythromycin antibiotic.

Effer-K potassium chloride replacement (Nomax Pharmaceutical, Inc.), see potassium chloride replacement.

Elavil antidepressant (Merck Sharp & Dohme), see amitriptyline antidepressant.

Elixicon bronchodilator (Berlex Laboratories, Inc.), see theophylline bronchodilator.

Elixomin bronchodilator (Cenci), see theophylline bronchodilator.

Elixophyllin bronchodilator (Forest Pharmaceuticals, Inc.), see theophylline bronchodilator.

Emcodeine analgesic (Major Pharmaceuticals), see Empirin with Codeine analgesic.

Emitrip antidepressant (Major Pharmaceuticals), see amitriptyline antidepressant.

Empirin with Codeine analgesic

Manufacturer: Burroughs Wellcome Co.
Ingredients: aspirin; codeine phosphate
Equivalent Products: Aspirin with Codeine, Halsey Drug Co., Inc.; Emcodeine, Major Pharmaceuticals
Dosage Form: Tablet (see Comments): aspirin, 325 mg and codeine phosphate (all are white)
Use: Relief of moderate to severe pain
Minor Side Effects: Bruising; confusion; constipation; dizziness; drowsiness; euphoria; flushing; headache; indigestion; itching; light-headedness; loss of appetite; nausea; slight blood loss; sweating; vomiting

Major Side Effects: Black, tarry stools; breathing difficulties; jaundice; palpitations; rapid or slow heartbeat; ringing in the ears; skin rash; tremors; ulcers; urine retention

Contraindication: This drug should not be used by people who are allergic to either of its ingredients. Consult your doctor immediately if this drug has been prescribed for you and you have such an allergy.

Warnings: This drug may cause drowsiness; avoid activities requiring alertness, including driving a motor vehicle or operating machinery. To prevent oversedation, avoid the use of other sedative drugs or alcohol. • This drug should be used cautiously by elderly or debilitated persons; pregnant women; and persons with head injuries, diseases of the abdomen, allergies, thyroid disease, peptic ulcer, liver or kidney disease, coagulation problems, or prostate problems. Be sure your doctor knows if any of these conditions applies to you. • This drug interacts with alcohol, ammonium chloride, methotrexate, steroids, 6-mercaptopurine, oral antidiabetics, phenytoin, oral anticoagulants, and gout medications (probenecid, sulfinpyrazone). If you are currently taking any drugs of these types, consult your doctor about their use. If you are unsure of the type or contents of your medications, ask your doctor or pharmacist. • Products containing narcotics (e.g., codeine) are usually not used for more than seven to ten days. This drug has the potential for abuse and must be used with caution. Tolerance may develop quickly; do not increase the dose of this drug without first consulting your doctor.

Comments: For this and other preparations containing codeine, the number which follows the drug name always refers to the amount of codeine present. Hence, #1 has 1/8 grain (7.5 mg); #2 has 1/4 grain (15 mg); #3 has 1/2 grain (30 mg); and #4 contains 1 grain (60 mg). These numbers are standard for amounts of codeine. • Take this drug with food or milk to lessen stomach upset. • If your ears feel strange, if you hear buzzing or ringing, or if your stomach hurts, your dosage may need adjustment; call your doctor. • Notify your doctor if you develop signs of jaundice (yellow eyes or skin; dark urine). • Side effects caused by this drug may be somewhat relieved by lying down. • While taking this drug, do not take any nonprescription medicine that contains aspirin.

Empracet with Codeine analgesic (Burroughs Wellcome Co.), see acetaminophen with codeine analgesic.

E-Mycin antibiotic (The Upjohn Company), see erythromycin antibiotic.

Endep antidepressant (Roche Products Inc.), see amitriptyline antidepressant.

Enduron diuretic and antihypertensive

Manufacturer: Abbott Laboratories
Ingredient: methyclothiazide
Equivalent Products: Aquatensen, Wallace Laboratories; Ethon, Major Pharmaceuticals; methyclothiazide, various manufacturers
Dosage Form: Tablet: 2.5 mg (orange); 5 mg (salmon)
Uses: Treatment of high blood pressure; removal of fluid from the tissues
Minor Side Effects: Constipation; cramps; diarrhea; dizziness; drowsiness; headache; heartburn; itching; loss of appetite; nausea; restlessness; sun sensitivity; vomiting
Major Side Effects: Blood disorders; blurred vision; bruising; chest pain; dry mouth; elevated blood sugar; elevated uric acid; fever; jaundice; mood

changes; muscle spasm; shortness of breath; skin rash; sore throat; thirst; tingling in the fingers and toes; weakness

Contraindications: This drug should not be taken by people who have severe kidney disease or by those who are allergic to this drug or sulfa drugs. Consult your doctor immediately if this drug has been prescribed for you and you have such a condition or such an allergy.

Warnings: This drug should be used cautiously by pregnant women and by people who have asthma or allergies, kidney or liver disease, or diabetes. Be sure your doctor knows if any of these conditions applies to you. • Nursing women who must take this drug should stop nursing. • This drug interacts with digitalis, lithium, nonsteroidal anti-inflammatories, oral antidiabetics, and steroids; if you are currently taking any drugs of these types, consult your doctor about their use. If you are unsure of the type or contents of your medications, ask your doctor or pharmacist. • This drug may affect the potency of, or your need for, other blood pressure drugs and antidiabetics; dosage adjustment may be necessary. • This drug must be used cautiously with digitalis; be sure your doctor knows if you are taking digitalis in addition to this drug. Watch for symptoms of increased toxicity (e.g., nausea, blurred vision, palpitations), and notify your doctor if they occur. • If you have high blood pressure, do not take any nonprescription item for weight control, cough, cold, or sinus problems without first checking with your doctor; such items may contain ingredients that can increase blood pressure. • While taking this product (as with many drugs that lower blood pressure), you should limit your consumption of alcoholic beverages in order to prevent dizziness or light-headedness. • This drug may influence the results of thyroid function tests; if you are scheduled to have such a test, remind your doctor that you are taking this drug. • This drug may cause gout, high blood levels of calcium, or the onset of diabetes that has been latent; periodic measurement of blood levels of sugar, calcium, uric acid, and potassium are advisable while you are using this drug.

Comments: This drug causes frequent urination. Expect this effect; it should not alarm you. Try to plan your dosage schedule to avoid taking this drug at bedtime. • Notify your doctor if you develop signs of jaundice (yellow eyes or skin; dark urine). • To avoid dizziness or light-headedness when you stand, contract and relax the muscles of your legs for a few moments before rising. Do this by pushing one foot against the floor while raising the other foot slightly, alternating feet so that you are "pumping" your legs in a pedaling motion. • To help avoid potassium loss while using this product, take your dose with a glass of fresh or frozen orange juice and eat a banana each day. The use of a salt substitute also helps prevent potassium loss. Do not change your diet, however, before discussing it with your doctor. Too much potassium may also be dangerous. Signs of potassium loss include dry mouth, thirst, weakness, muscle pain or cramps, nausea, and vomiting. Call your doctor if you notice such symptoms. • You should learn how to monitor your pulse and blood pressure while taking this drug. Discuss with your doctor what your normal values should be. • This drug must be taken exactly as directed. Do not skip a dose or take extra doses without first consulting your doctor.

Entex LA decongestant and expectorant

Manufacturer: Norwich Eaton Pharmaceuticals, Inc.
Ingredients: phenylpropanolamine hydrochloride; guaifenesin
Equivalent Products: Banex-LA, LuChem; Dura-Vent, Dura Pharmaceuticals, Inc; Rymed-TR, Edwards Pharmacal; Tega D & E, Ortega Pharmaceutical Company
Dosage Form: Sustained-release tablet (see Comments): phenylpropanolamine hydrochloride, 75 mg and guaifenesin, 400 mg (blue)

Use: For relief of cough and nasal congestion

Minor Side Effects: Dizziness; headache; insomnia; loss of appetite; nausea; nervousness; restlessness; stomach upset

Major Side Effects: Chest pain; difficulty in urinating; fainting; palpitations; tremor

Contraindications: This drug should not be used by persons with an allergy to either of its components or by persons with severe high blood pressure. This drug should not be used in conjunction with monoamine oxidase inhibitors. Contact your doctor immediately if this drug has been prescribed for you and any of these conditions applies. If you are unsure about the types or contents of your medications, consult your doctor or pharmacist. • This drug is not recommended for use in children under six years of age.

Warnings: This drug must be used cautiously by persons with high blood pressure, diabetes, certain types of heart disease, glaucoma, hyperthyroidism, or enlarged prostate and by pregnant or nursing women. Be sure your doctor knows if any of these conditions applies to you. • This drug interacts with monoamine oxidase inhibitors and sympathomimetic drugs. If you are currently taking drugs of these types, consult your doctor. If you are unsure about the types or contents of your medications, ask your doctor or pharmacist. • This drug may affect the results of certain laboratory tests. Be sure to remind your doctor you are taking this drug if you are scheduled for any tests.

Comments: This drug must be swallowed whole. Do not crush or chew the tablets. • While taking this drug, you should drink at least six to eight glasses of fluid each day. • To relieve dry mouth, chew gum or suck on ice chips or hard candy. • Contact your physician if chest pain, tremor, or dizziness occur while taking this medication. • Avoid the use of nonprescription cough and cold medicines in conjunction with this drug, unless recommended by your doctor or pharmacist; such items may contain similar ingredients to this drug. • Although Entex LA and Dura-Vent have similar actions and are used for the same purpose, Dura-Vent contains 200 mg more of the guaifenesin than does Entex LA. • This drug is also available in liquid and capsule forms under the name Entex, which must be dosed more frequently.

Epitol anticonvulsant (Lemmon Company), see Tegretol anticonvulsant.

Eramycin antibiotic (Wesley Pharmacal Co.), see erythromycin antibiotic.

Eryc antibiotic (Parke-Davis), see erythromycin antibiotic.

Erypar antibiotic (Parke-Davis), see erythromycin antibiotic.

EryPed antibiotic (Abbott Laboratories), see erythromycin antibiotic.

Ery-Tab antibiotic (Abbott Laboratories), see erythromycin antibiotic.

Erythrocin Stearate antibiotic (Abbott Laboratories), see erythromycin antibiotic.

erythromycin antibiotic

Manufacturer: various manufacturers
Ingredient: erythromycin
Equivalent Products: E.E.S., Abbott Laboratories; E-Mycin, The Upjohn Company; Eramycin, Wesley Pharmacal Co.; Eryc, Parke-Davis; Erypar, Parke-Davis; EryPed, Abbott Laboratories; Ery-Tab, Abbott Laboratories; Erythrocin Stearate, Abbott Laboratories; Ilosone, Dista Products Company; Ilotycin, Dista Products Company; PCE, Abbott Laboratories; Pediamycin, Ross Laboratories; Robimycin, A. H. Robins Company; Wyamycin, Wyeth-Ayerst Laboratories
Dosage Forms: Capsule; Chewable tablet; Drops; Liquid; Tablet (various dosages and various colors)
Use: Treatment of a wide variety of bacterial infections
Minor Side Effects: Abdominal cramps; black tongue; cough; diarrhea; fatigue; irritation of the mouth; loss of appetite; nausea; vomiting
Major Side Effects: Dark urine; fever; hearing loss; jaundice; pale stools; rash; rectal and vaginal itching; superinfection; weakness
Contraindication: This drug should not be taken by people who are allergic to it. Consult your doctor immediately if you have such an allergy.
Warnings: This drug should be used cautiously by people who have liver disease and by pregnant or nursing women. • This drug may affect the potency of theophylline; if you are currently taking theophylline, consult your doctor about its use. This drug may interact with digoxin, anticoagulants (blood thinners), and carbamazepine. If you are taking any of these medications, consult your doctor about their use. If you are unsure about the contents of your medications, ask your doctor or pharmacist.
Comments: It is best to take this drug on an empty stomach (one hour before or two hours after a meal); however, if stomach upset occurs, take this drug with food. Take each dose with a full glass of water. • It is best to take this medication at evenly spaced intervals around the clock. Your doctor or pharmacist will help you choose the best schedule. • Finish all the medication prescribed, even if your symptoms disappear after a few days. Stopping treatment early may lead to reinfection. • Call your doctor if diarrhea, vomiting, or stomach cramps persist or if your urine turns dark, your stools turn pale, or unusual weakness develops. • The liquid forms of this drug should be stored in the refrigerator. • Not all erythromycin products are chemically equivalent. However, most produce the same therapeutic effect. Discuss with your doctor or pharmacist which products are appropriate for you, and then choose among those recommended.

Esidrix diuretic and antihypertensive (Ciba Pharmaceutical Company), see hydrochlorothiazide diuretic and antihypertensive.

Ethon diuretic and antihypertensive (Major Pharmaceuticals), see Enduron diuretic and antihypertensive.

Etrafon phenothiazine and antidepressant (Schering Corp.), see Triavil phenothiazine and antidepressant.

Feldene anti-inflammatory

Manufacturer: Pfizer Laboratories Division
Ingredient: piroxicam
Dosage Form: Capsule: 10 mg (blue/maroon); 20 mg (maroon)
Use: Relief of pain and swelling due to arthritis

Minor Side Effects: Bloating; constipation; diarrhea; dizziness; drowsiness; gas; gastrointestinal upset; headache; insomnia; loss of appetite; mouth soreness; nausea; vomiting; weakness

Major Side Effects: Bleeding or bruising; blood disorders; blood in stools; blurred vision; breathing difficulties; confusion; difficulty in urinating; fluid retention; jaundice; ringing in the ears; skin rash; swelling of the feet and ankles; tightness in the chest; ulcer; weight gain

Contraindications: This drug should not be used by people who are allergic to it, to aspirin, or to other anti-inflammatory drugs. Contact your physician immediately if this drug has been prescribed for you and you have such an allergy.

Warnings: This drug should be used with extreme caution by patients with a history of ulcers or gastrointestinal disease. Peptic ulcers and gastrointestinal bleeding, sometimes severe, have been reported in persons taking this drug. Make sure your doctor knows if you have or have had either condition. Notify your doctor if you experience frequent indigestion or notice blood in your stools. • This drug should be used with caution by persons with anemia, certain types of heart disease, bleeding diseases, high blood pressure, liver disease, or kidney disease. Be sure your doctor knows if you have any of these conditions. • This drug should not be used by pregnant women or nursing mothers. It should be used cautiously in children. • Should any eye problems arise while taking this drug, notify your doctor immediately. • Use of this drug has been reported to bring about fluid retention, skin rash, and weight gain. If you notice any of these symptoms, you should immediately consult your doctor. • This drug should be used with caution if you are also taking anticoagulants, oral antidiabetics, barbiturates, diuretics, steroids, phenytoin, or aspirin. If you are currently taking any drugs of these types, consult your doctor about their use. If you are unsure of the type or contents of your medications, ask your doctor or pharmacist.

Comments: In numerous tests, this drug has been shown to be as effective as aspirin in the treatment of arthritis, but aspirin is still the drug of choice for the disease. This drug is often used when aspirin is no longer effective. • Do not take aspirin or alcohol while taking this drug without first consulting your doctor. • You should note improvement in your condition soon after you start using this drug; however, full benefit may not be obtained for one to two weeks. It is important not to stop taking this drug even though symptoms have diminished or disappeared. • This drug is not a substitute for rest, physical therapy, or other measures recommended by your doctor to treat your condition. • Notify your doctor if skin rash, itching, swelling of the hands or feet, or persistent headache occurs. • Notify your doctor if you develop signs of jaundice (yellow eyes or skin; dark urine). • Take this drug with food or milk to decrease stomach upset. • This drug acts very similarly to other anti-inflammatory drugs, such as Indocin, Motrin, and Tolectin, but has a longer duration of action, allowing it to be taken only once a day. If one of these anti-inflammatory drugs is not well tolerated, your doctor may have you try other ones in order to find the best drug for you.

Femazole antimicrobial and antiparasitic (Major Pharmaceuticals), see Flagyl antimicrobial and antiparasitic.

fenoprofen anti-inflammatory (various manufacturers), see Nalfon anti-inflammatory.

Fenylhist antihistamine (Mallard, Inc.), see Benadryl antihistamine.

Fiorgen PF analgesic (Goldline Laboratories), see Fiorinal analgesic.

Fiorgen with Codeine analgesic (Goldline Laboratories), see Fiorinal with Codeine analgesic.

Fiorinal analgesic

Manufacturer: Sandoz Pharmaceuticals
Ingredients: aspirin; butalbital; caffeine
Equivalent Products: butalbital compound, various manufacturers; Fiorgen PF, Goldline Laboratories; Isollyl (Improved), Rugby Laboratories; Lanorinal, The Lannett Company, Inc.; Marnal, Vortech Pharmaceutical, Ltd.
Dosage Forms: Capsule (bright green/light green); Tablet (white): aspirin, 325 mg; butalbital, 50 mg; caffeine, 40 mg
Use: Relief of headache pain associated with tension
Minor Side Effects: Dizziness; drowsiness; gas; insomnia; light-headedness; loss of appetite; nausea; nervousness; vomiting
Major Side Effects: Chest tightness; difficulty in urinating; jaundice; loss of coordination; palpitations; ringing in the ears; shortness of breath
Contraindications: This drug should not be taken by people who are allergic to aspirin or any of the other ingredients or by people who have porphyria. Consult your doctor immediately if this drug has been prescribed for you and you have such a condition or such an allergy.
Warnings: This drug should be used cautiously by people who have ulcers, coagulation problems, liver disease, gout, or kidney disease and by women who are pregnant or nursing. Be sure your doctor knows if you have any of these conditions. • Because of the butalbital (barbiturate) content, this drug may be habit-forming; do not take this drug unless absolutely necessary. This drug has the potential for abuse and must be used with caution. Tolerance may develop quickly; do not increase the dose without first consulting your doctor. • No more than six tablets or capsules of this drug should be taken in one day. • This drug may cause drowsiness; avoid tasks that require alertness. To prevent oversedation, avoid the use of alcohol or other drugs that have sedative properties. • The safety and effectiveness of this drug when used by children under the age of 12 has not been established. • This drug interacts with alcohol, aminophylline, theophylline, 6-mercaptopurine, anticoagulants, methotrexate, probenecid, sulfinpyrazone, central nervous system depressants, phenytoin, and antidepressants; if you are currently taking any drugs of these types, consult your doctor about their use. If you are unsure of the type or contents of your medications, ask your doctor or pharmacist.
Comments: Many headaches are believed to be caused by nervousness, tension, or prolonged contraction of the head and neck muscles. This drug is reported to relieve these conditions to help control headache. • Take this drug with food or milk. • If your ears feel strange, if you hear ringing or buzzing, or if your stomach hurts, your dosage may need adjustment. Call your doctor. • Notify your doctor if you develop signs of jaundice (yellow eyes or skin; dark urine). • Do not drive a motor vehicle or operate machinery while taking this drug, since this drug may cause drowsiness. • While using this medication, avoid the use of nonprescription medicines containing aspirin or caffeine and limit your consumption of caffeine-containing beverages.

Fiorinal with Codeine analgesic

Manufacturer: Sandoz Pharmaceuticals
Ingredients: aspirin; butalbital; caffeine; codeine phosphate

Equivalent Products: B-A-C #3, Mayrand, Inc.; Fiorgen with Codeine, Gold-line Laboratories

Dosage Form: Capsule #1 (red/yellow); #2 (grey/yellow); #3 (blue/yellow): aspirin, 325 mg; butalbital, 50 mg; caffeine, 40 mg; codeine phosphate (see Comments)

Use: Relief of pain associated with tension

Minor Side Effects: Blurred vision; bruising or bleeding; constipation; dizziness; drowsiness; flushing; headache; indigestion; insomnia; loss of appetite; nausea; nervousness; sweating; tiredness; vomiting; weakness

Major Side Effects: Abdominal pain; breathing difficulties; chest tightness; confusion; euphoria; jaundice; kidney disease; ringing in the ears; skin rash; sore throat; ulcer

Contraindications: This drug should not be taken by people who are allergic to any of its ingredients or to narcotic analgesics. Consult your doctor immediately if this drug has been prescribed for you and you have any such allergies.

Warnings: The use of this drug may be habit-forming, due to the presence of codeine and butalbital. This drug has the potential for abuse and must be used with caution. Tolerance to this drug may develop quickly; do not increase the dose of this drug without consulting your doctor. • No more than six capsules of this product should be taken in one day. • This drug should be used cautiously by pregnant or nursing women and by people who have ulcers, coagulation problems, liver disease, gout, brain disease, porphyria, thyroid disease, gallstones or gallbladder disease, or kidney disease. Be sure your doctor knows if any of these conditions applies to you. • This drug may cause drowsiness; avoid tasks that require alertness. To prevent oversedation, avoid the use of alcohol or other drugs that have sedative properties. • The safety and effectiveness of this drug when used by children under the age of 12 has not been established. • This drug interacts with alcohol, ammonium chloride, anticoagulants, methotrexate, oral antidiabetics, oral contraceptives, probenecid, quinidine, steroids, sulfinpyrazone, vitamin C, central nervous system depressants, griseofulvin, phenytoin, sulfonamides, tetracyclines, and antidepressants; if you are currently taking any drugs of these types, consult your doctor about their use. If you are unsure of the type or contents of your medications, ask your doctor or pharmacist.

Comments: For this and other preparations containing codeine, the number that follows the drug name always refers to the amount of codeine present. Hence, #1 has 1/8 grain (7.5 mg) codeine; #2 has 1/4 grain (15 mg); #3 has 1/2 grain (30 mg); #4 has 1 grain (60 mg). These numbers are standard for amounts of codeine contained in any codeine product. • Many headaches are believed to be caused by nervousness, tension, or prolonged contraction of the head and neck muscles. This drug is reported to relieve these conditions to help control headache. • Take this drug with food or milk. Nausea caused by this drug may be relieved by lying down. • If your ears feel strange, if you hear ringing or buzzing, or if your stomach hurts, your dosage may need adjustment. Call your doctor. • Notify your doctor if you develop signs of jaundice (yellow eyes or skin; dark urine). • Since this drug may cause drowsiness, do not drive a motor vehicle or operate machinery while taking this drug • While using this medication, avoid the use of nonprescription medicines containing aspirin or caffeine and limit your consumption of caffeine-containing beverages.

Flagyl antimicrobial and antiparasitic

Manufacturer: Searle & Co.
Ingredient: metronidazole
Equivalent Products: Femazole, Major Pharmaceuticals; Metizol, Glen-

wood, Inc.; metronidazole, various manufacturers; Metryl, Lemmon Company; Protostat, Ortho Pharmaceutical Corp.

Dosage Form: Tablet: 250 mg; 500 mg (both blue, film coated)

Use: Treatment of various infections

Minor Side Effects: Abdominal cramps; change in urine color; constipation; decreased sexual interest; diarrhea; dizziness; dry mouth; headache; insomnia; irritability; joint pain; loss of appetite; metallic taste in the mouth; nasal congestion; nausea; restlessness; vomiting

Major Side Effects: Confusion; convulsions; flushing; hives; itching; loss of control of urine; mouth sores; numbness and tingling in fingers and toes; rash; sense of pressure inside abdomen; superinfection in the mouth or vagina; unexplained sore throat or fever; unusual fatigue; unusual weakness; white furry growth on tongue

Contraindications: This drug should not be used by people with a history of blood disease or with active physical disease of the central nervous system. Be sure your doctor knows if either condition applies to you. In patients with trichomoniasis, this drug should not be used during the first three months of pregnancy. • This drug should not be taken by people who are allergic to it. Consult your doctor immediately if this drug has been prescribed for you and you have such an allergy.

Warnings: This drug should be used with caution during pregnancy. It should not be used, however, for the treatment of trichomoniasis during the first three months of pregnancy. Nursing mothers who must use this drug should stop nursing. • This drug should be used with caution by those with severe liver disease. • This drug should not be taken with anticoagulants or antialcoholic drugs. Alcohol should not be consumed when taking this drug because it may cause nausea, vomiting, stomach pains, and headache. If you are currently taking anticoagulants or antialcoholic drugs, consult your doctor about their use. Avoid taking nonprescription drugs containing alcohol while you are taking this medication. If you are unsure about the type or contents of your medications, ask your doctor or pharmacist. • Total and differential blood tests may be recommended before, during, and after prolonged therapy with this drug. • Known or previously unrecognized vaginal fungal infections may present more prominent signs during therapy with this drug.

Comments: Do not stop taking this drug earlier than recommended by your doctor. Stopping treatment early can lead to reinfection. Four to six weeks should elapse before a repeat course of treatment. • If this drug is being used to treat a sexually transmitted disease, your sexual partner may also need to be treated. You should refrain from sexual intercourse, unless a condom is used, while you are taking this product in order to prevent reinfection. • You should wash your hands before handling food and after using the bathroom. • This drug may cause darkening of the urine. Do not be alarmed. • If numbness or tingling of fingers or toes occurs, call your doctor. • Take this drug with food or milk if it upsets your stomach. • This drug may cause an unpleasant, metallic taste; this side effect is normal and not a cause for alarm. • For best results, take this drug at evenly spaced intervals around the clock.

Flexeril muscle relaxant and analgesic

Manufacturer: Merck Sharp & Dohme

Ingredient: cyclobenzaprine hydrochloride

Dosage Form: Tablet: 10 mg (yellow)

Use: Relief of muscle spasm

Minor Side Effects: Abdominal pain; black tongue; blurred vision; dizziness; drowsiness; dry mouth; fatigue; indigestion; insomnia; muscle pain; nausea; nervousness; sweating; unpleasant taste in the mouth; weakness

Major Side Effects: Confusion; depression; difficulty in urinating; disorientation; hallucinations; headache; increased heart rate; itching; numbness in fingers and toes; rash; swelling of the face and tongue; tremors

Contraindications: This drug should not be taken by people who are taking or have recently (within two weeks) taken monoamine oxidase inhibitors, by those who have certain heart or thyroid diseases, or by those who are allergic to it. Consult your doctor immediately if this drug has been prescribed for you and any of these conditions applies.

Warnings: This drug interacts with monoamine oxidase inhibitors, alcohol, barbiturates, and other central nervous system depressants; anticholinergics; and some antihypertensives. If you are currently taking any drugs of these types, consult your doctor about their use. If you are unsure of the type or contents of your medications, ask your doctor or pharmacist. • This drug should be used with extreme caution by people who have urinary retention, epilepsy, blood clots, narrow-angle glaucoma, congestive heart failure, arrhythmias, increased intraocular pressure, or thyroid disease. Be sure your doctor knows if you have any of these conditions. • This drug should be used cautiously by children under the age of 15 and by pregnant women. • This drug is not recommended for use by nursing mothers. • This drug may cause drowsiness; avoid tasks that require alertness. • Use of this drug for periods longer than two to three weeks is not recommended.

Comments: This drug is not useful for reducing muscle spasm associated with diseases of the central nervous system or spine, such as cerebral palsy. • This drug should not be taken as a substitute for rest, physical therapy, or other measures recommended by your doctor to treat your condition. • While taking this drug, do not take any nonprescription item for weight control, cough, cold, or sinus problems without first checking with your doctor. • Chew gum or suck on ice chips or a piece of hard candy to reduce mouth dryness.

Florvite vitamin and fluoride supplement (Everett Laboratories, Inc.), see Poly-Vi-Flor vitamin and fluoride supplement.

Fluocet topical steroid hormone (NMC Laboratories, Inc.), see Synalar topical steroid hormone.

fluocinolone acetonide topical steroid hormone (various manufacturers), see Synalar topical steroid hormone.

fluocinonide topical steroid hormone (various manufacturers), see Lidex topical steroid hormone.

Fluonid topical steroid hormone (Herbert Laboratories), see Synalar topical steroid hormone.

flurazepam sedative and hypnotic (various manufacturers), see Dalmane sedative and hypnotic.

Flurosyn steroid hormone (Rugby Laboratories), see Synalar topical steroid hormone.

Fumide diuretic and antihypertensive (Everett Laboratories, Inc.), see Lasix diuretic and antihypertensive.

Furadantin antibacterial (Norwich Eaton Pharmaceuticals, Inc.), see nitrofurantoin antibacterial.

Furalan antibacterial (The Lannett Company, Inc.), see nitrofurantoin antibacterial.

Furan antibacterial (American Urologicals), see nitrofurantoin antibacterial.

Furanite antibacterial (Major Pharmaceuticals), see nitrofurantoin antibacterial.

furosemide diuretic and antihypertensive (various manufacturers), see Lasix diuretic and antihypertensive.

Genahist antihistamine (Goldline Laboratories), see Benadryl antihistamine.

Gen-XENE antianxiety and anticonvulsant (Alra Laboratories, Inc.), see Tranxene antianxiety and anticonvulsant.

Geridium analgesic (Goldline Laboratories), see Pyridium analgesic.

Glucotrol oral antidiabetic

Manufacturer: Roerig
Ingredient: glipizide
Dosage Form: Tablet: 5 mg; 10 mg (both white)
Use: Treatment of diabetes mellitus not controlled by diet and exercise alone
Minor Side Effects: Diarrhea; dizziness; fatigue; headache; heartburn; loss of appetite; stomach upset; sun sensitivity; vomiting; weakness
Major Side Effects: Blood disorders; breathing difficulties; dark urine; itching; jaundice; light-colored stools; low blood sugar; muscle cramps; rash; sore throat and fever; tingling in the hands and feet; unusual bleeding or bruising
Contraindications: This drug should not be used for the treatment of juvenile (insulin dependent) or unstable diabetes. This drug should not be used by diabetics subject to acidosis or ketosis or those with a history of diabetic coma. Persons with severe liver, kidney, or thyroid disorders should not use this drug. Avoid using this drug if you are allergic to sulfonylureas. Be sure your doctor knows if any of these conditions applies to you. In the presence of infections, fever, or severe trauma, it may be necessary for you to use insulin instead of this medication—at least during the acute stage.
Warnings: This drug should be used cautiously during pregnancy. If you are currently pregnant or become pregnant while taking this drug, talk to your doctor about its use. • This drug should be used with caution by nursing women, children, and persons with liver, kidney, or thyroid disorders. • Thiazide diuretics and beta-blocking drugs commonly used to treat high blood pressure may interfere with your control of diabetes. • This drug interacts with steroids, estrogens, oral contraceptives, phenothiazines, phenytoin, isoniazid, thyroid hormones, aspirin, salicylates, diuretics, and certain antibiotics. If you are taking any drugs of these types, talk to your doctor about your use of Glucotrol. If you

are not sure about the types or contents of your medications, talk to your doctor or pharmacist. • Do not drink alcohol or take any other medications unless directed to do so by your doctor. Be especially careful with nonprescription cough and cold remedies. • Be sure you can recognize signs of low blood sugar and know what to do if you begin to experience these symptoms. Signs of low blood sugar include chills, cold sweat, drowsiness, headache, nausea, nervousness, rapid pulse, tremors, and weakness. If these symptoms develop, eat or drink something containing sugar and call your doctor. Poor diet, malnutrition, strenuous exercise, and alcohol may lead to low blood sugar.

Comments: Take this drug at the same time every day. It is usually taken 30 minutes before breakfast unless otherwise directed. • Avoid prolonged or unprotected exposure to sunlight while taking this drug, as it makes you more sensitive to the sun's burning rays. • While taking this drug, test your urine and/or blood as prescribed. It is important that you understand what the tests mean. • Studies have shown that a good diet and exercise program are extremely important in controlling diabetes. Discuss the use of this drug with your doctor. Persons taking this drug must carefully watch their diet and exercise program and should practice good personal hygiene. While taking this drug, call your doctor if you develop an infection, fever, sore throat, rash, excessive thirst or urination, unusual bleeding or bruising, dark urine, or light-colored stools. • You may have to switch to insulin therapy if you require surgery or if complications such as ketoacidosis, severe trauma, or infection develop. There are other drugs similar to this (see Orinase, Diabinese, Tolinase, Micronase) that vary slightly in their activity. Certain persons who do not benefit from one type of these oral antidiabetic agents may find another one more effective. Discuss this with your doctor. • Notify your doctor if you develop signs of jaundice (yellow eyes or skin; dark urine). • Do not discontinue taking this medication without consulting your doctor. • It is advised that persons taking this drug carry a medical alert card or wear a medical alert bracelet.

G-well pediculicide and scabicide (Goldline Laboratories), see Kwell pediculicide and scabicide.

Gyne-Lotrimin antifungal agent

Manufacturer: Schering Corp.
Ingredient: clotrimazole
Equivalent Product: Mycelex-G, Miles Pharmaceutical
Dosage Forms: Vaginal cream 1% (per applicator): 5 g. Vaginal tablet: 100 mg; 500 mg (both are white)
Use: Treatment of Candida ("yeast") infections of the vagina
Minor Side Effects: Redness; stinging sensation; vaginal burning; vaginal discharge
Major Side Effects: Abdominal cramps; blistering; bloating; irritation; painful urination; peeling of the skin
Contraindication: This drug should not be used by people who are allergic to it. Consult your doctor immediately if you have such an allergy.
Warnings: Although no ill effects from such use have been documented, this drug should be used cautiously during pregnancy. • If irritation occurs, stop using this product and call your doctor.
Comments: Insert the medication high into the vagina. Patient instructions are generally dispensed with the medication. • If no improvement is evident by the time you have used up your first prescription of this drug, you should see your doctor for rediagnosis. • Do not stop using this drug even if you do not notice improvement of your symptoms. Complete the full course of therapy, even

during your menstrual period. • If you have a fungal infection of the vagina, wear cotton panties rather than those made of nylon or other nonporous material while the infection is being treated. • Apply this product after cleaning the affected area unless directed otherwise by your doctor. • While taking this drug, avoid sexual intercourse or ask your partner to use a condom to help prevent reinfection. • Use a sanitary napkin to prevent the staining of clothing while taking this medication. • This medication is usually used at bedtime. The 500 mg tablet is indicated as a single-dose treatment. The cream and the 100 mg tablet are used for one to two weeks.

Halcion sedative and hypnotic

Manufacturer: The Upjohn Company
Ingredient: triazolam
Dosage Form: Tablet: 0.125 mg (lavender); 0.25 mg (blue)
Use: Short-term relief of insomnia
Minor Side Effects: Blurred vision; constipation; dizziness; drowsiness; headache; lethargy; light-headedness; loss of appetite; nausea; nervousness; relaxed feeling; vomiting
Major Side Effects: Confusion; depression; hallucinations; impaired coordination; memory loss; nightmares; rapid heartbeat; ringing in the ears; tremors; weakness
Contraindications: This drug should not be used by persons allergic to it or by pregnant women. Consult your doctor immediately if this drug has been prescribed for you and either condition applies.
Warnings: This drug should be used with caution by depressed people, nursing mothers, persons under the age of 18, elderly patients, and people with liver or kidney disease, narrow-angle glaucoma, or psychosis. Be sure your doctor knows if any of these conditions applies to you. • Because this drug has the potential for abuse, it must be used with caution, especially by those with a history of drug dependence. Tolerance may develop quickly; do not increase the dose or take this drug more often than prescribed without first consulting your physician. Do not abruptly discontinue taking this drug if you have been taking it for a long time. Your dosage may need to be decreased gradually. • This drug is safe when taken alone; when it is combined with other sedative drugs or alcohol, serious adverse reactions may develop. Avoid the use of alcohol, other sedatives, or central nervous system depressants. This drug may interact with anticonvulsants, antihistamines, and cimetidine. If you are currently taking any drugs of these types, consult your doctor about their use. If you are unsure of the type or contents of your medications, ask your doctor or pharmacist. • This drug causes drowsiness; avoid tasks that require alertness. • The elderly are more sensitive to this drug, so smaller doses are prescribed for them.
Comments: Take this drug one-half to one hour before bedtime unless otherwise prescribed. • After you stop taking this drug, your sleep may be disturbed for a few nights. • This drug is similar in action to Dalmane but has a shorter duration of action. Halcion is believed to cause less sluggishness and lethargy in the morning than does Dalmane.

Haldol antipsychotic agent

Manufacturer: McNeil Pharmaceutical
Ingredient: haloperidol
Equivalent Product: haloperidol, various manufacturers
Dosage Forms: Liquid concentrate (content per ml): 2 mg. Tablet: 0.5 mg (white); 1 mg (yellow); 2 mg (pink); 5 mg (green); 10 mg (aqua); 20 mg (salmon)

Uses: Treatment of certain psychotic disorders, certain symptoms of Gilles de la Tourette's syndrome in children and adults, and severe behavior problems in children; short-term treatment of hyperactive children

Minor Side Effects: Blurred vision; confusion; constipation; diarrhea; dizziness; drooling; drowsiness; dry mouth; fatigue; headache; heartburn; impotence; insomnia; jitteriness; loss of appetite; menstrual irregularities; milk production; nausea; photosensitivity; restlessness; sweating; vomiting; weakness

Major Side Effects: Aching joints and muscles; blood disorders; breast enlargement (in both sexes); breathing difficulties; convulsions; difficulty in urinating; eye changes; fluid retention; hair loss; hallucinations; heart attack; involuntary movements of the mouth, face, neck, and tongue; jaundice; liver damage; low blood pressure; mouth sores; palpitations; skin darkening; skin rash; sore throat; tremors

Contraindications: This drug should not be taken by people who are severely depressed, by those who have central nervous system depression due to alcohol or other centrally acting depressants, or by those who have Parkinson's disease. Be sure your doctor knows if any of these conditions applies to you. • This drug is not recommended for use in children under three years of age. • This drug should not be given to patients who are unconscious or comatose. • This drug should not be taken by people who are allergic to it. Consult your doctor immediately if this drug has been prescribed for you and you have such an allergy.

Warnings: This drug should be used with caution by pregnant and nursing women. • This drug should not be taken in combination with lithium. • Bronchopneumonia may result from usage of this drug. • Call your doctor if you feel lethargic, dehydrated, or short of breath or if you have difficulty breathing. • This drug may impair mental and/or physical abilities required for performance of potentially hazardous tasks such as operating machinery or driving a motor vehicle. • This drug should not be taken with alcohol. • This drug should be taken cautiously by patients with severe heart or blood vessel diseases, liver disease, anemia, glaucoma, enlarged prostate, ulcers, or kidney disease; by those receiving anticoagulant or anticonvulsant therapy; and by those with known allergies or thyroid disease. Be sure your doctor knows if you have any of these conditions or if you are taking any of these drug types or any of the following: alcohol, oral antacids, anticholinergics, depressants. If you are unsure about the type or contents of your medications, ask your doctor or pharmacist.

Comments: The effects of therapy with this drug may not be apparent for at least two weeks. • This drug has a persistent action; never take it more frequently than your doctor prescribes. A serious overdose may result. • Notify your doctor if you develop signs of jaundice (yellow eyes or skin; dark urine). • While taking this drug, do not take any nonprescription item for weight control, cough, cold, or sinus problems without first checking with your doctor. • Chew gum or suck on ice chips or a piece of hard candy to reduce mouth dryness. • To avoid dizziness or light-headedness when you stand, contract and relax the muscles of your legs for a few moments before rising. Do this by pushing one foot against the floor while raising the other foot slightly, alternating feet so that you are "pumping" your legs in a pedaling motion. • If this drug upsets your stomach, it may be taken with food or milk. • If you notice a sore throat, darkening of your vision, or any fine tremors of your tongue, call your doctor. • If you are taking this drug for a prolonged time, it may be advisable for you to stop for a while to see if you still need it. Talk to your doctor before stopping this drug. It may be necessary for you to reduce the dosage gradually. • Some of the side effects caused by this drug can be prevented by taking an antiparkinson drug. Talk to your doctor about this.

haloperidol antipsychotic agent (various manufacturers), see Haldol antipsychotic agent.

Haltran anti-inflammatory (The Upjohn Company), see ibuprofen anti-inflammatory.

hemorrhoidal HC steroid-hormone-containing anorectal product (various manufacturers), see Anusol-HC steroid-hormone-containing anorectal product.

Hi-Cor topical steroid (C & M Pharmacal, Inc.), see hydrocortisone topical steroid.

Hydrocet analgesic (Carnrick Laboratories, Inc.), see Vicodin analgesic.

Hydro-Chlor diuretic and antihypertensive (Vortech Pharmaceutical, Ltd.), see hydrochlorothiazide diuretic and antihypertensive.

hydrochlorothiazide diuretic and antihypertensive

Manufacturer: various manufacturers
Ingredient: hydrochlorothiazide
Equivalent Products: Diaqua, W. E. Hauck, Inc.; Esidrix, Ciba Pharmaceutical Company; Hydro-Chlor, Vortech Pharmaceutical, Ltd.; HydroDIURIL, Merck Sharp & Dohme; Hydromal, W. E. Hauck, Inc.; Hydro-T, Major Pharmaceuticals; Hydro-Z, Mayrand, Inc.; Mictrin, Econo Med, Inc.; Oretic, Abbott Laboratories; Thiuretic, Warner Chilcott Laboratories
Dosage Forms: Oral solution (content per ml): 10 mg; 100 mg. Tablet: 25 mg; 50 mg; 100 mg (various colors)
Uses: Treatment of high blood pressure; prevention of fluid accumulation
Minor Side Effects: Constipation; cramps; diarrhea; dizziness; drowsiness; headache; heartburn; itching; loss of appetite; nausea; restlessness; sun sensitivity; vomiting
Major Side Effects: Blood disorders; blurred vision; bruising; chest pain; elevated blood sugar; elevated uric acid; fever; jaundice; muscle spasm; palpitations; skin rash; sore throat; tingling in fingers and toes; weakness
Contraindications: This drug should not be used by people who are allergic to it or to sulfa drugs, by people with kidney disease, or by people who are unable to urinate. Consult your doctor immediately if this drug has been prescribed for you and any of these conditions applies.
Warnings: This drug should be used cautiously by pregnant women and by people who have diabetes, liver disease, a history of allergy, or asthma. Be sure your doctor knows if any of these conditions applies to you. • Nursing mothers who must take this drug should stop nursing. • This drug may affect the potency of, or your need for, other blood pressure drugs, antidiabetics, and some surgical muscle relaxants; dosage adjustment may be necessary. • This drug interacts with colestipol hydrochloride, digitalis, indomethacin, lithium, and steroids. If you are currently taking any drugs of these types, consult your doctor about their use. If you are unsure about the type or contents of your medications, ask your doctor or pharmacist. • This drug may affect thyroid and other laboratory tests; be sure your doctor knows that you are taking this drug if you are having any tests done. • This drug may cause gout, high blood levels of calcium, or the onset of diabetes that has been latent. To help prevent these problems, you should have blood tests done periodically while taking this drug. • This drug can cause potassium loss. Signs of such loss include dry mouth, thirst, weakness, muscle pain or cramps, nausea, and vomiting. Call your doc-

tor if you experience any of these symptoms. To help avoid potassium loss, take this product with a glass of fresh or frozen orange juice, or eat a banana every day. The use of a salt substitute also helps prevent potassium loss. Do not change your diet, however, without consulting your doctor. Too much potassium can also be dangerous. • While taking this product, limit your consumption of alcoholic beverages in order to prevent dizziness or light-headedness. • If you are taking digitalis in addition to this drug, watch carefully for symptoms of increased digitalis toxicity (e.g., nausea, blurred vision, palpitations) and notify your doctor immediately if they occur. • If you have high blood pressure, do not take any nonprescription item for weight control, cough, cold, or sinus problems without first checking with your doctor; such medications may contain ingredients that can increase blood pressure.

Comments: This product causes frequent urination. Expect this effect; it should not alarm you. Try to plan your dosage schedule to avoid taking this drug at bedtime. • Notify your doctor if you develop signs of jaundice (yellow eyes or skin; dark urine). • To avoid dizziness or light-headedness when you stand, contract and relax the muscles of your legs for a few moments before rising. Do this by pushing one foot against the floor while raising the other foot slightly, alternating feet so that you are "pumping" your legs in a pedaling motion. • This drug must be taken as directed. Do not take extra doses or skip a dose without first consulting your doctor. • You should learn how to monitor your pulse and blood pressure if you are taking this drug; discuss this with your doctor.

hydrocortisone oral steroid hormone

Manufacturer: various manufacturers
Ingredient: hydrocortisone (cortisol)
Equivalent Products: Cortef, The Upjohn Company; Hydrocortone, Merck Sharp & Dohme
Dosage Forms: Oral suspension (content per 5 ml teaspoon): 10 mg. Tablet: 5 mg; 10 mg; 20 mg
Uses: Treatment of endocrine or rheumatic disorders; asthma; blood diseases; certain cancers; eye disorders; gastrointestinal disturbances such as ulcerative colitis; respiratory diseases; inflammations such as arthritis, dermatitis, poison ivy
Minor Side Effects: Dizziness; headache; increased hair growth; increased susceptibility to infection; increased sweating; indigestion; insomnia; menstrual irregularities; muscle weakness; nervousness; reddening of the skin on the face; restlessness; thin skin; weight gain
Major Side Effects: Abdominal enlargement; blurred vision; bone loss; bruising; cataracts; convulsions; diabetes; euphoria; fluid retention; fracture; glaucoma; growth impairment in children; heart failure; high blood pressure; impaired healing of wounds; mood changes; mouth sores; muscle wasting; nightmares; peptic ulcer; potassium loss; salt retention; weakness
Contraindications: This drug should not be taken by people who are allergic to it or by those who have systemic fungal infections. Consult your doctor if this drug has been prescribed for you and either of these conditions applies.
Warnings: If you are using this drug for longer than a week, you may need to receive higher dosages if you are subjected to stress such as serious infection, injury, or surgery. • This drug may mask signs of an infection or cause new infections to develop. • This drug may cause glaucoma or cataracts, high blood pressure, high blood sugar, fluid retention, and potassium loss. Blood pressure, body weight, and vision should be checked at regular intervals if you are taking this drug for a prolonged period. • This drug should be used very cautiously by people who have had tuberculosis and by those who have thyroid disease, liver

disease, severe ulcerative colitis, diabetes, seizures, a history of ulcers, kidney disease, high blood pressure, a bone disease, or myasthenia gravis. Be sure your doctor knows if any of these conditions applies to you. • Stomach X rays are advised for persons with suspected or known peptic ulcers. • This drug has not been proven safe for use during pregnancy. • While you are taking this drug you should not be vaccinated or immunized. • If you have been taking this drug for more than a week, do not stop taking it suddenly. Never increase the dose or take the drug for a longer time than prescribed without consulting your doctor. • Report mood swings or depression to your doctor. • Growth of children may be affected by this drug. • This drug interacts with aspirin, barbiturates, diuretics, rifampin, cyclophosphamide, estrogens, indomethacin, oral anticoagulants, antidiabetics, and phenytoin; if you are currently taking any drugs of these types, consult your doctor about their use. If you are unsure of the type or contents of your medications, ask your doctor or pharmacist.

Comments: This drug is often taken on a decreasing-dosage schedule (four times a day for several days, then three times a day, etc.). Taking the entire daily dose at one time (about 8:00 A.M.) often gives the best results. Take this drug exactly as directed. Do not take extra doses or skip a dose without first consulting your doctor. For long-term treatment, taking the drug every other day is preferred. Ask your doctor about alternate-day dosing. • To help avoid potassium loss while using this drug, take your dose with a glass of fresh or frozen orange juice, or eat a banana each day. The use of a salt substitute also helps prevent potassium loss. Do not change your diet, however, before consulting your doctor. Too much potassium may also be dangerous. • If you are using this drug chronically, you should wear or carry a notice that you are taking a steroid. • To prevent stomach upset, take this drug with food or a snack.

hydrocortisone topical steroid

Manufacturer: various manufacturers
Ingredient: hydrocortisone acetate
Equivalent Products: Carmol HC, Syntex Laboratories, Inc.; Cortaid, The Upjohn Company; Cort-Dome, Miles Pharmaceutical; Cortef Acetate, The Upjohn Company; Cortizone-5, Thompson Medical; Cortril, Pfipharmecs Division; Delacort, Mericon; Dermacort, Reid-Rowell; DermiCort, Republic Drug; Dermolate, Schering Corp.; Dermtex HC, Pfieffer; Hi-Cor, C & M Pharmacal, Inc.; Hydro-Tex, Syosset Labs., Inc.; Hytone, Dermik Laboratories, Inc.; Nutracort, Owen/Allercreme; Penecort, Herbert Laboratories; Synacort, Syntex Laboratories, Inc.
Dosage Forms: Cream; Lotion; Ointment; Spray (in various strengths)
Uses: For temporary relief of skin inflammation, irritation, itching, and rashes associated with such conditions as dermatitis, eczema, and poison ivy
Minor Side Effects: Burning sensation; dryness; irritation; itching; rash
Major Side Effects: Blisters; increased hair growth; pain; redness; secondary infection; skin wasting
Contraindications: This drug should not be used in the presence of fungal infections, diseases that impair circulation, or tuberculosis of the skin. People with a perforated eardrum should not use this product in the ear. It should not be used by those with an allergy to hydrocortisone. Consult your doctor immediately if you have any of the conditions listed and this drug has been prescribed for you. • This drug should not be used in or near the eyes.
Warnings: This product is for external use only. • Avoid contact with the eyes. Wash your hands after applying this product. • Do not use this product for prolonged periods of time, and do not use it more frequently than directed on the label. If the condition does not improve after three days, discontinue use and consult your doctor or pharmacist. • If irritation (pain, itching, swelling, or

rash) occurs, discontinue use and consult your doctor. • Do not use on children under two years of age without consulting a physician. • Pregnant women should use this product cautiously. • This drug is not to be used on burns or infections, unless directed, as it may slow healing.

Comments: While this product relieves itching, it may take a couple of days for this relief to occur. Use this product as directed; meanwhile, apply rubbing alcohol or witch hazel diluted with an equal amount of water to the area to relieve itching. • Do not bandage or wrap the skin during treatment with this drug unless directed to do so by your physician. • If the affected area is extremely dry or is scaling, the skin may be moistened before applying the medication by soaking in water or by applying water with a clean cloth. The ointment form is preferred for use on dry skin. Lotions and aerosols are preferred for hairy areas. • Hydrocortisone-containing products are sold without a prescription in strengths of up to 0.5%. There are several brands on the market. Consult your pharmacist.

Hydrocortone steroid hormone (Merck Sharp & Dohme), see hydrocortisone oral steroid hormone.

HydroDIURIL diuretic and antihypertensive (Merck Sharp & Dohme), see hydrochlorothiazide diuretic and antihypertensive.

Hydrogesic analgesic (Edwards Pharmacal), see Vicodin analgesic.

Hydromal diuretic and antihypertensive (W. E. Hauck, Inc.), see hydrochlorothiazide diuretic and antihypertensive.

Hydro-T diuretic and antihypertensive (Major Pharmaceuticals), see hydrochlorothiazide diuretic and antihypertensive.

Hydro-Tex topical steroid (Syosset Labs., Inc.), see hydrocortisone topical steroid.

hydroxyzine hydrochloride antianxiety (various manufacturers), see Atarax antianxiety.

Hydro-Z diuretic and antihypertensive (Mayrand, Inc.), see hydrochlorothiazide diuretic and antihypertensive.

Hygroton diuretic and antihypertensive

Manufacturer: Rorer Pharmaceuticals
Ingredient: chlorthalidone
Equivalent Products: chlorthalidone, various manufacturers; Hylidone, Major Pharmaceuticals; Thalitone, Boehringer Ingelheim
Dosage Form: Tablet: 25 mg (peach); 50 mg (aqua); 100 mg (white)
Uses: Treatment of high blood pressure; removal of fluid from body tissues
Minor Side Effects: Constipation; cramps; diarrhea; dizziness; drowsiness; headache; heartburn; loss of appetite; nausea; restlessness; sun sensitivity; vomiting
Major Side Effects: Blood disorders; blurred vision; bruising; elevated blood sugar; elevated uric acid; fever; jaundice; mood changes; muscle spasm; palpi-

tations; rash; shortness of breath; sore throat; thirst; tingling in the fingers and toes; weakness; weak pulse

Contraindications: This drug should not be taken by persons suffering from anuria (inability to urinate). This drug should not be taken by people who are allergic to it or to sulfa drugs. Consult your doctor immediately if this drug has been prescribed for you and you have anuria or such an allergy.

Warnings: This drug should be used with caution by pregnant and nursing women and by persons with kidney disease, liver disease, diabetes, gout, allergies, or asthma. Be sure your doctor knows if any of these conditions applies to you. • This drug may cause low blood levels of potassium, gout, and diabetes that has been latent. To check for these effects, periodic blood tests are advisable while taking this drug. • Use of this drug may affect thyroid tests. If you are scheduled to have such tests, remind your doctor that you are taking this drug. • This drug may add to the actions of other blood pressure drugs; dosage adjustments may be necessary. This drug also interacts with digitalis, indomethacin, lithium, oral antidiabetics, steroids, and curare. If you are taking this drug and digitalis, watch carefully for signs of increased digitalis effects (e.g., nausea, blurred vision, palpitations), and notify your doctor immediately if symptoms occur. If you are currently taking any drugs of these types, consult your doctor about their use. If you are unsure of the type or contents of your medications, ask your doctor or pharmacist.

Comments: This drug causes frequent urination. Expect this effect; it should not alarm you. • This drug can cause potassium loss. Signs of such loss include dry mouth, thirst, weakness, muscle pain or cramps, nausea, and vomiting. If you experience such symptoms, call your doctor. To help avoid potassium loss, take this drug with a glass of fresh or frozen orange juice, or eat a banana each day. The use of a salt substitute can also help prevent potassium loss. Do not change your diet, however, without consulting your doctor. Too much potassium can also be dangerous. • Notify your doctor if you develop signs of jaundice (yellow eyes or skin; dark urine). • You should learn how to take your pulse and blood pressure while you are taking this drug; discuss this with your doctor. • Try not to take this drug at bedtime. This drug is best taken as a single dose in the morning, with food. This drug must be taken exactly as directed. Do not take extra doses or skip a dose without first consulting your doctor. • While taking this drug, as with many drugs that lower blood pressure, you should limit your consumption of alcoholic beverages in order to prevent dizziness or light-headedness. • To avoid dizziness or light-headedness when you stand, contract and relax the muscles of your legs for a few moments before rising. Do this by pushing one foot against the floor while raising the other foot slightly, alternating feet so that you are "pumping" your legs in a pedaling motion. • If you are allergic to a sulfa drug, you may likewise be allergic to this drug. • If you have high blood pressure, do not take any nonprescription item for weight control, cough, cold, or sinus problems without first checking with your doctor; such items may contain ingredients that can increase blood pressure.

Hylidone diuretic and antihypertensive (Major Pharmaceuticals), see Hygroton diuretic and antihypertensive.

Hyosophen sedative and anticholinergic (Rugby Laboratories), see Donnatal sedative and anticholinergic.

Hy-Phen analgesic (B. F. Ascher & Company, Inc.), see Viocodin analgesic.

Hytone topical steroid (Dermik Laboratories, Inc.), see hydrocortisone topical steroid.

Ibuprin anti-inflammatory (Thompson Medical), see ibuprofen anti-inflammatory.

ibuprofen anti-inflammatory

Manufacturer: various manufacturers

Ingredient: ibuprofen

Equivalent Products: Advil, Whitehall Laboratories, Inc.; Haltran, The Upjohn Company; Ibuprin, Thompson Medical; Ifen, Everett Laboratories, Inc.; Medipren, McNeil Consumer Products Co.; Midol 200, Glenbrook Laboratories; Motrin, The Upjohn Company; Nuprin, Bristol-Myers; Rufen, Boots Pharmaceuticals, Inc.; Trendar, Whitehall Laboratories, Inc.; (see Comments)

Dosage Form: Tablet: 200 mg; 300 mg; 400 mg; 600 mg; 800 mg

Uses: Reduction of pain and swelling due to arthritis; relief of menstrual pain, dental pain, postoperative pain, and musculoskeletal pain

Minor Side Effects: Bloating; constipation; cramps; diarrhea; dizziness; drowsiness; dry mouth; gas; headache; heartburn; indigestion; insomnia; itching; loss of appetite; nausea; nervousness; peculiar taste in mouth; stomach pain; vomiting

Major Side Effects: Anemia; bleeding; breast enlargement (in both sexes); blood in stools; chest tightness; convulsions; depression; difficulty in urinating; fever; fluid retention; hair loss; hallucinations; high blood pressure; jaundice; menstrual irregularities; palpitations; rash; ringing in the ears; shortness of breath; sore throat; ulcer; visual disturbances

Contraindications: This drug should not be taken by people who are allergic to it or to aspirin or similar drugs. Consult your doctor immediately if this drug has been prescribed for you and you have such an allergy.

Warnings: This drug should be used with extreme caution by patients with a history of ulcers or gastrointestinal disease. Peptic ulcers and gastrointestinal bleeding, sometimes severe, have been reported in persons taking this drug. Make sure your doctor knows if you have or have had either condition. Notify your doctor if you experience frequent indigestion or notice blood in your stools. • This drug should be used with caution by persons with anemia, certain types of heart disease, bleeding diseases, high blood pressure, liver disease, or kidney disease. Be sure your doctor knows if any of these conditions applies to you. • Should any eye problems arise while taking this drug, notify your doctor immediately. • This drug should not be used by pregnant women or nursing mothers. It should be used cautiously by children. • Use of this drug has been reported to bring about fluid retention, skin rash, and weight gain. If you notice any of these symptoms, immediately consult your doctor. • This drug should be used with caution if you are also taking anticoagulants, since this drug has been found to prolong bleeding time, even in normal subjects. • This drug interacts with anticoagulants, oral antidiabetics, barbiturates, diuretics, steroids, phenytoin, and aspirin. If you are currently taking any drugs of these types, consult your doctor about their use. If you are unsure of the type or contents of your medications, ask your doctor or pharmacist.

Comments: In numerous tests, this drug has been shown to be as effective as aspirin in the treatment of arthritis, but aspirin is still the drug of choice for the disease. • Do not take aspirin or alcohol while taking this drug without first consulting your doctor. • You should note improvement in your condition soon after you start using this drug; however, full benefit may not be obtained for one to two weeks. It is important not to stop taking this drug even though symptoms have diminished or disappeared. • This drug is not a substitute for rest, physical therapy, or other measures recommended by your doctor to treat your condition. • Notify your doctor if skin rash, itching, swelling of the hands or feet, or persistent headache occurs. • Notify your doctor if you develop signs of jaundice (yellow eyes or skin; dark urine). • Take this drug with food or milk to decrease stomach upset. • Ibuprofen 200 mg tablets are available without a prescription under the names of Aches-N-Pain, Advil, Genprin, Haltran, Ibuprin, Medipren, Midol 200, Nuprin, Pamprin-IB, and Trendar. Consult your doctor or pharmacist about their use.

Ifen anti-inflammatory (Everett Laboratories, Inc.), see ibuprofen anti-inflammatory.

Ilosone antibiotic (Dista Products Company), see erythromycin antibiotic.

Ilotycin antibiotic (Dista Products Company), see erythromycin antibiotic.

imipramine hydrochloride antidepressant (various manufacturers), see Tofranil antidepressant.

Imodium antidiarrheal

Manufacturer: Janssen Pharmaceutica Inc.
Ingredient: loperamide hydrochloride
Dosage Forms: Capsule: 2 mg (two-tone green). Liquid (content per 5 ml teaspoon): 1 mg (see Comments)
Uses: Treatment of severe diarrhea; use with ileostomies to reduce discharge
Minor Side Effects: Dizziness; drowsiness; dry mouth; fatigue; loss of appetite; nausea; vomiting
Major Side Effects: Abdominal bloating or pain; constipation; fever; rash; sore throat; stomach pain
Contraindications: This drug should not be used by persons allergic to it. Consult your doctor immediately if this drug has been prescribed for you and you have such an allergy. This drug should not be used by people who must avoid the possibility of constipation. This drug is not recommended for diarrhea that results from infection of the intestinal lining by amebas, viruses, or bacteria. Consult your doctor immediately if this drug has been prescribed for you and any of these conditions applies.
Warnings: This drug should be used with caution by people who have colitis, liver disease, or a history of drug dependency. This drug should be used cautiously by pregnant or nursing women. Consult your doctor immediately if this drug has been prescribed for you and any of these conditions applies. • This drug may cause drowsiness; avoid tasks that require alertness.
Comments: This drug is usually prescribed in conjunction with other drugs to treat severe diarrhea. It should be used for short periods only. If diarrhea continues after two days of taking this drug, consult your doctor. • This drug can be habit-forming if taken for longer than ten days. • No more than eight capsules of this product should be taken in 24 hours. • Notify your doctor if abdominal bloating, abdominal pain, or fever occurs. • Do not exceed prescribed dosage. • Chew gum or suck on ice chips or hard candy to relieve mouth dryness. • The liquid form of this drug is now available without a prescription under the name Imodium A-D (McNeil Consumer Products Company).

Inderal beta blocker (Wyeth-Ayerst Laboratories), see propranolol beta blocker.

Inderide diuretic and antihypertensive

Manufacturer: Wyeth-Ayerst Laboratories

Ingredients: propranolol; hydrochlorothiazide

Equivalent Product: propranolol and hydrochlorothiazide, various manufacturers

Dosage Forms: Sustained-action tablet (see Comments): propranolol, 80 mg and hydrochlorothiazide, 50 mg (beige with gold bands); propranolol, 120 mg and hydrochlorothiazide, 50 mg (beige/brown with gold bands); propranolol, 160 mg and hydrochlorothiazide, 50 mg (brown with gold bands). Tablet: propranolol, 40 mg and hydrochlorothiazide, 25 mg; propranolol, 80 mg and hydrochlorothiazide, 25 mg (both off-white)

Uses: Treatment of high blood pressure; removal of fluid from body tissues

Minor Side Effects: Abdominal cramps; blurred vision; constipation; drowsiness; fatigue; gas; headache; heartburn; insomnia; light-headedness; loss of appetite; muscle spasm; nasal congestion; nausea; restlessness; sweating; vomiting; weakness

Major Side Effects: Blood disorders; breathing difficulties; bruises; cold hands and feet; decreased sexual ability; depression; diarrhea; difficulty in urinating; dizziness; dry mouth; elevated uric acid; fever; hair loss; hallucinations; heart failure; jaundice; nightmares; rash; ringing in the ears; slow pulse; sore throat; sun sensitivity; tingling in the fingers; visual disturbances

Contraindications: This drug should not be used by persons with bronchial asthma, severe hay fever, certain types of heart problems, or allergies to either of the active ingredients of this medication or to sulfa drugs. Be sure your doctor knows if any of these conditions applies to you. • This drug should not be used concurrently with monoamine oxidase inhibitors or during the two week withdrawal period from such drugs. If you are currently taking any drugs of this type, consult your physician. If you are unsure of the types or contents of your medications, ask your doctor or pharmacist.

Warnings: This drug should be used with caution by persons undergoing major surgery and by persons with certain types of heart problems, thyroid disease, certain respiratory disorders, severe kidney disease, severe liver disease, diabetes, gout, or hypoglycemia. Be sure your doctor knows if any of these conditions applies to you. • This drug must be used with extreme caution in pregnancy. Discuss the risks and benefits with your doctor. • Nursing mothers who must take this drug should stop nursing. • This drug is a potent medication, and it should not be stopped abruptly. Chest pain — even heart attacks — can occur if this medication is stopped suddenly. • This drug may interact with reserpine, digitalis, cimetidine, theophylline, aminophylline, indomethacin, colestipol, lithium, and corticosteroids. If you are currently taking any drugs of these types, consult your doctor about their use. If you are unsure about the type or contents of your medications, ask your doctor or pharmacist. • This drug may affect thyroid and other laboratory tests; be sure your doctor knows that you are taking this drug if you are having any tests done. • Because this drug may add to the effect of other blood pressure drugs, the doses may need to be adjusted if taken concurrently. • If you are taking digitalis in addition to this drug, watch for symptoms of increased digitalis toxicity (e.g., nausea, blurred vision, palpitations), and notify your doctor immediately if they occur. • Because of the hydrochlorothiazide component, this drug may cause gout or increased blood levels of calcium. It may also cause the onset of diabetes that has been latent. • This drug can cause potassium loss. Some of the symptoms of potassium loss are thirst, dry mouth, and muscle cramps. Notify your doctor if you experience such symptoms. To help prevent potassium loss, take this drug with a glass of fresh or frozen orange juice, or eat a banana every day. The use of a salt substitute also helps prevent potassium loss. Do not change your diet, however, without consulting your doctor. Too much potassium may also be dangerous.

Comments: This drug causes increased urination. Expect this effect; it should not alarm you. • A doctor probably should not prescribe this drug or other "fixed dose" products as the first choice in treatment of high blood pressure. The patient should be treated first with each of the component drugs individually. If the response is adequate to the doses contained in this product, then this fixed dose product can be substituted. Combination products offer the advantage of increased convenience to the patient. • Notify your doctor if you develop signs of jaundice (yellow eyes or skin; dark urine). • Your doctor may want you to take your pulse and blood pressure every day while you are on this medication. Discuss this with your doctor. • Take this drug exactly as directed. Be sure to take your medication doses at the same time each day. Do not take extra doses or skip a dose without first consulting your doctor. The sustained-action tablets are designed for convenient once-a-day dosing; they are called Inderide LA. Do not crush or chew these tablets; they must be swallowed whole. • While you are taking Inderide, do not take any nonprescription drug for weight control, cough, cold, or sinus problems without first checking with your doctor or pharmacist; such items may contain ingredients that can increase blood pressure. • In order to prevent dizziness or light-headedness while taking this drug, limit your consumption of alcohol-containing beverages. To avoid dizziness or light-headedness when you stand, contract and relax the muscles of your legs for a few minutes before rising. Do this by pushing one foot against the floor while raising the other foot slightly, alternating feet so you are "pumping" your legs in a pedaling motion. • Notify your doctor if dizziness or diarrhea develops. • This drug may make you more sensitive to the cold. Dress warmly.

Indocin anti-inflammatory

Manufacturer: Merck Sharp & Dohme
Ingredient: indomethacin
Dosage Forms: Capsule: 25 mg; 50 mg (both are blue/white). Suppository: 50 mg. Suspension (content per 5 ml teaspoon): 25 mg. Sustained-release capsule (see Comments): 75 mg (blue/clear)
Uses: Reduction of pain, redness, and swelling due to arthritis, bursitis, or tendonitis
Minor Side Effects: Bloating; confusion; constipation; diarrhea; dizziness; drowsiness; gas; headache; heartburn; insomnia; loss of appetite; nausea; vomiting
Major Side Effects: Anemia; blood disorders; blood in stools, urine, or mouth; blurred vision; breathing difficulties; chest tightness; depression; difficulty in urinating; fatigue; fluid retention; high blood pressure; itching; jaundice; loss of hair; loss of hearing; numbness or tingling in fingers or toes; ringing in the ears; severe abdominal pain; skin rash; sore throat; ulcer; weight gain
Contraindications: This drug should not be used by people who are allergic to it or to aspirin or other nonsteroidal anti-inflammatory drugs. Consult your doctor immediately if this drug has been prescribed for you and you have such an allergy. • This drug should not be used by persons with nasal polyps associated with swelling. • The suppository form of this drug should not be used by persons with a history of proctitis or rectal bleeding. If you have either of these conditions and this drug has been prescribed for you, consult your doctor immediately.

Warnings: This drug should be used cautiously by elderly people; pregnant women; children under 14; people with a history of gastrointestinal disorders; and people with mental illness, epilepsy, Parkinson's disease, bleeding disorders, colitis, kidney or liver disease, high blood pressure, or heart failure. Be sure your doctor knows if any of these conditions applies to you. • Nursing women who must use this drug should stop nursing. • The severity of the side effects caused by this drug depends upon the dosage taken. Use the least amount possible and watch carefully for side effects. • This drug may irritate the stomach or intestines. Call your doctor if you experience stomach pain or if your stools are black and tarry. • If you notice changes in your vision or if you experience headaches while taking this drug, notify your doctor. • This drug may cause drowsiness; avoid tasks that require alertness. • Side effects are more likely to occur in the elderly. • This drug interacts with aspirin, probenecid, oral antidiabetics, lithium, anticoagulants, and furosemide. If you are currently taking any drugs of these types, consult your doctor about their use. If you are not sure about the type or contents of your medications, talk to your doctor or pharmacist.

Comments: This drug is potent and is not intended for general aches and pains. • Regular medical checkups, including blood tests, are required of persons taking this drug for prolonged periods. • This drug must be taken with food or milk, immediately after meals, or with antacids. Never take this drug on an empty stomach or with aspirin or alcohol. • If you are taking an anticoagulant (blood thinner), remind your doctor. • This drug may cause discoloration of the urine or feces. If you notice a change in color, call your doctor. • Notify your doctor if you develop signs of jaundice (yellow eyes or skin; dark urine). • It may take a month before you feel the full effect of this drug. • This drug should be taken regularly to control symptoms of arthritis. Do not take it only when you feel pain. This drug is not a substitute for rest, physical therapy, or other measures your doctor recommends to treat your condition. • The sustained-release capsules (Indocin SR) must be swallowed whole. Do not crush or chew them. These capsules are taken less frequently than Indocin. Talk to your doctor about their use. • This drug is similar in action to ibuprofen, Tolectin, Feldene, and other anti-inflammatory drugs. If one anti-inflammatory drug is not well tolerated, your doctor may prescribe another to find the best drug for you.

insulin antidiabetic

Manufacturer: various manufacturers
Ingredient: insulin
Equivalent Products: This drug is usually prescribed according to time of onset and duration of action, rather than by trade name.
Dosage Form: This drug is available only as an injectable. Various types of insulin provide different times of onset and duration of action. The types of insulin and their times of onset and duration are as follows:

	Onset (hr.)	Duration (hr.)
regular insulin	1/2	6-8
insulin zinc suspension, prompt (Semilente)	1	14
isophane insulin (NPH)	1	24
insulin zinc suspension (Lente)	1-2	24
protamine zinc insulin (PZI)	6	36
insulin zinc suspension, extended (Ultralente)	6	over 36

Use: Treatment of diabetes mellitus not controlled by diet alone
Minor Side Effect: Low blood sugar level, characterized by confusion,

CONSUMER GUIDE®

fatigue, headache, hunger, nausea, rapid pulse, sweaty skin, vision changes, and weakness

Major Side Effects: Difficulty breathing; rash

Contraindications: There are no specific contraindications to the use of insulin, but before you begin therapy, your doctor must determine your specific needs and carefully work out your dosage regimen.

Warnings: This drug should be used only under the direction of a doctor, and a prescribed diet should be followed precisely. • Do not substitute one type of this drug for another. Your doctor may put you on a regimen of two or more types of insulin to get the best effect. Stick to your prescribed regimen. • Roll insulin vial in hands to mix gently before withdrawing a dose in the syringe. • Purchase disposable syringes if possible, and remember to dispose of them properly. Once you have started using a particular brand of disposable insulin syringe and needle, do not switch brands without first talking with your doctor; a dosage error may occur. • When using this drug, be on guard for signs of low blood sugar — fatigue, nervousness, nausea, rapid heartbeat, and a cold sweat. If signs of low blood sugar are evident, eat a piece of candy or drink a glass of orange juice and try to contact your doctor who will instruct you on what to do in such a situation. • Also, be on the alert for signs of too much sugar. These signs include thirst, excess urination, and vision changes. Your urine test should show sugar in your urine if there is too much sugar in your blood. Call your doctor if you experience any of these symptoms. • Allergy to insulin is unusual, but it may happen. Symptoms of such an allergy are similar to those of other allergies, including rash and difficulty breathing. If these symptoms occur, call your doctor. • If you become ill — if you catch a cold or the flu or become nauseated, for example — your insulin requirement may change. Consult your doctor. • Injection sites for this drug should be rotated. It is important that this be done. Be sure to follow your doctor's instructions carefully. • This drug interacts with guanethidine, monoamine oxidase inhibitors, propranolol, steroids, tetracycline, and thyroid hormone. If you are currently taking any drugs of these types, consult your doctor about their use. If you are unsure of the type or contents of your medications, ask your doctor or pharmacist. • While taking this drug, do not take any nonprescription item for weight control, cough, cold, or sinus problems without first checking with your doctor.

Comments: It is best to store this drug in the refrigerator. Once the bottle has been opened, most forms (except U-500 strength) may be kept at room temperature if the contents are used within a month. Store in a cool, dry place. Avoid heat and sunlight. Do not freeze. • This drug comes in two different strengths. Be sure to buy the right strength of the drug and the right syringes. • Special injection kits are available for blind diabetics. Ask your doctor for help in obtaining them. • Doses of this drug may be prepared in advance. Ask your pharmacist for advice. • Most insulin products are composed of a mixture of both pork and beef insulins. However, products are available that contain all beef insulin or all pork insulin. Human insulin is also available. Never switch from one form to another unless your doctor tells you to do so. • For best results, it is important that you understand diabetes. Insulin is used in conjunction with a proper diet and exercise program. Frequent monitoring of your urine or blood to check sugar levels is important. Various tests are available. Find the one that best suits your needs (check with your doctor or pharmacist), and learn how to use it. • If you are diabetic, you should wear a medical I.D. alert bracelet or carry a medical I.D. alert card in your wallet.

Intal respiratory inhalant

Manufacturer: Fisons Corporation
Ingredient: cromolyn sodium

Equivalent Product: Nasalcrom, Fisons Corporation

Dosage Forms: Aerosal spray (per actuation): 800 mcg. Capsules for inhalation; Nasal solution (per 2 ml amp): 20 mg

Uses: Prevention and management of bronchial asthma and allergic symptoms

Minor Side Effects: Bad taste in mouth; cough; dizziness; dry throat; headache; increased frequency of urination; itchy nose; nasal congestion; nasal irritation; nausea; painful urination; postnasal drip; sneezing; teary eyes

Major Side Effects: Blood disorders; breathing difficulties; joint pain and swelling; nosebleed; rash; swelling of the hands and feet; wheezing

Contraindication: This drug should not be taken by anyone who is allergic to it.

Warnings: The safety of this drug for use in pregnant or nursing women has not been established. Discuss the risks and benefits with your doctor. • For best results, this drug must be taken continuously, at regular intervals throughout the day and night, even if you feel better. Do not stop taking this drug without consulting your doctor. • It may take two to four weeks for the full effect of this drug to become apparent. • The contents of the capsules are inhaled through a device called a spinhaler. DO NOT SWALLOW THE CAPSULES. To use the capsules, load them into the spinhaler device. Breath out deeply, then place the spinhaler between your lips. Inhale deeply and steadily, then hold your breath for a few seconds. Remove the spinhaler from your lips, then exhale. Repeat this procedure until all of the powder in the capsule is gone. Ask your doctor or pharmacist to demonstrate the proper use of the spinhaler; be sure you know how to use it correctly. Be sure to clean the spinhaler device weekly. • Before using the nasal solution, blow your nose to clear the nasal passages. To avoid contamination, be sure to replace the nasal solution every six months, even if you have not finished all of it.

Iophen-C antitussive and expectorant (various manufacturers), see Tussi-Organidin antitussive and expectorant.

Ipran beta blocker (Major Pharmaceuticals), see propranolol beta blocker.

Iso-Bid antianginal (Geriatric Pharmaceutical Corp.), see Isordil antianginal.

Isollyl (Improved) analgesic (Rugby Laboratories), see Fiorinal analgesic.

Isonate antianginal (Major Pharmaceuticals), see Isordil antianginal.

Isoptin antianginal and antihypertensive

Manufacturer: Knoll Pharmaceutical Company

Ingredient: verapamil hydrochloride

Equivalent Products: Calan, Searle & Co.; verapamil, various manufacturers

Dosage Forms: Sustained-release tablet (see Comments): 240 mg (light green). Tablet: 40 mg (light blue); 80 mg (yellow); 120 mg (white)

Uses: Prevention and control of angina pectoris (chest pain); management of high blood pressure

Minor Side Effects: Abdominal pain; blurred vision; constipation; dizziness; fatigue; fever; headache; sleeplessness; loss of balance; muscle cramps; nausea; sweating; tremors

Major Side Effects: Changes in menstruation; confusion; depression; fainting; hair loss; itching; limping; shortness of breath; slow or irregular heartbeat; swelling of the hands and feet; unusual weakness

Contraindications: This drug should not be taken by people who are allergic to it or by those who have certain types of heart disease or extremely low blood pressure. Contact your doctor immediately if this drug has been prescribed for you and any of these conditions applies. • Mothers who are breast-feeding should not take this drug. • Do not take this drug until at least two days after stopping the drug disopyramide (Norpace).

Warnings: This drug should be used with caution by people who have cardiogenic shock, AV block, sick sinus syndrome, congestive heart failure, or liver or kidney disease. • This drug may interact with beta blockers, antihypertensive drugs, digitalis, diuretics, calcium supplements, and quinidine. If you are currently using any of these types of drugs, consult your doctor about their use; dosage adjustments may be needed. If you are unsure about the type or contents of your medications, ask your doctor or pharmacist. • This medication causes dizziness, especially during the first few days of therapy. Avoid activities that require alertness and limit consumption of alcohol, which exaggerates this effect.

Comments: Your doctor may want to see you regularly when you first start taking this drug in order to check your response. Your doctor may also want you to monitor your pulse and blood pressure every day; discuss this with your doctor. • It may take several weeks before any effect from the drug is noticed. It is important that you continue to take the medication to prevent chest pain. This drug is not effective in treating an attack of angina already in progress. • Contact your doctor if this drug causes severe or persistent dizziness, constipation, nausea, swelling of hands and feet, shortness of breath, or irregular heartbeat. • Isoptin SR and Calan SR are sustained-release formulations that are usually taken only once a day with food. Do not crush or chew the sustained-release forms of this drug; they must be swallowed whole.

Isopto Carpine ophthalmic preparation

Manufacturer: Alcon Laboratories, Inc.

Ingredient: pilocarpine hydrochloride

Equivalent Products: Adsorbocarpine, Alcon Laboratories, Inc.; Akarpine, Akorn, Inc.; Ocusert Pilo-20, Alza Corporation; Ocusert Pilo-40, Alza Corporation; Pilocar, Iolab; pilocarpine hydrochloride, various manufacturers; Pilopine HS, Alcon Laboratories, Inc.

Dosage Forms: Drops: 0.25%; 0.5%; 1%; 2%; 3%; 4%; 5%; 6%; 8%; 10%. Gel: 4%. Ocular therapeutic system (see Comments): 20 mcg; 40 mcg

Use: Treatment of glaucoma

Minor Side Effects: Aching in the brow; blurred vision; headache; loss of night vision; twitching of eyelids

Major Side Effects: Diarrhea; difficulty in urinating; flushing; muscle tremors; nausea; nearsightedness or other changes in vision; palpitations; shortness of breath; stomach cramps; sweating

Contraindication: This drug should not be used by people who are allergic to pilocarpine. Consult your doctor immediately if this drug has been prescribed for you and you have such an allergy.

Warnings: This drug should be used cautiously by people who have heart damage, asthma, peptic ulcer, thyroid disease, spasms of the gastrointestinal tract, blockage of the urinary tract, seizures, or Parkinson's disease. Be sure your doctor knows if you have any of these conditions. • Be careful about the contamination of solutions used for the eyes. Wash your hands before using eye drops. Do not touch dropper to your eye. Do not wash or wipe the dropper before replacing it in the bottle. Close the bottle tightly to keep out moisture.

Comments: To administer eye drops, lie or sit down and tilt your head back. Carefully pull your lower eyelid down to form a pouch. Hold the dropper close to, but not touching, the eyelid, and place the prescribed number of drops into the pouch. Do not place the drops directly on the eyeball; you probably will blink and lose the medication. Close your eye and keep it shut for a few moments. • This drug may sting when first administered; this sensation usually goes away quickly. • The ocular therapeutic system (Ocusert Pilo) is an oval ring of plastic that contains pilocarpine. This ring is placed in the eye, and the drug is released gradually over a period of seven days. Use of these rings has made possible the control of glaucoma for some patients. If you are having trouble controlling glaucoma, ask your doctor about the possibility of using one of these devices.

Isordil antianginal

Manufacturer: Wyeth-Ayerst Laboratories
Ingredient: isosorbide dinitrate
Equivalent Products: Dilatrate-SR, Reed & Carnrick; Iso-Bid, Geriatric Pharmaceutical Corp.; Isonate, Major Pharmaceuticals; isosorbide dinitrate, various manufacturers; Isotrate Timecelles, W. E. Hauck, Inc.; Sorbitrate, ICI Pharma
Dosage Forms: Chewable tablet: 10 mg (yellow). Sublingual tablet: 2.5 mg (yellow); 5 mg (pink); 10 mg (white). Sustained-action capsule: 40 mg (blue/clear). Sustained-action tablet: 40 mg (green). Tablet: 5 mg (pink); 10 mg (white); 20 mg (green); 30 mg (blue); 40 mg (light green); see Comments
Use: Prevention (tablets and sustained-action forms only) and relief (chewable and sublingual tablets only) of chest pain (angina) due to heart disease
Minor Side Effects: Dizziness; flushing; headache; nausea; vomiting
Major Side Effects: Fainting spells; low blood pressure; palpitations; rash; restlessness; sweating; weakness
Contraindications: This drug should not be taken by people who are allergic to it or by people with low blood pressure or head injury. Sublingual tablets should not be used by persons who are recovering from a heart attack. Consult your doctor if this drug has been prescribed for you and any of these conditions applies.
Warnings: This drug interacts with nitroglycerin; if you are currently using nitroglycerin, consult your doctor about its use. • Before using this drug to relieve chest pain, be certain that pain arises from the heart and is not due to a muscle spasm or to indigestion. • If your chest pain is not relieved by use of this drug or if pain arises from a different location or differs in severity, consult your doctor immediately. • This drug should be used cautiously by those with glaucoma, severe anemia, thyroid disease, or frequent diarrhea.
Comments: Carefully discuss the possible benefits of the various dosage forms of this drug with your doctor before purchasing it. • With continued use, you may develop a tolerance to this drug; many adverse side effects disappear after two to three weeks of drug use, but you may also become less responsive to the drug's beneficial effects. Consult your doctor if you feel that the drug is losing its effectiveness. • The chewable tablets must be chewed to release the

medication they contain. Do not crush the chewable tablets before placing them in your mouth. • The sustained-action forms must be swallowed whole. • Sorbitrate also comes in a 5 mg chewable tablet, and isosorbide dinitrate is available in a 40 mg capsule. • Do not suddenly stop taking this medication without first consulting your doctor. • To take a sublingual tablet properly, place the tablet under your tongue, close your mouth, and hold the saliva in your mouth and under your tongue as long as you can before swallowing it. (If you have a bitter taste in your mouth after five minutes, the drug has not been completely absorbed. Wait five more minutes before drinking water.) It may be necessary to take another tablet in five minutes if the pain still exists. If you still have pain after using three tablets (one every five minutes) in a 15-minute period, call your doctor or go to a hospital. • To avoid dizziness or light-headedness when you stand, contract and relax the muscles of your legs for a few moments before rising. Do this by pushing one foot against the floor while raising the other foot slightly, alternating feet so that you are "pumping" your legs in a pedaling motion. • Alcoholic beverages should be avoided or used with caution, as they may enhance the severity of this drug's side effects. • In order to avoid loss of potency, the tablets and capsules should be stored in their original containers, and the containers should be kept tightly closed.

isosorbide dinitrate antianginal (various manufacturers), see Isordil antianginal.

Isotrate Timecelles antianginal (W. E. Hauck, Inc.), see Isordil antianginal.

Janimine antidepressant (Abbott Laboratories), see Tofranil antidepressant.

Kaochlor potassium chloride replacement (Adria Laboratories, Inc.), see potassium chloride replacement.

Kaon potassium chloride replacement (Adria Laboratories, Inc.), see potassium chloride replacement.

Kato potassium chloride replacement (ICN Pharmaceuticals, Inc.), see potassium chloride replacement.

Kay Ciel potassium chloride replacement (Forest Pharmaceuticals, Inc.), see potassium chloride replacement.

Kaylixir potassium chloride replacement (The Lannet Company, Inc.), see potassium chloride replacement.

Keflet antibiotic (Dista Products Company), see Keflex antibiotic.

Keflex antibiotic

Manufacturer: Dista Products Company
Ingredient: cephalexin
Equivalent Products: cephalexin, various manufacturers; Keflet, Dista Products Company; Keftab, Dista Products Company

Dosage Forms: Capsule: 250 mg (white/dark green); 500 mg (light green/dark green). Drop (content per ml): 100 mg. Liquid (content per 5 ml teaspoon): 125 mg; 250 mg. Tablet (see Comments): 250 mg; 500 mg; 1 g (all are green)

Use: Treatment of bacterial infections

Minor Side Effects: Abdominal pain; diarrhea; dizziness; fatigue; headache; heartburn; itching; loss of appetite; nausea; vomiting

Major Side Effects: Breathing difficulties; fever; rash; rectal and vaginal itching; severe diarrhea; sore mouth; stomach cramps; superinfection; tingling in the hands or feet; unusual bruising or bleeding

Contraindications: This drug should not be used by people who are allergic to it or to other antibiotics similar to it (such as penicillins; see Comments). Consult your doctor immediately if this drug has been prescribed for you and you have such an allergy.

Warnings: This drug should be used cautiously by women who are pregnant or nursing and by people with kidney disease. Be sure your doctor knows if any of these conditions applies to you. • This drug should be used cautiously in newborns. • Prolonged use of this drug may allow organisms that are not susceptible to it to grow wildly. Do not use this drug unless your doctor has specifically told you to do so. Be sure to follow directions carefully and report any unusual reactions to your doctor at once. • This drug should be used cautiously in conjunction with diuretics, probenecid, and aminoglycoside antibiotics. If you are unsure of the types or contents of your medications, ask your doctor or pharmacist. • This drug may interfere with some blood tests. Be sure your doctor knows you are taking it. • Diabetics using Clinitest urine test may get a false high sugar reading. Change to Clinistix urine test or Tes-Tape urine test to avoid this problem.

Comments: It is generally believed that about ten percent of all people who are allergic to penicillin will be allergic to an antibiotic like this as well. • Some infections can be adequately treated with penicillin, which is less expensive. Ask your doctor if you could take penicillin instead of this drug. You may be able to save money. • Take this drug with food or milk if stomach upset occurs. • The capsule and tablet forms of this drug should be stored at room temperature. The liquid form of this drug should be refrigerated and any unused portion should be discarded after 14 days. Shake well before using. This medication should never be frozen. • Take this drug as prescribed at evenly spaced intervals around the clock. Finish all the medication, even if you feel better, to ensure complete elimination of the infection. • The 250 mg and 500 mg tablet forms of this medication are available under the names Keflet and Keftab.

Keftab antibiotic (Dista Products Company), see Keflex antibiotic.

K-G potassium chloride replacement (Geneva Generics, Inc.), see potassium chloride replacement.

Klor-Con/EF potassium chloride replacement (Upsher-Smith Laboratories, Inc.), see potassium chloride replacement.

Klor-Con potassium chloride replacement (Upsher-Smith Laboratories, Inc.), see potassium chloride replacement.

K-Lor potassium chloride replacement (Abbott Laboratories), see potassium chloride replacement.

Klorvess potassium chloride replacement (Sandoz Pharmaceuticals), see potassium chloride replacement.

Klotrix potassium chloride replacement (Mead Johnson Nutritional), see potassium chloride replacement.

K-Lyte/Cl potassium chloride replacement (Mead Johnson Nutritional), see potassium chloride replacement.

K-Lyte DS potassium chloride replacement (Mead Johnson Nutritional), see potassium chloride replacement.

K-Lyte potassium chloride replacement (Mead Johnson Nutritional), see potassium chloride replacement.

Kolyum potassium chloride replacement (Pennwalt Pharmaceutical Division), see potassium chloride replacement.

K-Tab potassium chloride replacement (Abbott Laboratories), see potassium chloride replacement.

Kwell pediculicide and scabicide

Manufacturer: Reed & Carnrick
Ingredient: lindane (gamma benzene hexachloride)
Equivalent Products: G-well, Goldline Laboratories; Kwildane, Major Pharmaceuticals; lindane, various manufacturers; Scabene, Stiefel Laboratories, Inc.
Dosage Forms: Cream; Lotion; Shampoo: 1%
Uses: Elimination of crab lice, head lice and their nits, and scabies
Minor Side Effects: Rash; skin irritation
Major Side Effects: See Warnings
Contraindication: This drug should not be used by people who are allergic to it. Consult your doctor immediately if this drug has been prescribed for you and you have such an allergy.
Warnings: Side effects to this drug are rare if the directions for use are followed. However, convulsions and even death can result if the drug is swallowed or overused. If swallowed, do not take mineral oil; call the poison control center, your doctor, or your pharmacist immediately. • Do not use this drug with other skin products. • Special caution must be used in treating children, infants, and pregnant women with this drug. • If you get any of this product in your eyes, flush them immediately with water. • Do not use this product over a longer period or more often than recommended by your doctor. • Do not use this product on your face. • Be sure to rinse this product off completely, as is stated in the directions. • Avoid unnecessary skin contact.
Comments: Complete directions for the use of this drug are supplied by the manufacturer. Ask your pharmacist for these directions if they are not supplied with the drug. • Lice are easily transmitted from one person to another. All family members should be carefully examined. Personal items (clothing, towels) need only be machine-washed on the "hot" temperature cycle and dried. No unusual cleaning measures are required. Combs, brushes, and other such washable items may be soaked in boiling water for one hour. • After using this product you must remove the dead nits (eggs). Use a fine-tooth comb to remove them from your hair, or mix a solution of equal parts of water and vinegar and apply it to the affected area. Rub the solution in well. After several minutes, shampoo with your regular shampoo and then brush your hair. This process should remove all nits. • If required, a second application may be

repeated in seven to nine days. Do not use lindane products routinely as shampoo. • A lice infestation can be treated just as effectively with a nonprescription product as with this product. However, this product is effective for scabies; the nonprescription medication is not. Consult your pharmacist. • To equalize the doses, the lotion should be shaken before each dose is measured.

Kwildane pediculicide and scabicide (Major Pharmaceuticals), see Kwell pediculicide and scabicide.

Lanophyllin bronchodilator (The Lannet Company, Inc.), see theophylline bronchodilator.

Lanorinal analgesic (The Lannet Company, Inc.), see Fiorinal analgesic.

Lanoxicaps heart drug (Burroughs Wellcome Co.), see Lanoxin heart drug.

Lanoxin heart drug

Manufacturer: Burroughs Wellcome Co.
Ingredient: digoxin
Equivalent Products: digoxin, various manufacturers; Lanoxicaps, Burroughs Wellcome Co. (see Comments)
Dosage Forms: Capsule: 0.05 mg (red); 0.1 mg (yellow); 0.2 mg (green). Elixir, pediatric (content per ml): 0.05 mg. Tablet: 0.125 mg (yellow); 0.25 mg (white); 0.5 mg (green)
Use: To strengthen heartbeat and improve heart rhythm
Minor Side Effects: Apathy; diarrhea; drowsiness; headache; muscle weakness; weakness
Major Side Effects: Breast enlargement (in both sexes); depression; disorientation; hallucinations; loss of appetite; nausea; palpitations; slow heart rate; visual disturbances (such as blurred or yellow vision); vomiting
Contraindications: People who have suffered heart stoppage and people who are allergic to this drug should not take it. Consult your doctor immediately if this drug has been prescribed for you and either of these conditions applies.
Warnings: This drug should be used cautiously by people who have kidney disease, thyroid disease, certain heart diseases, lung disease, potassium depletion, or calcium accumulation. Be sure your doctor knows if any of these conditions applies to you. • This drug should be used cautiously in infants. • Some people develop toxic reactions to this drug. If you suffer any side effects that are prolonged or especially bothersome, contact your doctor. • The elderly may have more side effects from this drug than younger people and should therefore have regular checkups while taking it. • This drug interacts with aminoglycosides, antacids, antibiotics, amphotericin B, cholestyramine, colestipol hydrochloride, diuretics, phenylbutazone, propantheline, propranolol, and spironolactone; if you are currently taking any drugs of these types, consult your doctor about their use. If you are unsure of the type or contents of your medications, ask your doctor or pharmacist. • The pharmacologic activity of the different brands of this drug varies widely depending on how well the tablets or capsules dissolve in the stomach and bowels. Because of this variation, it is important not to change brands of the drug without consulting your doctor.
Comments: Dosages of this drug must be carefully adjusted to the needs and responses of the individual patient. Your doctor may find it necessary to adjust your dosage of this drug frequently. To do so, blood tests may be done to

measure the amount of the drug in your blood. Ask your doctor to explain the test and your results. • Your doctor may want you to take your pulse daily while you are using this drug. • Take this drug at the same time every day. Do not skip any doses, and do not stop taking this medication without consulting your doctor. • While taking this drug, do not take any nonprescription item for weight control, cough, cold, or sinus problems without first checking with your doctor. • There are no products exactly equivalent to Lanoxin heart drug. You should not switch to another brand of digoxin unless your doctor is monitoring your condition closely. Because this product is priced inexpensively, you will probably save little, if any, money by switching to another brand. • Notify your doctor if you experience a loss of appetite, pain in the stomach, nausea, vomiting, diarrhea, unusual tiredness or weakness, blurred or yellow vision, or mental depression.

Larotid antibiotic (Beecham Laboratories), see amoxicillin antibiotic.

Lasix diuretic and antihypertensive

Manufacturer: Hoechst-Roussel Pharmaceutical, Inc.
Ingredient: furosemide
Equivalent Products: Fumide, Everett Laboratories, Inc.; furosemide, various manufacturers; Luramide, Major Pharmaceuticals
Dosage Forms: Liquid (content per ml): 10 mg (see Comments). Tablet: 20 mg; 40 mg; 80 mg (all are white)
Uses: Treatment of high blood pressure; removal of fluid from body tissues
Minor Side Effects: Blurred vision; constipation; cramping; diarrhea; dizziness; headache; itching; loss of appetite; muscle spasm; nausea; sore mouth; stomach upset; sun sensitivity; vomiting; weakness
Major Side Effects: Anemia; blood disorders; bruising; dry mouth; gout; increase in blood sugar; jaundice; loss of appetite; low blood pressure; muscle cramps; palpitations; pancreatitis; rash; ringing in the ears; sore throat; thirst; tingling in the fingers and toes
Contraindications: This drug should not be used by pregnant women or women who may become pregnant, by persons with anuria (inability to urinate), or by people who are allergic to it. Consult your doctor immediately if this drug has been prescribed for you and any of these conditions applies.
Warnings: Use of this drug may cause gout, diabetes, hearing loss, and loss of potassium, calcium, water, and salt. Persons taking this drug should have periodic blood and urine tests to check for these effects. • Persons hypersensitive to sulfa drugs may also be hypersensitive to this drug. If this drug has been prescribed for you and you are allergic to sulfa drugs, consult your doctor immediately. • This drug should be used cautiously by persons with cirrhosis of the liver or other liver problems and by those with kidney disease. This drug should be used cautiously by children. Nursing mothers who must take this drug should stop nursing. Be sure your doctor knows if any of these conditions applies to you. • This drug has potent activity and should be used with caution in conjunction with other high blood pressure drugs. If you are taking other such medications, the dosages may require adjustment. • Use of this drug may activate the appearance of systemic lupus erythematosus. • Whenever adverse reactions to this drug are moderate to severe, this drug should be reduced or discontinued. Consult your doctor promptly if such side effects occur. • This drug interacts with aspirin, curare, indomethacin, digitalis, lithium carbonate, steroids, and cephaloridine. If you are currently taking any drugs of these types, consult your doctor about their use. If you are unsure of the type or contents of your medications, ask your doctor or pharmacist.

Comments: You should learn how to monitor your pulse and blood pressure while taking this medication; consult your doctor. • This drug can cause potassium loss. Signs of such loss include dry mouth, thirst, muscle cramps, weakness, and nausea or vomiting. If you experience any of these side effects, notify your doctor. To help avoid such loss, take this drug with a glass of fresh or frozen orange juice, or eat a banana each day. The use of a salt substitute helps prevent potassium loss. Do not change your diet, however, before discussing it with your doctor. Too much potassium may also be dangerous. • Notify your doctor if you develop signs of jaundice (yellow eyes or skin; dark urine). • When taking this drug (or other drugs for high blood pressure), limit the use of alcohol to avoid dizziness or light-headedness. To avoid dizziness or light-headedness when you stand, contract and relax the muscles of your legs for a few moments before rising. Do this by pushing one foot against the floor while raising the other foot slightly, alternating feet so that you are "pumping" your legs in a pedaling motion. • Persons taking this product and digitalis should watch carefully for symptoms of increased digitalis toxicity (e.g., nausea, blurred vision, palpitations), and notify their doctors immediately if symptoms occur. • If you have high blood pressure, do not take any nonprescription item for weight control, cough, cold, or sinus problems without first checking with your doctor; such items may contain ingredients that can increase blood pressure. • This drug causes frequent urination. Expect this effect; it should not alarm you. • Take this drug exactly as directed. It is usually taken in the morning with food. Avoid taking this medication near bedtime. Do not take extra doses or skip a dose without first consulting your doctor. • The liquid form of this drug should be stored in the refrigerator in a light-resistant container. • Furosemide liquid is also available in a 40 mg strength.

Ledercillin VK antibiotic (Lederle Laboratories), see penicillin potassium phenoxymethyl (penicillin VK) antibiotic.

Levothroid thyroid hormone (Rorer Pharmaceuticals), see Synthroid thyroid hormone.

levothyroxine sodium thyroid hormone (Lederle Laboratories), see Synthroid thyroid hormone.

Librax antianxiety

Manufacturer: Roche Products Inc.
Ingredients: chlordiazepoxide hydrochloride; clidinium bromide
Equivalent Products: Clindex, Rugby Laboratories; Clinoxide, Geneva Generics, Inc.; Clipoxide, Henry Schein, Inc.; Lidox, Major Pharmaceuticals
Dosage Form: Capsule: chlordiazepoxide hydrochloride, 5 mg and clidinium bromide, 2.5 mg (green)
Uses: In conjunction with other drugs for the treatment of peptic ulcer or irritable bowel syndrome; also used to relieve anxiety
Minor Side Effects: Blurred vision; change in sense of taste; confusion; constipation; depression; diarrhea; dizziness; drowsiness; dry mouth; fatigue; fluid retention; headache; increased sensitivity to light; insomnia; menstrual irregularities; nausea; reduced sweating; vomiting
Major Side Effects: Breathing difficulties; decreased sexual ability; difficulty in urinating; double vision; excitation; hallucinations; jaundice; palpitations; rash; sore throat; uncoordinated movements
Contraindications: This drug should not be taken by people who have glaucoma, enlarged prostate, or obstructed bladder or intestine. Consult your doctor

immediately if this drug has been prescribed for you and you have any of these conditions.

Warnings: This drug should be used cautiously by people who have severe heart or lung disease, liver or kidney disease, porphyria, high blood pressure, myasthenia gravis, epilepsy, thyroid disease, or colitis and by those who are pregnant or nursing. Be sure your doctor knows if any of these conditions applies to you. • This drug should not be used in conjunction with amantadine, haloperidol, other central nervous system depressants, phenothiazines, alcohol, or antacids; if you are currently taking any drugs of these types, consult your doctor about their use. If you are unsure of the type or contents of your medications, ask your doctor or pharmacist. • Call your doctor if you notice a rash, flushing, or pain in the eye. • This drug has a slight potential for abuse; if taken as directed, however, there is little danger. Do not increase or decrease the dose of this drug without first consulting your doctor. • Elderly patients generally should take the smallest effective dosage of this drug.

Comments: This drug is best taken one-half to one hour before meals. • This drug does not cure ulcers but may help them improve. • Chew gum or suck on ice chips or a piece of hard candy to reduce mouth dryness. • This drug always produces certain side effects, which may include dry mouth, blurred vision, reduced sweating, drowsiness, difficulty in urinating, constipation, increased sensitivity to light, and palpitations. • Avoid excessive work or exercise in hot weather and drink plenty of liquids. • Notify your doctor if you develop signs of jaundice (yellow eyes or skin; dark urine). • To prevent oversedation, avoid taking alcohol or other drugs that have sedative properties. Avoid tasks that require alertness. • If this drug makes it difficult for you to urinate, try to do so just before you take each dose.

Libritabs antianxiety (Roche Products Inc.), see Librium antianxiety.

Librium antianxiety

Manufacturer: Roche Products Inc.

Ingredient: chlordiazepoxide hydrochloride

Equivalent Products: chlordiazepoxide hydrochloride, various manufacturers; Libritabs, Roche Products Inc.; Lipoxide, Major Pharmaceuticals; Mitran, W.E. Hauck, Inc.; Reposans-10, Wesley Pharmacal Co.

Dosage Forms: Capsule: 5 mg (green/yellow); 10 mg (green/black); 25 mg (green/white). Tablet (see Comments): 5 mg; 10 mg; 25 mg (all are green)

Uses: Relief of anxiety, nervousness, tension, muscle spasms, and withdrawal symptoms of alcohol addiction

Minor Side Effects: Confusion; constipation; depression; dizziness; drooling; drowsiness; dry mouth; fainting; fatigue; fluid retention; headache; heartburn; insomnia; loss of appetite; menstrual irregularities; nausea; sweating

Major Side Effects: Blood disorders; blurred vision; breathing difficulties; decrease or increase in sex drive; difficulty in urinating; double vision; excitation; fever; hallucinations; jaundice; low blood pressure; rash; slow heart rate; slurred speech; sore throat; stimulation; tremors; weakness

Contraindications: This drug should not be used by people who are allergic to it or by pregnant or nursing women. Consult your doctor immediately if this drug has been prescribed for you and any of these conditions applies.

Warnings: This drug should be used cautiously by people who have liver or kidney disease; by those with acute, narrow-angle glaucoma; and by those who are depressed. Be sure your doctor knows if any of these conditions applies to you. • Elderly people should use this drug cautiously and take the smallest effective dose. • This drug has the potential for abuse and must be used with caution. • This drug is not recommended for use in children under six years of age. • Tolerance may develop quickly; do not increase the dose of this drug without first consulting your doctor. • Do not take it with other sedative drugs, central nervous system depressants, or alcohol; serious adverse reactions may develop. • This drug should be used cautiously in conjunction with phenytoin, cimetidine, lithium, levodopa, isoniazid, rifampin, and disulfiram. • This drug may cause drowsiness; avoid tasks that require alertness. • Consult your doctor if you wish to discontinue use of this drug; do not stop taking the drug suddenly. If you have been using the drug for an extended period of time, it will be necessary to reduce the dosage gradually, according to your doctor's instructions. • Unexpected excitement sometimes occurs in persons taking this drug. This effect is especially likely to occur in psychotics. If such an effect occurs, consult your doctor. • Persons taking this drug for a long period should have periodic blood counts and liver function tests.

Comments: This drug is effective in relieving nervousness, but it is important to try to remove the cause of the nervousness as well. Consult your doctor. • Notify your doctor if you develop signs of jaundice (yellow eyes or skin; dark urine). • Chew gum or suck on ice chips or a piece of hard candy to reduce mouth dryness. • Take this medication with food or a full glass of water if stomach upset occurs. Do not take it with an antacid; it may retard absorption of the drug. After taking this drug, wait 30 minutes before taking an antacid if one is needed. • The tablet forms of this drug are available under the name Libritabs.

Lidex topical steroid hormone

Manufacturer: Syntex Laboratories, Inc.
Ingredient: fluocinonide
Equivalent Product: fluocinonide, various manufacturers; see Comments
Dosage Forms: Cream; Gel; Ointment; Solution: 0.05%
Use: Relief of skin inflammation associated with conditions such as eczema and poison ivy
Minor Side Effects: Burning sensation; dryness; irritation of affected area; itching; rash
Major Side Effects: Blistering; increased hair growth; loss of skin color; secondary infection; skin wasting
Contraindications: This drug should not be taken by people who are allergic to it. This drug should not be used in the ear if the eardrum is perforated or by people who have viral or fungal skin disease, tuberculosis of the skin, or severe circulatory disorders. Consult your doctor immediately if this drug has been prescribed for you and any of these conditions applies.
Warnings: If irritation develops, consult your doctor. • If extensive areas are treated or if occlusive dressings are used, there will be increased systemic absorption of this drug; suitable precautions should be taken, especially in children and infants. If this drug is being used on a child's diaper area, avoid tight-fitting diapers or plastic pants, which can increase absorption of the drug. • This drug should be used cautiously by pregnant women. • This drug should not be used in the eyes.
Comments: The gel form may produce a cooling sensation on the skin. • If the affected area is dry or is scaling, the skin may be moistened before applying the product by soaking in water or by applying water with a clean cloth. The ointment form is probably the better product for dry skin. • Do not use these products with an occlusive wrap of transparent plastic film unless directed to do so by your doctor. If it is necessary for you to use this drug under a wrap, follow your doctor's directions exactly. Do not leave the wrap in place for a longer time than specified. • Lidex-E topical steroid hormone is also manufactured by Syn-

tex Laboratories, Inc. It contains fluocinonide in a cream form similar to Lidex but has more skin-softening ingredients. For all practical purposes, Lidex and Lidex-E are the same. • Use this product to treat only the condition for which it was prescribed. Using topical steroids to treat an infection may worsen the infection.

Lidox antianxiety (Major Pharmaceuticals), see Librax antianxiety.

lindane pediculicide and scabicide (various manufacturers), see Kwell pediculicide and scabicide.

Lipoxide antianxiety (Major Pharmaceuticals), see Librium antianxiety.

Liquid Pred prednisone steroid hormone (Muro Pharmaceutical, Inc.), see prednisone steroid hormone.

Lixolin bronchodilator (Mallard, Inc.), see theophylline bronchodilator.

Lodrane bronchodilator (Poythress Laboratories, Inc.), see theophylline bronchodilator.

Lofene antidiarrheal (The Lannett Company, Inc.), see Lomotil antidiarrheal.

Logen antidiarrheal (Goldline Laboratories), see Lomotil antidiarrheal.

Lomotil antidiarrheal

Manufacturer: Searle & Co.
Ingredients: diphenoxylate hydrochloride with atropine sulfate
Equivalent Products: Diphenatol, Rugby Laboratories; diphenoxylate hydrochloride with atropine sulfate, various manufacturers; Lofene, The Lannett Company, Inc.; Logen, Goldline Laboratories; Lonox, Geneva Generics, Inc.; Lo-Trol, Vangard Laboratories; Low-Quel, Halsey Drug Co., Inc.; Nor-Mil, Vortech Pharmaceutical, Ltd.
Dosage Forms: Liquid (content per 5 ml teaspoon); Tablet (white): atropine sulfate, 0.025 mg and diphenoxylate hydrochloride, 2.5 mg
Use: Treatment of diarrhea
Minor Side Effects: Blurred vision; constipation; dizziness; drowsiness; dry mouth; fever; flushing; headache; increased heart rate; itching; loss of appetite; nervousness; sedation; sweating; swollen gums
Major Side Effects: Abdominal pain; bloating; breathing difficulties; coma; depression; difficulty in urinating; euphoria; fever; hives; numbness in fingers or toes; palpitations; rash; severe nausea; vomiting; weakness
Contraindications: This drug should not be taken by children under the age of two or by people who have jaundice or drug-induced diarrhea or by those who are allergic to it. Consult your doctor immediately if this drug has been prescribed for you and any of these conditions applies.
Warnings: This drug should be used cautiously by children, by pregnant or nursing women, by women of childbearing age, and by people who have liver

or kidney disease, lung disease, glaucoma, high blood pressure, myasthenia gravis, gallstones, enlarged prostate, thyroid disease, certain types of heart disease, or ulcerative colitis. Be sure your doctor knows if any of these conditions applies to you. • This drug has the potential for abuse and must be used with caution. Tolerance to this drug may develop quickly; do not increase the dose of this drug without first checking with your doctor. • This drug may add to the effect of alcohol and other drugs that have sedative properties. Do not use them without first checking with your doctor. • This drug interacts with amantadine, haloperidol, phenothiazines, and monoamine oxidase inhibitors; if you are currently taking any drugs of these types, consult your doctor about their use. If you are unsure of the type or contents of your medications, ask your doctor or pharmacist.

Comments: While taking this drug, drink at least eight glasses of water a day. • This drug may cause dry mouth. To relieve this, chew gum or suck on ice chips or a piece of hard candy. • This drug may interfere with your ability to perform potentially hazardous tasks such as driving or operating machinery. • Unless your doctor prescribes otherwise, do not take this drug for more than five days. • If diarrhea does not subside within two to three days, consult your doctor. • If you take this drug with you when traveling to a foreign country, do not use it unless absolutely necessary. Make sure that the diarrhea is not just a temporary occurrence (two to three hours). • Call your doctor if you notice a rash or if fever or heart palpitations develop.

Lonox antidiarrheal (Geneva Generics, Inc.), see Lomotil antidiarrheal.

Lopressor beta blocker

Manufacturer: Geigy Pharmaceuticals
Ingredient: metoprolol tartrate
Dosage Form: Tablet: 50 mg (pink); 100 mg (light blue)
Uses: Management of high blood pressure or chest pain (angina); prevention of irregular heartbeat after heart attack
Minor Side Effects: Abdominal cramps; constipation; diarrhea; drowsiness; dry eyes; dry mouth; gas; gastric pain; headache; heartburn; insomnia; loss of appetite; nasal congestion; nausea; slow heart rate
Major Side Effects: Bruising; cold extremities; confusion; depression; dizziness; fainting; fever; hallucinations; heart failure; itching; nightmares; numbness or tingling in the hands and feet; palpitations; rash; reversible loss of hair; ringing in the ears; shortness of breath; slurred speech; sore throat; tiredness; visual disturbances; weak pulse; wheezing
Contraindications: This drug should not be used by people with certain types of heart disease (such as bradycardia, overt cardiac failure, heart block, or cardiogenic shock) or certain lung diseases. Consult your doctor if this drug has been prescribed for you and any of these conditions applies.
Warnings: This drug should be used with caution by people with thyroid disease (certain types), impaired kidney or liver function, asthma, bronchospasm, or diabetes. Be sure your doctor knows if any of these conditions applies to you. • Diabetics should be aware that this drug may mask signs of hypoglycemia, such as changes in pulse rate and blood pressure. • Persons about to undergo surgery should use this drug with caution. • Pregnant women, nursing mothers, and children should take this drug only when clearly needed. • Extra care is needed if this drug is used with reserpine, phenytoin, terbutaline, aminophylline, theophylline, digitalis, phenobarbital, or cimetidine. If you are currently taking any drugs of these types, consult your doctor about their use. If

you are unsure of the type or contents of your medications, ask your doctor or pharmacist. • This drug should not be stopped abruptly (unless your doctor advises you to do so). Chest pain and even heart attacks have occurred when this drug has been stopped suddenly.

Comments: It is best to take this drug with food. • While taking this drug, do not take any nonprescription item for weight control, cough, cold, or sinus problems without first checking with your doctor; such items may contain ingredients that can increase blood pressure. • Your doctor may want you to take your pulse and blood pressure every day while you are taking this drug. Discuss this with your doctor. • Be sure to take the doses of this drug at the same time each day. • Notify your doctor if dizziness, diarrhea, rash, or breathing difficulty develops. • This drug may cause you to be sensitive to the cold. Dress warmly. • There are many beta blockers available. Your doctor may want you to try different ones in order to find the one that works best for you.

Lopurin antigout drug (Boots Pharmaceuticals, Inc.), see Zyloprim antigout drug.

Loraz antianxiety and sedative (Quantum Pharmics), see Ativan antianxiety and sedative.

lorazepam antianxiety and sedative (various manufacturers), see Ativan antianxiety and sedative.

Lorcet analgesic (UAD Laboratories, Inc.), see Vicodin analgesic.

Lorelco antihyperlipidemic

Manufacturer: Merrell Dow Pharmaceuticals, Inc.
Ingredient: probucol
Dosage Form: Tablet: 250 mg; 500 mg (both white)
Use: In conjunction with diet to reduce elevated blood cholesterol levels
Minor Side Effects: Altered senses of taste and smell; blurred vision; diarrhea; dizziness; flatulence; headache; indigestion; itching; loss of appetite; nausea; stomach cramps; stomach upset; sweating; vomiting
Major Side Effects: Blood disorders; fainting; impotence; ringing in the ears; swelling of ankles and feet; tingling of the hands or feet
Contraindication: This drug should not be taken by anyone who is allergic to it. Consult your doctor immediately if this drug has been prescribed for you and you have such an allergy.
Warnings: This drug must be used with caution in pregnant or nursing women. Discuss the benefits and risks with your doctor if either condition applies to you. • This drug is not recommended for use in children. • Persons with certain types of heart disease (arrhythmias, for example) must be monitored closely while taking this drug.
Comments: Diet therapy is considered the initial treatment of choice for high blood cholesterol levels. This drug should be used only after diet therapy has been tried. This drug is not a substitute for a proper diet. For maximum effectiveness, this drug must be used in conjunction with a diet that is low in saturated fat and cholesterol. You may be referred to a nutritionist for diet counseling. • The full effects of this drug may not be evident for up to three months. Your doctor will want to monitor the effects of this drug by doing periodic blood tests. Ask your doctor to explain what your cholesterol levels mean and what your therapy goals are. Learn to monitor your progress. • For best results, take this drug with meals. • Do not stop taking this drug suddenly unless instructed to do

so by your doctor. • Diarrhea, gas, abdominal pain, nausea, and vomiting may occur when first taking this drug. These effects usually disappear with continued use. Notify your doctor if they persist or worsen.

Lortab 5 analgesic (Russ, Inc.), see Vicodin analgesic.

Lotrimin antifungal agent

Manufacturer: Schering Corp.
Ingredient: clotrimazole
Equivalent Product: Mycelex, Miles Pharmaceutical; see Comments
Dosage Forms: Cream (content per gram); Lotion; Solution (content per ml): 1%
Use: Treatment of superficial fungal infections of the skin
Minor Side Effects: Redness; stinging sensation
Major Side Effects: Blistering; irritation; peeling of skin; swelling
Contraindication: This drug should not be used by people who are allergic to it. Consult your doctor immediately if this drug has been prescribed for you and you have such an allergy.
Warnings: This drug should be used with caution by pregnant women. • Do not use this drug in or near the eyes. • If irritation occurs, stop using this product and call your doctor.
Comments: Apply this product after cleansing the area, unless your doctor has directed otherwise. This drug should be gently rubbed into the affected area and the surrounding skin. • Do not use a dressing over this drug unless instructed to do so by your doctor. • Improvement in your condition may not be seen for one week after beginning treatment with this drug. Nevertheless, be sure to complete a full course of therapy. If the condition has not improved after four weeks, or if it worsens, consult your doctor. • This drug is also available in vaginal cream and vaginal tablet forms to treat certain fungal infections of the vagina. Mycelex-G (Miles Pharmaceutical) and Gyne-Lotrimin (Schering Corp.) antifungal agents are trademarked products of this type.

Lotrisone steroid hormone and antifungal

Manufacturer: Schering Corp.
Ingredients: betamethasone; clotrimazole
Dosage Form: Cream: betamethasone, 0.05% and clotrimazole, 1%
Use: Treatment of certain skin infections
Minor Side Effects: Burning sensation; irritation; itching; redness of skin
Major Side Effects: Blistering; peeling of skin; rash; secondary infection; swelling of extremities
Contraindications: This drug should not be used by persons sensitive to either of its ingredients or to corticosteroids. Consult your doctor immediately if this drug has been prescribed for you and you have any such allergies. • This drug is not to be used in the eyes, nor in the ear canals of persons with a perforated eardrum.
Warnings: Prolonged use of large amounts of this drug should be avoided, especially in areas where the skin is damaged, as with extensive burns. If extensive areas are treated or if an occlusive dressing is used to cover the area, there will be increased absorption of this drug into the bloodstream leading to systemic side effects. Suitable precautions should be taken, especially with children, who have a greater tendency to absorb the drug. Use this drug sparingly, especially on children, and do not use an occlusive dressing unless

directed to do so by your physician. Follow your doctor's directions closely, and do not leave the dressing in place longer than specified. When using this drug on children, avoid tight-fitting diapers or plastic pants, which can act as occlusive dressings. • This drug must be used cautiously by pregnant or nursing women and by children under two years of age.

Comments: Use this drug for as long as prescribed and only for the condition for which it was prescribed. Do not use it more often since the chance of side effects increases. Continue using it for the complete period prescribed even if symptoms disappear within that time. Notify your doctor if no improvement is seen after a few days or if symptoms worsen. • If irritation develops, discontinue use and notify your doctor.

Lo-Trol antidiarrheal (Vangard Laboratories), see Lomotil antidiarrheal.

Low-Quel antidiarrheal (Halsey Drug Co., Inc.), see Lomotil antidiarrheal.

Lozol diuretic and antihypertensive

Manufacturer: Rorer Pharmaceuticals
Ingredient: indapamide
Dosage Form: Tablet: 2.5 mg (white)
Uses: Treatment of high blood pressure and removal of fluid from tissues
Minor Side Effects: Altered sense of taste; cough; diarrhea; dizziness; dry mouth; fatigue; headache; insomnia; light-headedness; loss of appetite; muscle pain; nausea; somnolence; stomach upset; sweating
Major Side Effects: Anxiety; blood disorders; breathing difficulties; chest pain; depression; impotence; itching; jaundice; muscle cramps; palpitations; rash; sore throat; tingling in the hands and feet; vomiting
Contraindication: This drug should not be taken by anyone who is allergic to it.
Warnings: This drug must be used cautiously by pregnant or nursing women, by persons with kidney disease, and by diabetics. Be sure your doctor knows if any of these conditions applies to you. • This drug may cause potassium loss, so it is often prescribed in conjunction with a potassium supplement. Your doctor may periodically test your blood to check the potassium level. Watch for signs of potassium loss (dry mouth, thirst, weakness, muscle pain or cramps, nausea, and vomiting). Call your doctor if you develop any of these signs. To help prevent potassium loss, take this drug with a glass of fresh or frozen orange juice, or eat a banana each day. The use of salt substitutes, which contain potassium, can also help prevent the loss of potassium. Do not change your diet, however, without first consulting your doctor. Too much potassium can also be dangerous. • If you are taking digitalis in addition to this drug, watch carefully for increased digitalis effects (e.g. nausea, blurred vision, palpitations), and notify your doctor immediately if they occur. • Persons taking this drug along with other antihypertensive medications may need to have their dosages adjusted.
Comments: Side effects from this drug are usually mild and transient. During the first few days of therapy, you may experience light-headedness, which should subside with continued use. If side effects continue or become bothersome, consult your doctor. • Notify your doctor if you develop signs of jaundice (yellow eyes or skin; dark urine). • To avoid dizziness or light-headedness when you stand, contract and relax the muscles of your legs for a few minutes before rising. Do this by pushing one foot against the floor while raising the

other foot slightly, alternating feet so that you are "pumping" your legs in a pedaling motion. ● Do not take any nonprescription items for weight control, cough, cold, or sinus problems without first consulting your doctor; such items may contain ingredients that can increase blood pressure. ● Take this drug exactly as prescribed. Do not take extra doses or skip a dose without first consulting your doctor. ● This drug causes frequent urination. Expect this effect; it should not alarm you. ● Learn how to monitor your pulse and blood pressure; discuss this with your doctor.

Ludiomil antidepressant

Manufacturer: Ciba Pharmaceutical Company
Ingredient: maprotiline hydrochloride
Dosage Form: Tablet: 25 mg; 50 mg (both dark orange); 75 mg (white)
Uses: Treatment of depression and of anxiety associated with depression
Minor Side Effects: Abdominal cramps; bitter taste in mouth; black tongue; bloating; blurred vision; constipation, diarrhea; dizziness; drooling; drowsiness; dry mouth; false sense of well-being; headache; increased appetite; increased or decreased sex drive; increased salivation; irregular heartbeat; loss of memory; nasal congestion; nausea; nervousness; nightmares; pupil dilation; restlessness; sensitivity to sunlight; shaking; stomach distress; sweating; trouble in sleeping; vomiting; weight loss or gain
Major Side Effects: Anxiety; breast enlargement (in both sexes); confusion; convulsions; dark-colored urine; difficulty swallowing; disturbed concentration; eye pain; fever; frequent or difficult urination; hair loss; hallucinations; impotence; itching; menstrual irregularities; palpitations; panic; ringing in the ears; severe mental disorders; severe weakness; skin rash; sore throat; sores on the skin or mouth; swelling of the testicles; tingling in the hands or feet; yellowing of the skin or eyes
Contraindications: This drug should not be taken by anyone who is allergic to it. This drug should not be taken by persons who have seizure disorders, persons who have recently had a heart attack, or persons who are taking or who have recently taken monoamine oxidase inhibitors. Consult your doctor immediately if this drug has been prescribed for you and any of these conditions applies. ● Children and adolescents should not take this drug.
Warnings: This drug should be used with caution by persons with certain types of heart disease, high blood pressure, thyroid problems, glaucoma, urinary tract problems, stomach or intestinal problems, an enlarged prostate, schizophrenia, or liver or kidney disease and by persons with a history of suicidal tendencies, alcoholism, or electroshock treatments. This drug should be used cautiously by those about to undergo surgery. Be sure your doctor knows if any of these conditions applies to you. ● This drug should be used cautiously by pregnant or nursing women. ● This drug may cause changes in blood sugar levels. ● This drug interacts with anticholinergic or sympathomimetic drugs, amphetamines, oral contraceptives, epinephrine, phenylephrine, antiparkinson drugs, methylphenidate, barbiturates, phenothiazines, oral anticoagulants, beta blockers, antiarrhythmics, thyroid drugs, blood pressure medications, and some painkillers and sedatives. If you are using any drugs of these types, consult your doctor about their use. If you are unsure of the type or contents of your medications, consult your doctor or pharmacist. ● Avoid drinking alcohol while taking this drug. ● Report any mood changes to your doctor.
Comments: It may take one to two weeks before the therapeutic effect of this drug is evident. Your doctor may adjust your dose frequently during the first few months of therapy to find the best dose for you. ● If this drug causes stomach upset, take it with food. ● This drug increases your sensitivity to sunlight; wear protective clothing and sunglasses and use an effective sunscreen when

outdoors. • Chew gum or suck on ice chips or a piece of hard candy to reduce mouth dryness. • If you take this drug for a prolonged period of time, you will need to see your doctor regularly for blood cell counts and liver function tests. • Do not stop taking this drug suddenly and do not increase the dose without first consulting your doctor. • If this drug makes you feel dizzy or drowsy, avoid activities that require alertness, such as driving a vehicle or operating machinery. To minimize dizziness and light-headedness, rise slowly from a sitting or reclining position. • This drug is similar in action to other antidepressants. If one antidepressant is not effective or well tolerated, your doctor may have you try others in order to find the one that's best for you.

Luramide diuretic and antihypertensive (Major Pharmaceuticals), see Lasix diuretic and antihypertensive.

Macrodantin antibacterial (Norwich Eaton Pharmaceuticals, Inc.), see nitrofurantoin antibacterial.

Malatal sedative and anticholinergic (Mallard, Inc.), see Donnatal sedative and anticholinergic.

Mallergan VC with Codeine expectorant (W.E. Hauck, Inc.), see Phenergan VC, Phenergan VC with Codeine expectorants.

Marnal analgesic (Vortech Pharmaceutical, Ltd.), see Fiorinal analgesic.

Maxolon gastrointestinal stimulant (Beecham Laboratories), see Reglan gastrointestinal stimulant.

Maxzide diuretic and antihypertensive

Manufacturer: Lederle Laboratories
Ingredients: hydrochlorothiazide; triamterene
Dosage Form: Tablet: Maxzide: hydrochlorothiazide, 50 mg and triamterene, 75 mg (yellow); Maxzide-25 mg: hydrochlorothiazide, 25 mg and triamterene, 37.5 mg (light green)
Uses: Treatment of high blood pressure and removal of fluid from body tissues
Minor Side Effects: Anxiety; constipation; diarrhea; dizziness; drowsiness; dry mouth; fatigue; headache; itching; loss of appetite; nausea; restlessness; sun sensitivity; upset stomach; vomiting; weakness
Major Side Effects: Blood disorders; breathing difficulties; bruising; confusion; cracking at the corners of the mouth; elevated blood sugar; fever; jaundice; kidney stones; mood changes; mouth sores; muscle cramps or spasms; palpitations; rash; sore throat; tingling in fingers or toes; weak pulse
Contraindications: This drug should not be used by persons with severe liver or kidney disease, hyperkalemia (high blood levels of potassium), or anuria (inability to urinate). Be sure your doctor knows if any of these conditions applies to you. • This drug is generally not used during pregnancy, since mother and fetus may be exposed to possible hazards. • This drug should not be used by persons allergic to it or to sulfa drugs. Consult your doctor immediately if this drug has been prescribed for you and you have such an allergy.
Warnings: Unlike some other medications of this type, this drug usually does

not cause the loss of potassium. Do not take potassium supplements while taking this drug unless directed to do so by your doctor. • This drug should be used cautiously by pregnant women, by children, and by people with diabetes, allergies, asthma, liver disease, anemia, blood diseases, high calcium levels, or gout. Be sure your doctor knows if any of these conditions applies to you. • Nursing mothers who must take this drug should stop nursing. • This drug may affect the results of thyroid function tests. Be sure your doctor knows you are taking this drug if you are scheduled to have such tests. • Regular blood tests should be performed if you must take this drug for a long time. You should also be tested for kidney function. • If you develop a sore throat, bleeding, bruising, dry mouth, weakness, or muscle cramps, call your doctor. • Persons taking this drug and digitalis should watch for signs of increased digitalis effects (e.g. nausea, blurred vision, palpitations), and notify their doctor if such signs develop. • If you must undergo surgery, remind your doctor that you are taking this drug. • This drug interacts with curare, digitalis, lithium carbonate, oral antidiabetics, potassium salts, steroids, and spironolactone. If you are currently taking any drugs of these types, consult your doctor about their use. If you are unsure of the type or contents of your medications, consult your doctor or pharmacist.

Comments: This drug causes frequent urination. Expect this effect; it should not alarm you. • Take this drug with food or milk. • Take this drug exactly as directed. Do not skip a dose or take extra doses without first consulting your doctor. • While taking this drug (as with many drugs that lower blood pressure), you should limit your consumption of alcoholic beverages in order to prevent dizziness or light-headedness. To avoid dizziness or light-headedness when you stand, contract and relax the muscles of your legs for a few minutes before rising. Do this by pushing one foot against the floor while raising the other foot slightly, alternating feet so that you are "pumping" your legs in a pedaling motion. • While taking this drug, you should learn how to monitor your pulse and blood pressure; consult your doctor. • Notify your doctor if you develop signs of jaundice (yellow eyes or skin; dark urine). • While taking this drug, do not take any nonprescription item for weight control, cough, cold, or sinus problems without first consulting your doctor; such items may contain ingredients that can increase blood pressure. • A doctor probably should not prescribe this drug or other "fixed dose" products as the first choice in the treatment of high blood pressure. The patient should receive each of the individual ingredients singly, and if the response is adequate to the fixed dose contained in Maxzide, it can then be substituted. The advantage of a combination product such as this drug is increased convenience to the patient. • This medication has the same ingredients as Dyazide but the strengths of the two drugs are different. Maxzide and Dyazide cannot be used interchangeably unless your doctor adjusts the dosage.

meclizine hydrochloride antinauseant (various manufacturers), see Antivert antinauseant.

meclofenamate anti-inflammatory (various manufacturers), see Meclomen anti-inflammatory.

Meclomen anti-inflammatory

Manufacturer: Parke-Davis
Ingredient: meclofenamate sodium
Equivalent Product: meclofenamate, various manufacturers
Dosage Form: Capsule: 50 mg (orange and peach); 100 mg (orange and beige); see Comments

Uses: Treatment of symptoms of acute or chronic arthritis; relief of mild to moderate pain

Minor Side Effects: Bloating; confusion; constipation; diarrhea; dizziness; drowsiness; gas; headache; heartburn; insomnia; loss of appetite; nausea; vomiting

Major Side Effects: Anemia; blood disorders; blood in stools, urine, or mouth; blurred vision; breathing difficulties; chest tightness; depression; difficulty in urinating; fatigue; fluid retention; high blood pressure; itching; jaundice; loss of hair; loss of hearing; numbness or tingling in fingers or toes; ringing in the ears; severe abdominal pain; sore throat; ulcer; weight gain

Contraindications: This drug should not be used by people who are allergic to it or to aspirin or other nonsteroidal anti-inflammatory drugs. Consult your doctor immediately if this drug has been prescribed for you and you have such an allergy. • This drug should not be used by children under the age of 14.

Warnings: This drug should be used cautiously by elderly people; by pregnant women; by people with a history of gastrointestinal disorders; and by people with mental illness, epilepsy, Parkinson's disease, infections, bleeding disorders, colitis, kidney or liver disease, high blood pressure, or heart failure. Be sure your doctor knows if any of these conditions applies to you. • Nursing women who must use this drug should stop nursing. • The severity of the side effects caused by this drug depends upon the dosage taken. Use the least amount possible and watch carefully for side effects. • This drug may irritate the stomach or intestines. Call your doctor if you experience stomach pain, if your stools are black and tarry, or if diarrhea becomes severe. • If you notice changes in your vision or experience headaches while taking this drug, notify your doctor. • This drug may cause drowsiness; avoid tasks that require alertness. • Side effects are more likely to occur in the elderly. • This drug interacts with aspirin, probenecid, lithium, oral antidiabetics, anticoagulants, anticonvulsants, sulfa drugs, beta blockers, and diuretics. If you are currently taking any drugs of these types, talk to your doctor about their use. If you are not sure about the type or contents of your medications, talk to your doctor or pharmacist.

Comments: Regular medical checkups, including blood tests, are required of persons taking this drug for a prolonged period. • This drug may be taken with food or milk; immediately after meals; or with antacids, but not sodium bicarbonate. Never take this drug on an empty stomach or with aspirin or alcohol. • If you are taking an anticoagulant (blood thinner), remind your doctor. • This drug may cause discoloration of the urine or feces. If you notice a change in color, call your doctor. • It may take a month before you feel the full effect of this drug. • This drug is not a substitute for rest, physical therapy, or other measures recommended by your doctor to treat your condition. • It is important to continue taking this medication even if symptoms diminish or disappear. Do not discontinue taking it without consulting your doctor. • This drug is a potent pain reliever and is not to be used for general aches and pains. It is usually reserved for use after other anti-inflammatory agents have failed. • Generic meclofenamate is also available in 50 mg and 100 mg tablets.

Medipren anti-inflammatory (McNeil Consumer Products Co.), see ibuprofen anti-inflammatory.

Medrol steroid hormone

Manufacturer: The Upjohn Company
Ingredient: methylprednisolone

Equivalent Products: Meprolone, Major Pharmaceuticals; methylpred-nisolone, various manufacturers

Dosage Form: Tablet: 2 mg (pink); 4 mg (white); 8 mg (peach); 16 mg (white); 24 mg (yellow); 32 mg (peach); 21-day Dosepak

Uses: Treatment of endocrine or rheumatic disorders; asthma; blood diseases; certain cancers; eye disorders; gastrointestinal disturbances such as ulcerative colitis; respiratory diseases; and inflammations such as arthritis, dermatitis, and poison ivy

Minor Side Effects: Dizziness; false sense of well-being; headache; increased appetite; increased susceptibility to infection; increased sweating; indigestion; menstrual irregularities; muscle weakness; reddening of the skin on the face; restlessness; thin skin

Major Side Effects: Abdominal enlargement; bone loss; bruising; cataracts; convulsions; diabetes; fluid retention; glaucoma; growth impairment in children; heart failure; high blood pressure; impaired healing of wounds; mood changes; muscle wasting; peptic ulcer; potassium loss; salt retention; weakness

Contraindications: This drug should not be taken by people who are allergic to it or by those who have systemic fungal infections. Consult your doctor if this drug has been prescribed for you and either of these conditions applies.

Warnings: If you are using this drug for longer than a week and are subjected to stress such as serious infection, injury, or surgery, you may need to receive higher dosages. • This drug may mask signs of an infection or cause new infections to develop. • This drug may cause glaucoma or cataracts, high blood pressure, high blood sugar, fluid retention, and potassium loss. • This drug has not been proven safe for use during pregnancy. • While you are taking this drug you should not be vaccinated or immunized. • This drug should be used very cautiously by people who have had tuberculosis and by those who have thyroid disease, liver disease, severe ulcerative colitis, a history of ulcers, kidney disease, high blood pressure, a bone disease, or myasthenia gravis. Be sure your doctor knows if any of these conditions applies to you. • If you have been taking this drug for more than a week, do not stop taking it suddenly. Talk to your doctor about tapering off slowly. Never increase the dose or take the drug for a longer time than prescribed without consulting your doctor. • Report mood swings or depression to your doctor. • Growth of children may be affected by this drug. • This drug interacts with aspirin, barbiturates, diuretics, estrogens, indomethacin, oral anticoagulants, antidiabetics, and phenytoin; if you are currently taking any drugs of these types, consult your doctor about their use. If you are unsure of the type or contents of your medications, ask your doctor or pharmacist. • Blood pressure, body weight, and vision should be checked at regular intervals if you are taking this drug for a prolonged period. Stomach X rays are advised for persons with suspected or known peptic ulcers.

Comments: This drug is often taken on a decreasing-dosage schedule (four times a day for several days, then three times a day, etc.). • Often, taking the entire dose at one time (about 8:00 A.M.) gives the best results. Ask your doctor. • Take this drug exactly as directed. Do not take extra doses or skip a dose without first consulting your doctor. For long-term treatment, this drug may be taken on an alternate-day dosing schedule to minimize side effects. Talk to your doctor about this. • To help avoid potassium loss while using this drug, take your dose with a glass of fresh or frozen orange juice, or eat a banana each day. The use of a salt substitute also helps prevent potassium loss. Do not change your diet, however, without consulting your doctor. Too much potassium may also be dangerous. • If you are using this drug chronically, you should wear or carry a notice that you are taking a steroid. • To prevent stomach upset, take this drug with food or a snack. • It is best to limit alcohol consumption while taking this drug. Alcohol may aggravate stomach problems.

Mellaril antipsychotic

Manufacturer: Sandoz Pharmaceuticals
Ingredient: thioridazine hydrochloride
Equivalent Products: Millazine, Major Pharmaceuticals; thioridazine, various manufacturers
Dosage Forms: Liquid concentrate (content per ml): thioridazine hydrochloride, 30 mg and alcohol, 3%; thioridazine hydrochloride, 100 mg and alcohol, 4.2%. Suspension: Mellaril-S (content per 5 ml teaspoon): 25 mg; 100 mg. Tablet: 10 mg (chartreuse); 15 mg (pink); 25 mg (tan); 50 mg (white); 100 mg (green); 150 mg (yellow); 200 mg (pink)
Uses: Relief of certain types of psychoses and depression; control of agitation, aggressiveness, and hyperactivity in children
Minor Side Effects: Blurred vision; constipation, decreased sweating; dizziness; drooling; drowsiness; dry mouth; fatigue; headache; impotence; insomnia; jitteriness; loss of appetite; menstrual irregularities; milk production; nasal congestion; nausea; photosensitivity; restlessness; tremors; weakness
Major Side Effects: Arthritis; asthma; blood disorders; breast enlargement (in both sexes); breathing difficulties; convulsions; eye changes; fever; fluid retention; heart attack; involuntary movements of the mouth, face, neck, and tongue; liver damage; low blood pressure; rash; skin darkening; sore throat
Contraindications: This drug should not be taken by persons with severe heart disease, central nervous system depression, or bone marrow disease or by those who are allergic to it. Be sure your doctor knows if any of these conditions applies to you.
Warnings: When taking this drug, you should be monitored closely, since convulsions, blood disorders, and eye disease have been known to occur. • This drug should be used with caution by pregnant women. • Tasks requiring mental alertness should be avoided since this drug may cause drowsiness • This drug may cause discoloration of the urine; this is harmless. • To prevent oversedation, avoid the use of alcohol or other drugs with sedative properties. • This drug is not recommended for use by children under two years of age. • This drug should be used cautiously by people who have glaucoma, kidney disease, nervous system disorders, ulcers, or an enlarged prostate. • This drug may interact with anticholinergics, antihypertensive drugs, barbiturates, lithium, oral antidiabetics, oral anticoagulants, and oral contraceptives. If you are currently taking any drugs of this type, consult your doctor about their use. If you are unsure of the type or contents of your medications, ask your doctor or pharmacist. • This drug may cause motor restlessness, uncoordinated movements, or involuntary muscle spasms. If you notice these effects, contact your doctor. Your dosage may need to be adjusted or use of the drug may need to be discontinued.
Comments: The effects of this drug may not be apparent for at least two weeks. • This drug has persistent action; never take it more frequently than your doctor prescribes. A serious overdose may result. • Your doctor may adjust your dose frequently during the first few months of therapy to determine the best dose for you. • While taking this drug, do not take any nonprescription item for weight control, cough, cold, or sinus problems without first checking with your doctor. • Chew gum or suck on ice chips or a piece of hard candy to reduce mouth dryness. • To avoid dizziness or light-headedness when you stand, contract and relax the muscles of your legs for a few moments before rising. Do this by pushing one foot against the floor while raising the other foot slightly, alternating feet so that you are "pumping" your legs in a pedaling motion. • Because this drug decreases sweating, avoid excessive work or exercise in hot weather and drink plenty of fluids. • The liquid concentrate form of this drug should be added to 60 ml (¼ cup) or more of water, milk, juice, cof-

fee, tea, or carbonated beverages or to pulpy foods (applesauce, etc.) just prior to administration. • If you get a sore throat or notice that your vision is darkening or that your tongue is moving involuntarily, call your doctor. • Antacids may prevent the absorption of this drug. Don't take them at the same time as you take this drug; space their dosing by at least two hours. • This drug may interfere with certain laboratory tests. Remind your doctor that you are taking this medication before undergoing any tests. • This drug may make you more sensitive to the sun. Avoid prolonged sun exposure, and wear protective clothing and a sunscreen when outdoors.

Meprolone steroid hormone (The Upjohn Company), see Medrol steroid hormone.

Metaprel bronchodilator (Sandoz Pharmaceuticals), see Alupent bronchodilator.

methyclothiazide diuretic and antihypertensive (various manufacturers), see Enduron diuretic and antihypertensive.

methyldopa and hydrochlorothiazide diuretic and antihypertensive (various manufacturers), see Aldoril diuretic and antihypertensive.

methyldopa antihypertensive (various manufacturers), see Aldomet antihypertensive.

methylphenidate hydrochloride central nervous system stimulant (various manufacturers), see Ritalin central nervous system stimulant.

methylprednisolone steroid hormone (various manufacturers), see Medrol steroid hormone.

Meticorten steroid hormone (Schering Corp.), see prednisone steroid hormone.

Metizol antimicrobial and antiparasitic (Glenwood, Inc.), see Flagyl antimicrobial and antiparasitic.

metoclopramide gastrointestinal stimulant (various manufacturers), see Reglan gastrointestinal stimulant.

metronidazole antimicrobial and antiparasitic (various manufacturers), see Flagyl antimicrobial and antiparasitic.

Metryl antimicrobial and antiparasitic (Lemmon Company), see Flagyl antimicrobial and antiparasitic.

Mevacor antihyperlipidemic

Manufacturer: Merck Sharp & Dohme
Ingredient: lovastatin

Dosage Form: Tablet: 20 mg (light blue)

Use: In conjunction with diet to reduce elevated blood cholesterol levels

Minor Side Effects: Abdominal pain; altered sense of taste; constipation; cramps; diarrhea; dizziness; flatulence; heartburn; itching; nausea; rash; stomach upset

Major Side Effects: Blurred vision; clouding of the eye; fever; liver disorders; malaise; muscle aches, cramps, pain, or weakness; tingling in the fingers or toes

Contraindications: This drug should not be used by persons who are allergic to it, by those with active liver disease, or by pregnant women. Consult your doctor if this drug has been prescribed for you and any of these conditions applies.

Warnings: This drug must be used cautiously in persons with a history of liver disease. Periodic liver function tests are recommended during long-term therapy to assure that the drug is not affecting the liver. • This drug must be used with caution by persons who have developed a severe infection, uncontrolled seizures, or a severe blood disorder and by those who are undergoing major surgery or trauma. The drug may be temporarily discontinued during these situations. • This drug may cause muscle pain, tenderness, or weakness associated with fever and fatigue. If you develop these symptoms while taking lovastatin, contact your doctor. These symptoms are most common in persons who are also taking immunosuppressive drugs, gemfibrozil, or nicotinic acid. Consult your doctor about concurrent use of these drugs. • This drug is not recommended for use in nursing women or in children. • There are reports that this drug may cause a clouding of the lens in the eye during long-term therapy. An eye examination is recommended before therapy is begun and then once each year thereafter. • This drug may interact with the anticoagulant warfarin. If you are currently taking warfarin, your dose may be monitored more frequently and an adjustment may be required. Make sure your doctor knows you are taking warfarin.

Comments: This drug should be used only after diet therapy has proven ineffective. This drug is not a substitute for proper diet, exercise, and weight control. For maximum results, this drug must be used in conjunction with a diet that is low in saturated fat and cholesterol. You may be referred to a nutritionist for diet counseling. • The full effects of this drug may not be evident for four to six weeks. Your doctor will want to monitor the effects of this drug by doing periodic blood tests. Ask your doctor to explain your cholesterol level and the goals of your therapy. Learn to monitor your progress. • This drug is best taken as a single dose with the evening meal. • When first taking this drug, you may experience stomach upset and gas. These effects usually disappear with continued use. Notify your doctor if they persist or worsen.

Micro-K potassium chloride replacement (A. H. Robins Company), see potassium chloride replacement.

Micronase oral antidiabetic

Manufacturer: The Upjohn Company

Ingredient: glyburide

Equivalent Product: DiaBeta, Hoechst-Roussel Pharmaceutical, Inc.

Dosage Form: Tablet: 1.25 mg (white); 2.5 mg (pink); 5 mg (blue)

Use: Treatment of diabetes mellitus not controlled by diet and exercise alone

Minor Side Effects: Diarrhea; dizziness; fatigue; headache; heartburn; loss of appetite; stomach upset; sun sensitivity; vomiting; weakness

Major Side Effects: Blood disorders; breathing difficulties; dark urine; itching; jaundice; light-colored stools; low blood sugar; muscle cramps; rash; sore throat and fever; tingling in the hands and feet; unusual bleeding or bruising

Contraindications: This drug should not be used for the treatment of juvenile (insulin dependent) or unstable diabetes. This drug should not be used by diabetics subject to acidosis or ketosis or by diabetics with a history of diabetic coma. • Persons with severe liver, kidney, or thyroid disorders should not use this drug. • Avoid using this drug if you are allergic to sulfonylureas. Be sure your doctor knows if you have such an allergy. • In the presence of infections, fever, or severe trauma, it may be necessary for you to use insulin instead of this medication—at least during the acute stage.

Warnings: This drug should be used cautiously during pregnancy. If you are currently pregnant, or become pregnant while taking this drug, talk to your doctor about its use. • This drug should be used with caution by nursing women; children; and persons with liver, kidney or thyroid disorders. • Thiazide diuretics and beta-blocking drugs commonly used to treat high blood pressure may interfere with your control of diabetes. • This drug interacts with steroids, estrogens, oral contraceptives, phenothiazines, phenytoin, isoniazid, thyroid hormones, and diuretics. If you are taking any drugs of these types, talk to you doctor about your use of glyburide. If you are not sure about the types or contents of your medications, consult your doctor or pharmacist. • Do not drink alcohol or take any other medications unless directed to do so by your doctor. Be especially careful with nonprescription cough and cold remedies. • Be sure you can recognize signs of low blood sugar and know what to do if you begin to experience these symptoms. Signs of low blood sugar include chills, cold sweat, drowsiness, headache, nausea, nervousness, rapid pulse, tremors, and weakness. If these symptoms develop, eat or drink something containing sugar and call your doctor. Poor diet, malnutrition, strenuous exercise, and alcohol consumption may lead to low blood sugar.

Comments: Take this drug at the same time every day. It is usually taken 30 minutes before breakfast unless directed otherwise. • Avoid prolonged or unprotected exposure to sunlight while taking this drug, as it makes you more sensitive to the sun's burning rays. • While taking this drug, test your urine and/or blood as prescribed. It is important that you understand what the results mean. • Studies have shown that a good diet and exercise program are extremely important in controlling diabetes. Discuss the use of this drug with your doctor. Persons taking this drug must carefully watch their diet and exercise program and avoid infection through good personal hygiene. • While taking this drug, call your doctor if you develop an infection, fever, sore throat, rash, excessive thirst or urination, unusual bleeding or bruising, dark urine, light-colored stools, or yellow eyes or skin. • There are other drugs similar to this (Orinase, Diabinese, Tolinase, Glucotrol) that vary slightly in their activity. Certain persons who do not benefit from one type of these oral antidiabetic agents may find another one more effective. Discuss this with your doctor. • Do not discontinue use without consulting your doctor. • Persons taking this drug should carry a medical alert card or wear a medical alert bracelet.

Microx diuretic and antihypertensive (Pennwalt Pharmaceutical Division), see Zaroxolyn diuretic and antihypertensive.

Mictrin diuretic and antihypertensive (Econo Med, Inc.), see hydrochlorothiazide diuretic and antihypertensive.

Midol 200 anti-inflammatory (Glenbrook Laboratories), see ibuprofen anti-inflammatory.

Millazine antipsychotic (Major Pharmaceuticals), see Mellaril antipsychotic.

Minipress antihypertensive

Manufacturer: Pfizer Laboratories Division
Ingredient: prazosin hydrochloride
Equivalent Product: Minizide, Pfizer Laboratories Division (see Comments)
Dosage Form: Capsule: 1 mg (white); 2 mg (pink/white); 5 mg (blue/white)
Use: Treatment of high blood pressure
Minor Side Effects: Abdominal pain; constipation; diarrhea; dizziness; drowsiness; dry mouth; frequent urination; headache; impotence; itching; loss of appetite; nasal congestion; nausea; nervousness; sweating; tiredness; vivid dreams; vomiting; weakness
Major Side Effects: Blurred vision; chest pain; constant erection; depression; difficulty in urinating; fainting; fast pulse; fluid retention; hallucinations; loss of hair; nosebleed; palpitations; rash; ringing in the ears; shortness of breath; tingling in the fingers or toes
Contraindication: This drug should not be taken by people who are allergic to it. Consult your doctor if this drug has been prescribed for you and you have such an allergy.
Warnings: This drug should be used with caution in conjunction with other antihypertensive drugs and with beta-blocker drugs such as propranolol. If you are currently taking either of these drug types, consult your doctor about their use. If you are unsure of the type or contents of your medications, ask your doctor or pharmacist. • This drug should be used very cautiously by pregnant women and children. • Because initial therapy with this drug may cause dizziness and fainting, your doctor will probably start you on a low dose and gradually increase your dosage.
Comments: The effects of this drug may not be apparent for at least two weeks. • Mild side effects (e.g., nasal congestion) are most noticeable during the first two weeks of therapy and become less bothersome after this period. • Do not drive or operate machinery for four hours after taking the first dose of this drug. It is best to take the first dose at bedtime. • Do not discontinue this medication unless your doctor directs you to do so. • Take this drug exactly as directed. Do not take extra doses or skip a dose without consulting your doctor first. • While taking this drug, do not take any nonprescription item for weight control, cough, cold, or sinus problems without first checking with your doctor; such items may contain ingredients that can increase blood pressure. • While taking this drug, you should limit your consumption of alcoholic beverages in order to prevent dizziness or light-headedness. To avoid dizziness or lightheadedness when you stand, contract and relax the muscles of your legs for a few moments before rising. Do this by pushing one foot against the floor while raising the other foot slightly, alternating feet so that you are "pumping" your legs in a pedaling motion. • If you are taking this drug and begin therapy with another antihypertensive drug, your doctor will probably reduce the dosage of Minipress, then recalculate your dose over the next couple of weeks. Dosage adjustments will be made based on your response. • Learn how to monitor your pulse and blood pressure while taking this drug; discuss this with your doctor. • Minizide is a combination antihypertensive and diuretic agent. It contains the diuretic polyzide in addition to prazosin.

Minizide antihypertensive (Pfizer Laboratories Division), see Minipress antihypertensive.

Minocin antibiotic

Manufacturer: Lederle Laboratories
Ingredient: minocycline hydrochloride
Dosage Forms: Capsule: 50 mg (orange); 100 mg (purple/orange). Syrup (content per 5 ml teaspoon): 50 mg. Tablet: 50 mg; 100 mg (both orange)
Use: Treatment of a wide variety of bacterial infections
Minor Side Effects: Diarrhea; dizziness; drowsiness; increased sensitivity to sunlight; loss of appetite; nausea; upset stomach; vomiting
Major Side Effects: Anemia; breathing difficulties; irritation of the mouth; itching; rash; rectal and vaginal itching; sore throat; superinfection
Contraindication: Anyone who has demonstrated an allergy to any of the tetracyclines should not take this drug. Consult your doctor immediately if this drug has been prescribed for you and you have such a history.
Warnings: This drug should be used cautiously by people who have liver or kidney diseases; by children under the age of eight; and by women who are pregnant or nursing. Be sure your doctor knows if any of these conditions applies to you. • This drug may impair your ability to perform tasks that require alertness, such as driving and operating machinery. • This drug can cause permanent discoloration of the teeth when taken by children under eight. When taken during the last half of pregnancy, it can cause permanent discoloration of the fetus's teeth. • Call the doctor if you develop a fever, headache, sore throat, or nausea while taking this drug. • This drug interacts with penicillin, lithium, oral antidiabetics, steroids, and anticoagulants. If you are currently taking any drugs of these types, consult your doctor about their use. If you are unsure of the type or contents of your medications, ask your doctor or pharmacist. • Prolonged use of this drug may allow organisms that are not susceptible to it to grow wildly. • Do not use this drug unless your doctor has specifically told you to do so. Be sure to follow the directions carefully and report any unusual reactions to your doctor at once. • Complete blood cell counts and liver and kidney function tests should be done if you take this drug for a prolonged period. • Do not take this drug within two hours of the time you take an antacid or within three hours of taking an iron preparation; both of these drugs interact with minocycline and make it ineffective. • This drug may affect tests for syphilis. Make sure your doctor knows you are taking this drug if you are scheduled for this test.
Comments: Try to take this drug on an empty stomach (one hour before or two hours after a meal) with at least eight ounces of water. If you find the drug upsets your stomach, you may try taking it with food. • While taking this drug, you may sunburn easily; avoid prolonged exposure to sunlight. • This drug is taken once or twice a day at evenly spaced intervals around the clock. Never increase the dosage unless your doctor tells you to do so. • When used to treat strep throat, this drug should be taken for at least ten days, even if the symptoms have disappeared. Stopping treatment early may lead to reinfection. • Make sure that your prescription is marked with the drug's expiration date. Do not use this drug after the expiration date has passed. Any unused medication should be discarded.

Mitran antianxiety (W.E. Hauck, Inc.), see Librium antianxiety.

Moduretic diuretic and antihypertensive

Manufacturer: Merck Sharp & Dohme
Ingredients: amiloride; hydrochlorothiazide
Dosage Form: Tablet: amiloride, 5 mg and hydrochlorothiazide, 50 mg (peach)

Uses: Treatment of high blood pressure; removal of fluid from body tissues

Minor Side Effects: Anxiety; constipation; diarrhea; dizziness; drowsiness; fatigue; headache; itching; joint pain; loss of appetite; nausea; nervousness; restlessness; sun sensitivity; upset stomach; vomiting; weakness

Major Side Effects: Blood disorders; blurred vision; breathing difficulties; confusion; dry mouth; elevated blood sugar; excessive thirst; impotence; jaundice; kidney stones; mood changes; muscle cramps or spasms; palpitations; rash; sore throat; tingling in fingers or toes; unusual bleeding or bruising; weak pulse

Contraindications: This drug should not be used by persons with severe liver or kidney disease, hyperkalemia (high blood levels of potassium), or anuria (inability to urinate). Be sure your doctor knows if you have any of these conditions. • This drug is generally not used during pregnancy, since mother and fetus may be exposed to possible hazards. • This drug should not be used by persons allergic to it or to sulfa drugs. Consult your doctor immediately if this drug has been prescribed for you and you have such an allergy.

Warnings: Unlike most diuretics, this drug usually does not cause the loss of potassium. Do not take potassium supplements while taking this drug unless directed to do so by your doctor. • This drug should be used cautiously by pregnant women; children; and people with diabetes, allergy, asthma, liver disease, anemia, blood diseases, high calcium levels, or gout. Nursing mothers who must take this drug should stop nursing. Be sure your doctor knows if any of these conditions applies to you. • This drug may affect the results of thyroid function tests. Be sure your doctor knows you are taking this drug if you must have such tests. • Regular blood tests should be performed if you must take this drug for a long time. You should also be tested for kidney function. • If you develop a sore throat, bleeding, bruising, dry mouth, weakness, or muscle cramps, call your doctor. • Persons who take this drug with digitalis should watch for signs of increased digitalis effects (e.g., nausea, blurred vision, palpitations). Call your doctor if such symptoms develop. • If you must undergo surgery, remind your doctor that you are taking this drug. • This drug interacts with curare, digitalis, lithium carbonate, oral antidiabetics, potassium salts, steroids, and spironolactone. If you are currently taking any drugs of these types, consult your doctor about their use. If you are unsure of the type or contents of your medications, ask your doctor or pharmacist.

Comments: This drug causes frequent urination. Expect this effect; it should not alarm you. • Take this drug with food or milk. • Take this drug exactly as directed. Do not skip a dose or take extra doses without first consulting your doctor. • While taking this drug (as with many drugs that lower blood pressure), you should limit your consumption of alcoholic beverages in order to prevent dizziness or light-headedness. To avoid dizziness or light-headedness when you stand, contract and relax the muscles of your legs for a few minutes before rising. Do this by pushing one foot against the floor while raising the other foot slightly, alternating feet so that you are "pumping" your legs in a pedaling motion. • While taking this drug, do not take any nonprescription item for weight control, cough, cold, or sinus problems without first checking with your doctor; such items may contain ingredients that can increase blood pressure. • Notify your doctor if you develop signs of jaundice (yellow eyes or skin; dark urine). • A doctor should probably not prescribe this drug or other "fixed dose" products as the first choice in the treatment of high blood pressure. The patient should receive each of the individual ingredients singly, and if the response is adequate to the fixed doses contained in Moduretic, it can then be substituted. The advantage of a combination product such as this drug is increased convenience to the patient.

Monistat antifungal agent

Manufacturer: Ortho Pharmaceutical Corp.

Ingredient: miconazole nitrate

Dosage Forms: Vaginal cream: 2%. Vaginal suppository: 100 mg; 200 mg
Use: Treatment of fungal infections of the vagina
Minor Side Effects: Burning; irritation; itching; vaginal discharge
Major Side Effects: Headache; hives; pelvic cramps; skin rash
Contraindication: This drug should not be used by people who are allergic to it. Consult your doctor immediately if this drug has been prescribed for you and you have such an allergy.
Warnings: This drug should be used with caution by pregnant women in the first three months of their pregnancy. Be sure your doctor knows if you are pregnant. • Notify your doctor immediately if sensitization, burning, itching, or irritation occurs during use of this drug.
Comments: This drug is effective in the treatment of fungal infections in pregnant and nonpregnant women, as well as in women taking oral contraceptives. However, because small amounts of the drug may be absorbed through the vaginal wall, this drug generally should not be used during the first three months of pregnancy. • This drug should be used until the prescribed amount is gone. Be sure to complete a full course of therapy, even during your menstrual period. • Avoid sexual intercourse or ask your partner to use a condom until treatment is complete in order to avoid reinfection. • Wear cotton panties rather than those made of nylon or other nonporous materials while treating fungal infections. • This medication is usually used at bedtime. • Apply this product after cleansing the area unless otherwise directed by your doctor. • Insert suppositories high into the vagina. Patient instructions are usually dispensed with this medication. If you don't receive them, ask your pharmacist for a copy. • Use a sanitary napkin to prevent staining of clothing. • Unless otherwise instructed by your doctor, do not douche during treatment with this drug or for two to three weeks thereafter. • The 200 mg suppositories are usually used for three days; the 100 mg suppositories and the vaginal cream are usually used for one to two weeks.

Motrin anti-inflammatory (The Upjohn Company), see ibuprofen anti-inflammatory.

Myapap with Codeine analgesic (My-K Labs), see acetaminophen with codeine analgesic.

Mycelex antifungal agent (Miles Pharmaceutical), see Lotrimin antifungal agent.

Mycelex-G antifungal agent (Miles Pharmaceutical), see Gyne-Lotrimin antifungal agent.

Mycogen II topical steroid hormone and anti-infective (Goldline Laboratories), see Mycolog II topical steroid hormone and anti-infective.

Mycolog II topical steroid hormone and anti-infective

Manufacturer: E. R. Squibb & Sons, Inc.
Ingredients: nystatin; triamcinolone acetonide
Equivalent Products: Mycogen II, Goldline Laboratories; Myco-Triacet II, Lemmon Company; Mykacet, NMC Laboratories, Inc.; Mytrex, Savage Laboratories; N.G.T., Geneva Generics, Inc.; triamcinolone and nystatin, various manufacturers

Dosage Forms: Cream; Ointment (content per gram): nystatin, 100,000 units and triamcinolone acetonide, 0.1%

Use: Relief of skin inflammations associated with conditions such as dermatitis, eczema, and poison ivy.

Minor Side Effects: Burning sensation; dryness; irritation; itching

Major Side Effects: Allergy; blistering; increased hair growth; loss of hearing; loss of skin color; rash; secondary infection; skin wasting

Contraindications: This drug should not be used for viral diseases of the skin, for most fungal lesions of the skin, or in circumstances when circulation is markedly impaired. Be sure your doctor knows if any of these conditions applies to you. • This drug should not be used in the eyes or in the external ear canals of patients with perforated eardrums. • This drug should not be used by people who are allergic to either of its ingredients. Consult your doctor immediately if this drug has been prescribed for you and you have such an allergy.

Warnings: Prolonged use of large amounts of this drug should be avoided in the treatment of skin infections following extensive burns and other conditions where absorption of neomycin is possible. Prolonged use of this drug may result in secondary infection. Use this drug only for the reason prescribed. • If extensive areas are treated or if an occlusive bandage is used, the possibility exists of increased absorption of this drug into the bloodstream. Do not use this product with an occlusive wrap or transparent plastic film unless instructed to do so by your doctor. If it is necessary for you to use this drug under a wrap, follow your doctor's directions exactly. Do not leave the wrap in place for a longer time than specified. • If this drug is prescribed for use on a child's diaper area, avoid tight-fitting diapers or plastic pants, which may increase absorption of the drug. • If irritation develops, discontinue use of this drug and notify your doctor immediately. • This drug should not be used extensively, in large amounts, or for prolonged periods on pregnant women.

Comments: If the affected area is extremely dry or is scaling, the skin may be moistened before applying the medication by soaking in water or by applying water with a clean cloth and then drying thoroughly. The ointment form is probably better for dry skin. • Apply a thin layer of this product to the affected area and rub in gently.

Mycostatin antifungal agent

Manufacturer: E. R. Squibb & Sons, Inc.

Ingredient: nystatin

Equivalent Products: Mykinac, NMC Laboratories, Inc.; Nilstat, Lederle Laboratories; nystatin, various manufacturers; Nystex, Savage Laboratories; O-V Statin, E. R. Squibb & Sons, Inc.

Dosage Forms: Cream; Ointment; Powder (per gram): 100,000 units. Oral suspension (per ml): 100,000 units. Oral tablet: 500,000 units. Oral troches: 200,000 units. Vaginal tablet: 100,000 units

Use: Treatment of fungal infections

Minor Side Effects: Oral forms: diarrhea; nausea; vomiting. Topical and vaginal forms: irritation; itching

Major Side Effect: Rash

Contraindication: This drug should not be used by people who are allergic to it. Contact your doctor immediately if this drug has been prescribed for you and you have such an allergy.

Warnings: If you suffer a rash or irritation from taking this drug, consult your doctor; use of the drug will probably be discontinued. • Avoid use around the eyes.

Comments: If you are using the powder form of this drug to treat a foot infection, sprinkle the powder liberally into your shoes and socks. • Moist lesions or sores are best treated with the powder form of this drug. • If you are using an oral form of this drug to treat an infection in the mouth, rinse the drug around in your mouth as long as possible before swallowing. Do not crush or chew the oral tablets or troches; let them dissolve slowly in your mouth. The oral suspension must be shaken well before use. It need not be refrigerated. • If you are using this drug to treat a vaginal infection, avoid sexual intercourse or ask your partner to wear a condom until treatment is completed; these measures will help prevent reinfection. • The vaginal tablets are supplied with an applicator that should be used to insert the tablets high into the vagina. • Unless instructed otherwise by your doctor, do not douche during the treatment period or for two to three weeks following your use of the vaginal tablets. Use the vaginal tablets continuously, including during your menstrual period, until your doctor tells you to stop. Be sure to complete a full course of therapy. • Wear cotton panties rather than those made of nylon or other nonporous materials while fungal infections of the vagina are being treated. • You may wish to wear a sanitary napkin while using the vaginal tablets to prevent soiling of your underwear. • If you are using the topical cream or ointment form of this drug, apply it after cleaning the area unless otherwise specified by your doctor. • If irritation develops while you are using a topical form of nystatin, discontinue use and call your doctor.

Myco-Triacet II topical steroid hormone and anti-infective (Lemmon Company), see Mycolog II topical steroid hormone and anti-infective.

Mykacet topical steroid hormone and anti-infective (NMC Laboratories, Inc.), see Mycolog II topical steroid hormone and anti-infective.

My-K Elixir potassium chloride replacement (My-K Labs), see potassium chloride replacement.

Mykinac antifungal agent (NMC Laboratories, Inc.), see Mycostatin antifungal agent.

Mytrex topical steroid hormone and anti-infective (Savage Laboratories), see Mycolog II topical steroid hormone and anti-infective.

Naldecon decongestant and antihistamine

Manufacturer: Bristol Laboratories
Ingredients: chlorpheniramine maleate; phenylephrine hydrochloride; phenylpropanolamine hydrochloride; phenyltoloxamine citrate
Equivalent Products: Amaril "D", Vortech Pharmaceutical, Ltd.; Decongestabs, various manufacturers; Naldelate, various manufacturers; Nalgest, Major Pharmaceuticals; New-Decongest, Goldline Laboratories; Phentox Compound, My-K Labs; Tri-Phen-Chlor, Rugby Laboratories; Vasominic T.D., A.V.P. Pharmaceuticals, Inc.
Dosage Forms: Pediatric drops (content per ml); Pediatric syrup (content per 5 ml teaspoon): chlorpheniramine maleate, 0.5 mg; phenylephrine hydrochloride, 1.25 mg; phenylpropanolamine hydrochloride, 5.0 mg; phenyltoloxamine citrate, 2.0 mg. Sustained-action tablet: chlorpheniramine maleate,

5 mg; phenylephrine hydrochloride, 10 mg; phenylpropanolamine hydrochloride, 40 mg; phenyltoloxamine citrate, 15 mg (white with red specks). Syrup (content per 5 ml teaspoon): chlorpheniramine maleate, 2.5 mg; phenylephrine hydrochloride, 5.0 mg; phenylpropanolamine hydrochloride, 20 mg; phenyltoloxamine citrate, 7.5 mg

Uses: Relief of symptoms of hay fever and other allergies, ear infections, sinusitis, and upper respiratory tract congestion

Minor Side Effects: Blurred vision; confusion; constipation; diarrhea; dizziness; drowsiness; dry mouth; headache; heartburn; insomnia; loss of appetite; nasal congestion; nausea; reduced sweating; restlessness; sensitivity to sunlight; vomiting; weakness

Major Side Effects: Breathing difficulties; chest pain; difficulty in urinating; hallucinations; high blood pressure; low blood pressure; palpitations; rash; severe abdominal pain; sore throat; unusual bleeding or bruising

Contraindications: This drug should not be taken by people who are allergic to any of its components or by people who have severe high blood pressure, severe heart disease, glaucoma (certain types), urinary retention, ulcers, or asthma. Consult your doctor immediately if this drug has been prescribed for you and any of these conditions applies. • This drug should not be used in conjunction with guanethidine or monoamine oxidase inhibitors; if you are currently taking any drugs of these types, consult your doctor about their use. If you are unsure of the type or contents of your medications, ask your doctor or pharmacist.

Warnings: This drug should be used cautiously by children; by pregnant or nursing women; and by people who have high blood pressure, heart disease, diabetes, urinary tract or intestinal blockage, epilepsy, thyroid disease, glaucoma, vessel disease, or enlarged prostate. Be sure your doctor knows if any of these conditions applies to you. • This drug interacts with beta blockers and certain drugs used to treat high blood pressure. If you are unsure about the type of drugs you take, ask your doctor or pharmacist. • Do not take any nonprescription items for weight control, cough, cold, or sinus problems without first checking with your doctor or pharmacist. • This drug may cause drowsiness; avoid tasks that require alertness. To prevent oversedation, avoid the use of alcohol or other drugs that have sedative properties.

Comments: Because this drug reduces sweating, avoid excessive work or exercise in hot weather and drink plenty of fluids. • There are other types of Naldecon products available for specific uses; some are formulated especially for children, for adults, or for the elderly. • The tablet form of this drug has sustained action; never increase your dose or take it more frequently than your doctor prescribes. A serious overdose could result. • The tablet form of this drug must be swallowed whole. • Chew gum or suck on ice chips or a piece of hard candy to reduce mouth dryness.

Naldelate decongestant and antihistamine (various manufacturers), see Naldecon decongestant and antihistamine.

Nalfon anti-inflammatory

Manufacturer: Dista Products Company
Ingredient: fenoprofen calcium
Equivalent Product: fenoprofen, various manufacturers
Dosage Forms: Capsule: 200 mg (white/ocher); 300 mg (yellow/ocher). Tablet: 600 mg (yellow); see Comments
Uses: Relief of pain and swelling due to arthritis; relief of menstrual pain, dental pain, postoperative pain, and musculoskeletal pain

Minor Side Effects: Abdominal pain; bloating; confusion; constipation; cramps; diarrhea; dizziness; drowsiness; dry mouth; gas; headache; heartburn; insomnia; itching; loss of appetite; nausea; nervousness; peculiar taste in mouth; rapid heart rate; sweating; vomiting; weakness

Major Side Effects: Anemia; blood in stools; breathing difficulties; bruising; chest tightness; difficulty in urinating; fluid retention; hair loss; hearing loss; jaundice; kidney disease; menstrual irregularities; nightmares; palpitations; rash; ringing in the ears; seizures; tremors; ulcer; visual disturbances

Contraindications: This drug should not be taken by persons with kidney disease or by those who are allergic to this drug or to aspirin or other drugs like it. Consult your doctor immediately if this drug has been prescribed for you and you have kidney disease or such an allergy.

Warnings: This drug should be taken with caution by patients with a history of upper gastrointestinal tract disease. Gastrointestinal bleeding, sometimes severe, has been reported in persons receiving this drug. Be sure your doctor knows if this condition applies to you. • This drug should be used cautiously by persons with peptic ulcer, anemia, heart disease, high blood pressure, bleeding diseases, liver disease, or kidney disease. Be sure your doctor knows if any of these conditions applies to you. • This drug should be used with caution by pregnant women, nursing mothers, and children. • Since this drug may cause drowsiness, tasks requiring alertness should be avoided while taking this drug. • Patients with impaired hearing who take this drug for a long time should have periodic tests of auditory function. • Use of this drug may prolong bleeding times, so persons taking anticoagulants (blood thinners) in addition to this drug should use this drug with extreme caution. • It is desirable to have periodic eye tests while receiving this drug. • This drug interacts with aspirin, diuretics, anticoagulants, oral antidiabetics, phenobarbital, phenytoin, and sulfonamides. If you are currently taking any drugs of these types, consult your doctor about their use. If you are unsure of the type or contents of your medications, ask your doctor of pharmacist.

Comments: In numerous tests, this drug has been shown to be as effective as aspirin in the treatment of arthritis, but aspirin is still the drug of choice for the disease. This drug is often prescribed when aspirin is no longer effective. • Do not take aspirin or alcohol while taking this drug without first consulting your doctor. • You should note improvement in your condition soon after you start using this drug; however, full benefit may not be obtained for one to two weeks. It is important not to stop taking this drug even though symptoms have diminished or disappeared. • This drug is not a substitute for rest, physical therapy, or other measures recommended by your doctor to treat your condition. • This drug is best taken on an empty stomach, but it may be taken with food or milk to reduce stomach upset. • Notify your doctor if skin rash, yellow eyes or skin, itching, black tarry stools, dark urine, swelling of the hands or feet, or persistent headache occurs. • This drug is similar in action to other anti-inflammatory drugs, such as Indocin, ibuprofen, and Tolectin. If one of these medications is not well tolerated, your doctor may have you try other ones in order to find the best drug for you. • Fenoprofen is also available in 600 mg capsules and in 200 mg and 300 mg tablets. To reduce dizziness when you stand, rise slowly from a sitting or reclining position.

Nalgest decongestant and antihistamine (Major Pharmaceuticals), see Naldecon decongestant and antihistamine.

Napamide antiarrhythmic (Major Pharmaceuticals), see Norpace antiarrhythmic.

Naprosyn anti-inflammatory

Manufacturer: Syntex Laboratories, Inc.
Ingredient: naproxen
Equivalent Product: Anaprox, Syntex Laboratories, Inc. (see Comments)
Dosage Forms: Oral suspension (content per 5 ml teaspoon): 125 mg.
Tablet: 250 mg (yellow); 375 mg (peach); 500 mg (yellow)
Uses: Relief of pain and swelling due to rheumatoid arthritis, tendonitis, bursitis, and acute gout; relief of mild to moderate pain; relief of menstrual pain
Minor Side Effects: Abdominal pain; bloating; bruising; constipation; diarrhea; dizziness; drowsiness; dry mouth; headache; heartburn; insomnia; itching; loss of appetite; nausea; nervousness; peculiar taste in mouth; sore mouth; sweating; vomiting; weakness
Major Side Effects: Blood in stools; breast enlargement (in both sexes); breathing difficulties; chest tightness; depression; difficulty in urinating; fluid retention; hair loss; hallucinations; hearing loss; jaundice; kidney disease; menstrual irregularities; palpitations; rash; ringing in the ears; sore throat; tingling in hands or feet; ulcers; visual disturbances
Contraindications: This drug should not be taken by people who are allergic to it or to aspirin or similar drugs. Consult your doctor immediately if this drug has been prescribed for you and you have such an allergy.
Warnings: This drug should be used with caution by pregnant women, nursing mothers, and children and by persons with anemia, ulcers, bleeding disorders, high blood pressure, liver disease, heart disease, or kidney disease. Be sure your doctor knows if any of these conditions applies to you. • Patients prone to upper gastrointestinal tract disease should take this drug only under close supervision. Gastrointestinal bleeding, sometimes severe, has been reported in patients receiving this drug. • It is recommended that persons taking this drug for a long time have eye tests performed periodically. • This drug may cause drowsiness, dizziness, or depression; avoid activities that require alertness. • This drug may prolong bleeding times, so persons also taking anticoagulants (blood thinners) should use this drug with extreme caution. • This drug interacts with anticoagulants, diuretics, aspirin, oral antidiabetics, phenytoin, and sulfonamides. If you are currently taking any drugs of these types, consult your doctor about their use. If you are unsure of the type or contents of your medications, ask your doctor or pharmacist.
Comments: In numerous tests, this drug has been shown to be as effective as aspirin in the treatment of arthritis, but aspirin is still the drug of choice for the disease. This drug is often prescribed when aspirin is no longer effective. • You should note improvement in your condition soon after you start using this drug; however, full benefit may not be obtained for one to two weeks. It is important not to stop taking this drug even though symptoms have diminished or disappeared. • This drug is not a substitute for rest, physical therapy, or other measures recommended by your doctor to treat your condition. • Do not take aspirin or alcohol while taking this drug without first consulting your doctor. • This drug is best taken on an empty stomach, but it may be taken with food or milk to reduce stomach upset. • Syntex Laboratories, Inc. also produces a related drug (naproxen sodium) called Anaprox. This drug is converted in the body to naproxen. The two drugs should not be taken together. • Notify your doctor if skin rash, yellow eyes or skin, itching, black tarry stools, dark urine, swelling of the hands or feet, or persistent headache occurs. • This drug is similar in action to other anti-inflammatory medications, such as Indocin, ibuprofen, and Tolectin. If one of these medications is not well tolerated, your doctor may have you try other ones in order to find the best drug for you.

Nasalcrom respiratory inhalant (Fisons Corporation), see Intal respiratory inhalant.

Nasalide topical steroid

Manufacturer: Syntex Laboratories, Inc.
Ingredient: flunisolide
Dosage Form: Nasal solution: 0.025%
Use: For relief of symptoms of stuffy nose, runny nose, and sneezing
Minor Side Effects: Change in senses of taste and smell; sneezing; sore throat; temporary nasal burning and stinging; watery eyes
Major Side Effects: Headache; nasal congestion; nasal infection; nasal irritation; nausea; vomiting
Contraindications: This drug should not be used by persons allergic to it or by persons who have an untreated nasal infection. Consult your doctor immediately if this drug has been prescribed for you and you have either of these conditions.
Warnings: This drug must be used cautiously by persons receiving oral steroid therapy and persons being switched from oral therapy to Nasalide. Report any increase in symptoms or feelings of weakness to your physician. A dosage adjustment may be necessary. • This drug must be used cautiously by persons with tuberculosis, viral infections, ocular herpes simplex, or nasal ulcers and by persons recovering from nasal trauma or surgery. Be sure your doctor knows if any of these conditions applies to you. • Take this drug exactly as prescribed. For maximum effect, it must be taken at regular intervals. It is not effective for immediate relief of symptoms. Although symptoms will improve in a few days, full relief may not be obtained for one to two weeks with continued use of this drug. Do not increase the dose. Taking more than prescribed leads to increased incidence of side effects. Adults should not exceed eight sprays in each nostril per day. The maximum recommended dose for children is four sprays per nostril per day. • If symptoms do not improve or if they worsen with continued use, contact your doctor. • This drug is to be used in pregnant or nursing women only when clearly necessary. Discuss the benefits and risks with your doctor. • This drug is not recommended for use in children under six.
Comments: If you are also using a decongestant spray, it is best to use the decongestant prior to the Nasalide. The decongestant will clear nasal passages, ensuring adequate penetration of Nasalide. • For best results, clear nasal passages of all secretions prior to using this drug. • Patient instructions explaining proper use of the nasal pump unit are available. Read and follow the instructions carefully for best results. • Each Nasalide pump unit contains approximately 200 sprays.

Navane antipsychotic

Manufacturer: Roerig
Ingredient: thiothixene
Equivalent Product: thiothixene, various manufacturers
Dosage Forms: Capsule: 1 mg (orange/yellow); 2 mg (blue/yellow); 5 mg (orange/white); 10 mg (blue/white); 20 mg (blue/green). Oral concentrate (content per ml): 5 mg
Use: Management of certain types of psychoses
Minor Side Effects: Blurred vision; constipation; dizziness; drowsiness; dry mouth; fatigue; impotence; increased sensitivity to the sun; increased sweating; increased thirst; insomnia; light-headedness; loss of appetite; nasal congestion; nausea; restlessness; vomiting; weakness; weight gain
Major Side Effects: Blood disorders; breast enlargement (in both sexes); fainting; involuntary movements of the face or tongue; itching; palpitations; skin rash

Contraindications: This drug should not be taken by anyone who is allergic to it or by persons with certain blood disorders or circulatory problems. Be sure your doctor knows if any of these conditions applies to you.

Warnings: This drug must be used with caution by pregnant or nursing women. Discuss the benefits and risks with your doctor. • This drug is not recommended for use in children under 12 years of age. • This drug may cause motor restlessness, uncoordinated movements, or involuntary muscle spasms, especially in the muscles of the face. If you notice any of these effects, contact your doctor. Your dosage may need to be adjusted, or the drug may need to be discontinued. • This drug must be used cautiously in persons with certain heart problems. • When taking this drug for prolonged periods, you should be monitored closely for blood disorders and eye changes, which have been reported to occur. • This drug has been known to interact with anticonvulsant medications, sedatives, alcohol, and other depressants. If you are currently taking any drugs of these types, contact your doctor. If you are unsure of the type or contents of your medications, ask your doctor or pharmacist. • This drug may cause dizziness, light-headedness, or drowsiness, especially during the first few days of therapy. Avoid driving and other tasks that require alertness during this time. If these symptoms persist or become bothersome, consult your doctor. To prevent oversedation, avoid the use of alcohol and other drugs that have sedative effects.

Comments: It may be two to four weeks before the full effects of this drug become evident. This drug is usually started at a low dose and then gradually increased in order to find the best dose for the individual patient. Do not be concerned if your doctor adjusts your dose frequently when you first begin taking this medication. • This drug has persistent action. Never take it more frequently than prescribed; a serious overdose could result. • While taking this drug, do not take any nonprescription items for weight control, cough, cold, or sinus problems without first checking with your doctor or pharmacist. • Chew gum or suck on ice chips or a piece of hard candy to relieve mouth dryness. • Because this drug decreases sweating, avoid excessive work or exercise in hot weather and drink plenty of fluids. • This drug may make you more sensitive to the sun. Avoid prolonged sun exposure and wear protective clothing and a sunscreen when outdoors. • To avoid dizziness or light-headedness when you stand, contract and relax the muscles of your legs for a few minutes before rising. Do this by pushing one foot against the floor while raising the other foot slightly, alternating feet so that you are "pumping" your legs in a pedaling motion. • To avoid stomach irritation, take the capsule form of this drug with a meal or with a glass of milk. • The oral concentrate must be diluted immediately before you take it. Carefully measure the prescribed amount and dilute it in one-half cup of milk, carbonated beverage, applesauce, or pudding. Do not dilute this drug in coffee, tea, or apple juice; they can make the drug less effective. • Do not stop taking this drug suddenly unless instructed to do so by your doctor. Nausea, vomiting, stomach upset, headache, tremors, and increased heart rate may occur if this drug is stopped suddenly. • Some of the side effects of this drug may be prevented by taking an antiparkinson drug. Discuss the use of an antiparkinson drug with your doctor.

Neocidin ophthalmic antibiotic preparation (Major Pharmaceuticals), see Neosporin Ophthalmic antibiotic preparation.

Neomycin Sulfate-Polymyxin B Sulfate-Gramicidin ophthalmic antibiotic preparation (Rugby Laboratories), see Neosporin Ophthalmic antibiotic preparation.

Neosporin Ophthalmic antibiotic preparation

Manufacturer: Burroughs Wellcome Co.

Ingredients: gramicidin (solution only); neomycin sulfate; polymyxin B sulfate; alcohol (solution only); thimerosal (solution only); bacitracin (ointment only)

Equivalent Products: AK-Spore ointment, Akorn, Inc.; Neocidin, Major Pharmaceuticals; Neomycin Sulfate-Polymyxin B Sulfate-Gramicidin, Rugby Laboratories

Dosage Forms: Ointment (content per gram): bacitracin, 400 units; neomycin sulfate, 3.5 mg; polymyxin B sulfate, 10,000 units. Solution (content per ml): gramicidin, 0.025 mg; neomycin sulfate, 1.75 mg; polymyxin B sulfate, 10,000 units; alcohol, 0.5%; thimerosal, 0.001%

Use: Short-term treatment of superficial bacterial infections of the eye

Minor Side Effects: Burning; blurred vision; red eyes; skin rash; stinging

Major Side Effects: None

Contraindication: This drug should not be taken by people with known sensitivity to any of its ingredients. Make sure your doctor knows if you have such a sensitivity.

Warnings: Prolonged use of this drug may result in secondary infection. • Tests should be performed during treatment to be sure the drug is working. • This drug should be used cautiously by people who have an injured cornea, kidney disease, inner ear disease, myasthenia gravis, or Parkinson's disease.

Comments: Minor side effects will go away quickly. • If symptoms do not improve within a few days, contact your doctor. • Continue using this drug for the full period prescribed even if symptoms have subsided. • Be careful about the contamination of solutions used for the eyes. Wash your hands before administering eye drops. Do not touch the dropper to your eye. Do not wash or wipe the dropper before replacing it in the bottle. Close the bottle tightly to keep out moisture. • See the chapter called Administering Medication Correctly for instructions on using eye drops.

New-Decongest decongestant and antihistamine (Goldline Laboratories), see Naldecon decongestant and antihistamine.

N.G.T. topical steroid hormone and anti-infective (Geneva Generics, Inc.), see Mycolog II topical steroid hormone and anti-infective.

Nicorette smoking deterrent

Manufacturer: Merrell Dow Pharmaceuticals, Inc.

Ingredient: nicotine resin complex

Dosage Form: Chewing gum (content per piece): 2 mg (beige)

Use: An aid to stop smoking

Minor Side Effects: Constipation; diarrhea; dizziness; dry mouth; gas pains; headache; hiccups; hoarseness; insomnia; jaw ache; light-headedness; mouth sores; sneezing; sore throat

Major Side Effects: Breathing difficulties; cold sweats; euphoria; faintness; flushing; heart palpitations; visual disturbances

Contraindications: Nonsmokers; people who have recently suffered a heart attack; people with certain heart conditions, such as chest pain or severe arrhythmias; and pregnant and nursing women should consult their doctor if this drug has been prescribed for them.

Warnings: This drug must be used with caution by persons with certain types of heart disease, thyroid disease, diabetes, hypertension, or peptic ulcer disease. If any of these conditions applies to you, discuss the use of this drug with your doctor. • Nursing mothers should stop nursing while taking this drug. • Use of this drug in adolescents or children who smoke has not been evaluated. • Dental problems may be exacerbated while using this drug. • Nicorette contains nicotine, as do cigarettes; therefore, concurrent use can lead to overdose. • Because nicotine is known to be addictive, this drug is not recommended to be used for longer than six months. After three months of therapy, your doctor may want to gradually reduce the amount of Nicorette that you chew. • This drug interacts with caffeine, theophylline, imipramine, pentazocine, furosemide, propranolol, glutethimide, and propoxyphene. If you are taking any of these medicines, consult your doctor or pharmacist about their use. If you are unsure of the types or contents of your medications, ask your doctor or pharmacist.

Comments: Nicotine is similar in action to caffeine. Try to limit your consumption of coffee, tea, cola, chocolate, and other caffeine-containing products while taking this drug. • Patient information sheets are available for Nicorette. If one is not dispensed with your prescription, ask your pharmacist for one. Read the information carefully before taking this drug. • To be most effective, this drug is to be used in conjunction with a smoking cessation program by persons who have a desire to stop smoking. • The gum should be chewed slowly. Chewing the gum too quickly can cause symptoms similar to oversmoking (nausea, hiccups, and throat irritation). • Take this drug as directed by your doctor. Do not use more than recommended. You should not be chewing more than 30 pieces of gum a day—most people require about ten pieces a day during the first month of use. • Remember to keep this gum out of the reach of children; it is medicine, not candy.

Nilstat antifungal agent (Lederle Laboratories), see Mycostatin antifungal agent.

Nitro-Bid sustained-release antianginal (Marion Laboratories, Inc.), see nitroglycerin sustained-release antianginal.

Nitro-Bid topical antianginal (Marion Laboratories, Inc.), see nitroglycerin topical antianginal.

Nitrocap T.D. sustained-release antianginal (Vortech Pharmaceutical, Ltd.), see nitroglycerin sustained-release antianginal.

Nitrocine transdermal antianginal (Schwarz Pharma Kremers-Urban), see nitroglycerin transdermal antianginal.

Nitrodisc transdermal antianginal (Searle & Co.), see nitroglycerin transdermal antianginal.

Nitro-Dur transdermal antianginal (Key Pharmaceuticals, Inc.), see nitroglycerin transdermal antianginal.

nitrofurantoin antibacterial

Manufacturer: various manufacturers
Ingredient: nitrofurantoin

Equivalent Products: Furadantin, Norwich Eaton Pharmaceuticals, Inc.; Furalan, The Lannett Company, Inc.; Furan, American Urologicals; Furanite, Major Pharmaceuticals; Macrodantin, Norwich Eaton Pharmaceuticals, Inc. (see Comments)

Dosage Forms: Capsule: 25 mg (Macrodantin only); 50 mg; 100 mg. Liquid (content per 5 ml teaspoon): 25 mg. Tablet: 50 mg; 100 mg

Use: Treatment of bacterial urinary tract infections such as pyelonephritis, pyelitis, or cystitis

Minor Side Effects: Abdominal cramps; change in urine color; diarrhea; dizziness; drowsiness; headache; loss of appetite; nausea; vomiting

Major Side Effects: Anemia; breathing difficulties; chest pain; chills; cough; fever; hair loss; hepatitis; irritation of the mouth; low blood pressure; muscle aches; numbness and tingling in face; rash; rectal and vaginal itching; superinfection; symptoms of lung infection; weakness; yellowing of eyes and skin

Contraindications: This drug should not be used by persons with severe kidney disease or little or no urine production. Be sure your doctor knows if either condition applies to you. • This drug should not be used by pregnant women at term or in infants under one month of age. • This drug should not be used by people who are allergic to it. Consult your doctor immediately if this drug has been prescribed for you and you have such an allergy.

Warnings: This drug should be taken cautiously; it has been associated with lung problems. If such problems occur, your doctor will discontinue this drug and appropriate measures will be taken. Report to your doctor any symptoms such as chest pain, shortness of breath, or cough. • This drug should be used with caution by blacks and by ethnic groups of Mediterranean and Near Eastern origin, since cases of hemolytic anemia have been known to be brought about in a percentage of such persons while using this drug. • If you experience fever, pallor, weakness, or jaundice, stop taking this drug and consult your doctor. The problem usually ceases when the drug is withdrawn. • This drug should be used with caution by pregnant women, by women who may become pregnant, and by nursing mothers. • This drug should be used cautiously by people with kidney disease, anemia, diabetes, vitamin-B imbalance, electrolyte imbalance, and certain other debilitating diseases. Be sure your doctor knows if any of these conditions applies to you. • This drug may interact with nalidixic acid, probenecid, magnesium trisilicate, and sulfinpyrazone. If you are currently taking any drugs of these types, consult your doctor. If you are unsure about the type or contents of your medications, ask your doctor or pharmacist. • This drug may cause nerve damage and liver disease. If this drug is taken for prolonged periods, tests to monitor for these effects are recommended. • This drug may interfere with certain blood and urine laboratory tests. Remind your doctor that you are taking this drug if you are scheduled for any tests.

Comments: Not all nitrofurantoin preparations are generic equivalents; consult your pharmacist about the use of generics. Macrodantin contains macrocrystals of nitrofurantoin, which are better tolerated. It causes less nausea and less stomach distress than other nitrofurantoin products. • If you have a urinary tract infection, you should drink at least nine or ten glasses of water each day. • To reduce nausea and vomiting, take this drug with a meal or glass of milk. • This drug may cause false results with urine sugar tests. • This drug may cause your urine to become dark in color. Do not be alarmed. • Notify your doctor if fever, chills, cough, rash, yellow eyes or skin, breathing difficulties, or tingling of the fingers or toes occurs. • It is best to take this medication at evenly spaced intervals around the clock. Ask your doctor or pharmacist to help you establish a practical dosing schedule. • This drug should be taken for as long as prescribed; stopping treatment early may result in reinfection.

nitroglycerin sublingual antianginal

Manufacturer: Eli Lilly & Co.
Ingredient: nitroglycerin
Equivalent Product: Nitrostat, Parke-Davis
Dosage Form: Sublingual tablet: 0.15 mg; 0.3 mg; 0.4 mg; 0.6 mg (all are white)
Use: Relief of chest pain (angina) due to heart disease
Minor Side Effects: Dizziness; flushing of the face; headache; nausea; vomiting
Major Side Effects: Fainting; palpitations; sweating
Contraindications: This drug should not be used by people who are allergic to it; by those who have low blood pressure, glaucoma, or severe anemia; or by those who have suffered a head injury or recent heart attack. Consult your doctor immediately if this drug has been prescribed for you and you have any of these conditions.
Warnings: Do not swallow this drug. The tablets must be placed under the tongue. Do not drink water or swallow for five minutes after taking this drug. • If you use too much of this product, you are likely to get a severe headache. • This drug should be used cautiously by pregnant women. Be sure your doctor knows if you are pregnant. • If you develop blurred vision or dry mouth, contact your doctor. • This drug interacts with alcohol and other vasodilators. Consult your doctor about their use. If you are unsure of the type or contents of your medications, ask your doctor or pharmacist. • If you require more tablets than usual to relieve chest pain, contact your doctor. You may have developed a tolerance to the drug, or the drug may not be working effectively because of interference with other medication. • If this drug does not relieve pain or if pain arises from a different location or differs in severity, call your doctor immediately. • Before using this drug to relieve pain, be certain that the pain arises from the heart and is not due to a muscle spasm or indigestion.
Comments: Frequently chest pain will be relieved in two to five minutes simply by sitting down. • When you take this drug, sit down, lower your head, and breathe deeply. (See the chapter called Administering Medication Correctly to be sure you are taking this drug properly.) If relief is not obtained in five minutes, take another tablet. Repeat in five minutes if necessary. Take no more than three tablets in 15 minutes. If relief still does not occur or if pain increases, call your doctor immediately or go to the nearest emergency treatment facility. • Side effects caused by this drug are most bothersome the first two weeks after starting therapy; they should subside as therapy continues. • This drug must be stored in a tightly capped glass container. Store the bottle in a cool, dry place. Never store the tablets in a metal box, plastic vial, or in the refrigerator or the bathroom medicine cabinet, as the drug may lose potency. The tablet should cause a slight stinging sensation when placed under the tongue. If this does not occur, it indicates loss of potency and a new bottle of pills is necessary. To ensure potency, discard unused tablets six months after the original container is opened. Replace with a fresh bottle. • Nitroglycerin is available in many different dosage forms. Discuss the various products with your doctor or pharmacist.

nitroglycerin sustained-release antianginal

Manufacturer: various manufacturers
Ingredient: nitroglycerin
Equivalent Products: Nitro-Bid, Marion Laboratories, Inc.; Nitrocap T.D., Vortech Pharmaceutical, Ltd.; Nitroglyn, Key Pharmaceuticals, Inc.; Nitrolin, Henry Schein, Inc.; Nitrong, Wharton Laboratories, Inc.; Nitrospan, Rorer Pharmaceuticals

Dosage Forms: Time-release capsule: 2.5 mg; 6.5 mg; 9 mg. Time-release tablet (Nitrong only): 2.6 mg; 6.5 mg; 9 mg

Use: Prevention of chest pain (angina) due to heart disease

Minor Side Effects: Dizziness; flushing of the face; headache; nausea; vomiting; weakness

Major Side Effects: Fainting; palpitations; rash; sweating

Contraindications: This drug should not be taken by people who have a head injury, low blood pressure, severe anemia, or glaucoma or by those who are allergic to this drug. Consult your doctor immediately if this drug has been prescribed for you and any of these conditions applies.

Warnings: This drug is not effective against an attack of angina that is already in progress. It must be taken consistently to prevent chest pain. ● This drug may not continue to relieve chest pain after one to three months because tolerance to nitroglycerin develops quickly. If this drug begins to seem less effective, consult your doctor. ● The time-release forms of this drug must be swallowed whole; do not crush or break the capsules or tablets. ● This medication should be used cautiously by persons who have recently suffered a heart attack, by those with low blood pressure, and by pregnant or nursing women. ● This drug should be used cautiously in conjunction with antihypertensive drugs.

Comments: Side effects generally disappear after two to three weeks of continued therapy. ● Headache is a common side effect. It occurs after taking a dose and lasts a short time. However, the headaches should be less noticeable with continued treatment. If they persist, contact your doctor. ● If you develop blurred vision or dry mouth, contact your doctor. ● Do not stop taking this medication abruptly or without consulting your doctor. ● It is best to take the capsule form on an empty stomach with a full glass of water. ● To avoid dizziness or light-headedness when you stand, contract and relax the muscles of your legs for a few moments before rising. Do this by pushing one foot against the floor while raising the other foot slightly, alternating feet so that you are "pumping" your legs in a pedaling motion. ● Do not drink alcohol unless your doctor has told you that you may.

nitroglycerin topical antianginal

Manufacturer: various manufacturers

Ingredient: nitroglycerin

Equivalent Products: Nitro-Bid, Marion Laboratories, Inc.; Nitrol, Adria Laboratories, Inc.; Nitrong, Wharton Laboratories, Inc.; Nitrostat, Parke-Davis

Dosage Form: Ointment: 2%

Use: Prevention of angina (chest pain) attacks due to heart disease

Minor Side Effects: Dizziness; flushing; headache; skin irritation; vomiting; weakness

Major Side Effects: Fainting; palpitations; rash; sweating

Contraindications: This drug should not be taken by people who have a head injury, low blood pressure, severe anemia, or glaucoma or by those who are allergic to it. Consult your doctor immediately if this drug has been prescribed for you and any of these conditions applies.

Warnings: If you develop blurred vision or dry mouth, contact your doctor. ● This drug is not effective against an attack of angina that is already in progress. It must be used consistently to prevent chest pain. ● This drug may not continue to relieve chest pain after one to three months because tolerance to nitroglycerin develops quickly. If this drug begins to seem less effective, consult your doctor. ● This medication should be used cautiously by persons who have recently suffered a heart attack, by those with low blood pressure, and by pregnant or nursing women. ● This drug should be used cautiously in conjunction with antihypertensive drugs.

Comments: Side effects usually disappear after two to three weeks of continued therapy. • Headache is a common side effect. It generally lasts only a short time. However, the headaches should be less noticeable with continued treatment. If they persist, contact your doctor. • Do not stop using this medication abruptly or without consulting your doctor. • The ointment should be applied using the special applicators. Measure the prescribed dose onto the applicator and spread it in a thin, even layer over the skin. Do not rub it into the skin. Use an occlusive wrap only if instructed to do so by your doctor. • To avoid dizziness or light-headedness when you stand, contract and relax the muscles of your legs for a few moments before rising. Do this by pushing one foot against the floor while raising the other foot slightly, alternating feet so that you are "pumping" your legs in a pedaling motion. • Do not drink alcohol unless your doctor has told you that you may. • Nitroglycerin is also available in a transdermal patch dosage form (see nitroglycerin transdermal antianginal) that may be more convenient for you than the ointment. Discuss the use of such patches with your doctor.

nitroglycerin transdermal antianginal

Manufacturer: various manufacturers
Ingredient: nitroglycerin
Equivalent Products: Deponit, Wyeth-Ayerst Laboratories; Nitrocine, Schwarz Pharma Kremers-Urban; Nitrodisc, Searle & Co.; Nitro-Dur, Key Pharmaceuticals, Inc.; Transderm-Nitro, Ciba Pharmaceutical Company
Dosage Form: Transdermal patch systems: various strengths
Use: Prevention of angina (chest pain) attacks
Minor Side Effects: Dizziness; flushing of face; headache; light-headedness; nausea; skin irritation
Major Side Effects: Blurred vision; fainting; skin rash; vomiting; weakness
Contraindications: This product should not be used by people who are allergic to nitrates or by those who have anemia, certain types of glaucoma, or head injuries. Consult your doctor if this drug has been prescribed for you and any of these conditions applies.
Warnings: This drug should be used with caution by people who have had a recent heart attack and by those with severe heart failure. Be sure your doctor knows if either of these conditions applies to you. • If you develop blurred vision or a rash, contact your doctor. • Do not stop using these patches suddenly. If you have been using them for a prolonged period, your doctor will reduce your dose gradually.
Comments: Side effects generally disappear after two to three weeks of continued therapy. If they persist or worsen, call your doctor. • To avoid dizziness or light-headedness when you stand, contract and relax the muscles of your legs for a few moments before rising. Do this by pushing one foot against the floor while raising the other foot slightly, alternating feet so that you are "pumping" your legs in a pedaling motion. • Do not drink alcohol unless your doctor has told you that you may. • This drug may interact with antihypertensive drugs. If you are currently taking drugs of this type, the dosages may have to be adjusted. Consult your doctor. If you are unsure about the type or contents of your medications, ask your doctor or pharmacist. • This drug is supplied as a transdermal patch. Each patch is designed to continually release nitroglycerin over a 24-hour period. It may be necessary to clip hair prior to using these patches; hair may interfere with patch adhesion. • Do not apply patch to lower parts of arms or legs. Application sites should be changed slightly with each use to avoid skin irritation. Avoid placing patch on irritated or damaged skin. • You can shower or bathe while the patch is in place. If it loosens, apply a new patch. • It is recommended that you apply a new patch 30 minutes before

removing the old one, if possible; this will ensure constant protection. ● Store the patches in a cool, dry place. Do not refrigerate. ● Patient instructions for application of these patches are available. Ask your pharmacist for them if they are not provided with your prescription. For maximum benefit, read and follow the instructions carefully.

Nitroglyn sustained-release antianginal (Key Pharmaceuticals, Inc.), see nitroglycerin sustained-release antianginal.

Nitrolin sustained-release antianginal (Henry Schein, Inc.), see nitroglycerin sustained-release antianginal.

Nitrol topical antianginal (Adria Laboratories, Inc.), see nitroglycerin topical antianginal.

Nitrong sustained-release antianginal (Wharton Laboratories, Inc.), see nitroglycerin sustained-release antianginal.

Nitrong topical antianginal (Wharton Laboratories, Inc.), see nitroglycerin topical antianginal.

Nitrospan sustained-release antianginal (Rorer Pharmaceuticals), see nitroglycerin sustained-release antianginal.

Nitrostat sublingual antianginal (Parke-Davis), see nitroglycerin sublingual antianginal.

Nitrostat topical antianginal (Parke-Davis), see nitroglycerin topical antianginal.

Norcet analgesic (Holloway Labs, Inc.), see Vicodin analgesic.

Nordryl antihistamine (Vortech Pharmaceutical, Ltd.), see Benadryl antihistamine.

Norgesic, Norgesic Forte analgesics

Manufacturer: Riker Laboratories, Inc.
Ingredients: aspirin; caffeine; orphenadrine citrate
Equivalent Products: Norgesic: Orphengesic, various manufacturers. Norgesic Forte: Orphengesic Forte, various manufacturers
Dosage Form: Norgesic: Tablet: aspirin, 385 mg; caffeine, 30 mg; orphenadrine citrate, 25 mg. Norgesic Forte: Tablet: aspirin, 770 mg; caffeine, 60 mg; orphenadrine citrate, 50 mg (both trilayered green/white/yellow)
Use: Relief of mild to moderate pain in muscles or joints
Minor Side Effects: Blurred vision; confusion; constipation; diarrhea; dilation of pupils; dizziness; drowsiness; dry mouth; headache; indigestion; insomnia; nausea; nervousness; slight blood loss; vomiting; weakness
Major Side Effects: Abdominal pain; blood in the stools; breathing difficulties; chest tightness; hearing loss; palpitations; rapid heartbeat; rash; ringing in the ears; urinary hesitancy or retention

Contraindications: This drug should not be used by patients with glaucoma, intestinal obstruction, difficulty in swallowing, enlarged prostate, obstructions of the bladder, or myasthenia gravis. Be sure your doctor knows if any of these conditions applies to you. • This drug should not be taken by persons who are allergic to any of its ingredients. Contact your doctor immediately if this drug has been prescribed for you and you have such an allergy.

Warnings: This drug may cause drowsiness; avoid activities that require alertness, such as operating machinery or driving a motor vehicle. • To prevent oversedation, avoid the use of alcohol or other drugs that have sedative properties. • This drug should be used cautiously by pregnant or nursing women and by women of childbearing age. It is not recommended for use by children under 12 years of age. This drug should be used with caution by persons with peptic ulcers, anemia, gout, liver disease, kidney disease, or coagulation problems. Be sure your doctor knows if any of these conditions applies to you. • If this drug is prescribed for a long period, periodic monitoring of blood, urine, and liver function is recommended. • This drug interacts with central nervous system depressants, propoxyphene (Darvon analgesic, for example), anticoagulants, methotrexate, 6-mercaptopurine, phenytoin, oral antidiabetics, and gout medications (probenecid, sulfinpyrazone). If you are currently taking any drugs of these types, ask your doctor about their use. If you are unsure about the type or contents of your medications, ask your doctor or pharmacist. • Avoid the use of aspirin and aspirin-containing products while taking this drug.

Comments: This drug is not a substitute for rest, physical therapy, or other measures recommended by your doctor to treat your condition. • This drug may be taken with food or milk to lessen stomach upset. • If you hear buzzing or ringing, if your ears feel strange, or if your stomach hurts, your dosage may need adjustment. Call your doctor. • Chew gum or suck on ice chips or a piece of hard candy to reduce mouth dryness.

Nor-Mil antidiarrheal (Vortech Pharmaceutical, Ltd.), see Lomotil antidiarrheal.

Normodyne antihypertensive

Manufacturer: Schering Corp.
Ingredient: labetalol hydrochloride
Equivalent Product: Trandate, Allen & Hanburys
Dosage Form: Tablet: 100 mg (light brown); 200 mg (white); 300 mg (blue)
Use: Treatment of high blood pressure
Minor Side Effects: Abdominal pain; altered sense of taste; bloating; blurred vision; constipation; drowsiness; dry eyes; dry mouth; gas; headache; heartburn; insomnia; loss of appetite; nasal congestion; nausea; scalp tingling; slowed heart rate; sweating
Major Side Effects: Blood disorders; change in vision; decreased sexual ability; depression; difficulty in urinating; dizziness; fever; impotence; jaundice; mouth sores; numbness in fingers and toes; shortness of breath; skin rash; sore throat; swelling in hands and feet
Contraindications: This drug should not be used by persons allergic to it or by those with a sensitivity to beta blockers. This drug should not be used by persons with bronchial asthma or certain types of heart disease (severe heart failure, bradycardia, shock). Consult your doctor immediately if this drug has been prescribed for you and any of these conditions applies.
Warnings: This drug must be used cautiously by persons with certain respiratory diseases, certain heart problems, diabetes, or liver disease. Be sure your doctor knows if any of these conditions applies to you. • This drug should be

used with caution by pregnant or nursing women. • If you undergo major surgery while taking this drug, your blood pressure must be monitored closely. • This drug must be used cautiously in conjunction with cimetidine, beta blockers, nitroglycerin, anesthetic agents, and other antihypertensive agents. If you are currently taking any drugs of these types, consult your doctor about their use. If you are unsure about the type or contents of your medications, ask your doctor or pharmacist. • Do not suddenly stop taking this drug without first consulting your doctor. Chest pain — even heart attacks — may occur if this drug is suddenly stopped after prolonged use. • Diabetics should be aware that this drug can mask signs of hypoglycemia, such as changes in heart rate and blood pressure. Routinely monitor urine or blood glucose while taking this drug.

Comments: Initially this drug may cause dizziness or light-headedness, which should disappear as therapy continues. If it persists or worsens, notify your doctor. To prevent light-headedness when standing, change positions slowly. Contract and relax the muscles of your legs for a few minutes before rising. Do this by pushing one foot against the floor while raising the other foot slightly, alternating feet so that you are "pumping" your legs in a pedaling motion. While taking this drug, limit your consumption of alcoholic beverages to minimize dizziness and light-headedness. • Learn how to monitor your pulse and blood pressure while taking this drug; discuss this with your doctor. • Transient scalp tingling has been reported by persons when the drug is first taken. This effect should disappear as therapy continues. • If you have high blood pressure, do not take any nonprescription item for weight control, cough, cold, or sinus problems without first checking with your doctor; such items may contain ingredients that can increase blood pressure. • Notify your doctor if you develop a sore throat, fever, bruising, shortness of breath, yellow eyes or skin, dark urine, or difficulty in urinating while taking this drug. • Take this drug as prescribed. Do not skip doses or take extra doses without your doctor's approval. • This drug may be taken with food to prevent stomach upset.

Noroxin antibiotic

Manufacturer: Merck Sharp & Dohme
Ingredient: norfloxacin
Dosage Form: Tablet: 400 mg (dark pink)
Use: Treatment of urinary tract infections in adults
Minor Side Effects: Abdominal pain; blurred vision; constipation; dizziness; drowsiness; dry mouth; fatigue; flatulence; headache; heartburn; nausea; stomach upset
Major Side Effects: Depression; fever; skin rash; vomiting
Contraindications: This drug should not be taken by anyone who is allergic to it. Be sure your doctor knows if you have such an allergy. • This drug is not recommended for use in children or pregnant women.
Warnings: This drug must be used with caution by nursing women. Discuss the benefits and risks with your doctor. • Persons with certain kidney problems should use this drug cautiously. Lower than normal doses may be necessary. • This drug has been shown to interact with nitrofurantoin, probenecid, and antacids. Do not take this drug within two hours of taking an antacid. If you are currently taking any drugs of these types, consult your doctor or pharmacist about their use. If you are unsure of the type or contents of your medications, ask your doctor or pharmacist.
Comments: This drug is best if taken one hour before or two hours after a meal at evenly spaced intervals throughout the day and night. Ask your doctor or pharmacist to help you devise a dosing schedule. • Take this drug for as long as prescribed, even if symptoms disappear before that time. If you stop

taking the drug too soon, resistant bacteria are given a chance to continue growing, and the infection could recur. • Drink plenty of fluids while taking this drug. Try to drink eight to ten glasses of water, orange juice, or cranberry juice each day. • This drug may cause dizziness, especially during the first few days of therapy. Use caution when driving or operating machinery during this time.

Norpace antiarrhythmic

Manufacturer: Searle & Co.

Ingredient: disopyramide phosphate

Equivalent Products: disopyramide phosphate, various manufacturers; Napamide, Major Pharmaceuticals

Dosage Forms: Capsule: 100 mg (white/orange); 150 mg (brown/orange). Controlled-release capsule: 100 mg (light green/white); 150 mg (light green/brown)

Use: Treatment of some heart arrhythmias

Minor Side Effects: Abdominal pain; aches and pains; blurred vision; constipation; diarrhea; dizziness; dry mouth; dry nose, eyes, throat; fatigue; gas; headache; impotence; increased sensitivity to sunlight; loss of appetite; muscle pain; muscle weakness; nausea; nervousness; rash; vomiting

Major Side Effects: Chest pain; difficulty in urinating; edema and weight gain; fainting; fever; heart failure; jaundice; low blood pressure; low blood sugar; numbness or tingling sensation; palpitations; psychosis; severe mental disorders; shortness of breath; sore throat

Contraindications: This drug should not be taken by persons who have certain types of severe heart disease or by those who are allergic to it. Consult your doctor immediately if this drug has been prescribed for you and either condition applies.

Warnings: This drug should be used with caution, since its use may cause low blood pressure and heart failure. • This drug should be used cautiously in conjunction with certain other agents such as quinidine or procainamide, phenytoin, rifampin, beta blockers, and alcohol. If you are currently taking any drugs of these types, consult your doctor about their use. If you are unsure of the type or contents of your medications, ask your doctor or pharmacist. • Patients receiving more than one antiarrhythmic drug must be carefully monitored. Your doctor may want you to monitor your pulse and blood pressure while you are taking this medication; discuss this with your doctor. • This drug should be used with caution by pregnant or nursing women and by persons with glaucoma, myasthenia gravis, enlarged prostate, low blood sugar (hypoglycemia), malnutrition, urinary retention, low blood potassium (hypokalemia), liver disease, or kidney disease. Be sure your doctor knows if any of these conditions applies to you. • This drug should be used with caution in children.

Comments: This drug is similar in action to procainamide and to quinidine sulfate. All of these medications are used to help control the heart's rhythm. • While taking this drug, do not take any nonprescription item for weight control, cough, cold or sinus problems without first checking with your doctor. • This drug must be taken exactly as directed. Do not take extra doses or skip a dose. Do not stop taking this drug unless advised to do so by your physician. • Chew gum or suck on ice chips or a piece of hard candy to reduce mouth dryness. • To minimize dizziness, rise from a lying or sitting position slowly. • Side effects such as dry mouth, constipation, blurred vision, and difficulty in urinating should be temporary. If these symptoms persist, call your doctor. • Notify your doctor if you develop signs of jaundice (yellow eyes or skin; dark urine). • The controlled-release form of this drug is taken less frequently during the day. It must be swallowed whole. Discuss the use of this form with your doctor.

Norpramin antidepressant

Manufacturer: Merrell Dow Pharmaceuticals, Inc.

Ingredient: desipramine hydrochloride

Equivalent Product: Pertofrane, Rorer Pharmaceuticals

Dosage Forms: Capsule: 25 mg (pink); 50 mg (maroon/pink). Tablet: 10 mg (blue); 25 mg (yellow); 50 mg (green); 75 mg (orange); 100 mg (peach); 150 mg (white)

Use: For relief of depression

Minor Side Effects: Agitation; anxiety; blurred vision; confusion; constipation; cramps; diarrhea; dizziness; drowsiness; dry mouth; fatigue; headache; heartburn; increased sensitivity to light; insomnia; loss of appetite; nausea; peculiar tastes; restlessness; sweating; vomiting; weakness; weight gain or loss

Major Side Effects: Bleeding; bruising; chest pain; convulsions; difficulty in urinating; enlarged or painful breasts (in both sexes); fainting; fever; fluid retention; hair loss; hallucinations; high or low blood pressure; impotence; jaundice; loss of balance; mood changes; mouth sores; nervousness; nightmares; numbness in fingers or toes; palpitations; psychosis; ringing in the ears; seizures; skin rash; sleep disorders; sore throat; stroke; tremors; uncoordinated movements

Contraindications: This drug should not be taken by people who are allergic to it; by those who have recently had a heart attack; or by those who are taking monoamine oxidase inhibitors (ask your pharmacist if you are unsure). Consult your doctor immediately if this drug has been prescribed for you and any of these conditions applies.

Warnings: This drug is not recommended for use by children under the age of 12. • This drug should be used cautiously by people who have glaucoma (certain types), heart disease (certain types), high blood pressure, enlarged prostate, epilepsy, urine retention, liver disease, or hyperthyroidism and by pregnant or nursing women. Be sure your doctor knows if any of these conditions applies to you. • This drug should be used cautiously by patients who are receiving electroshock therapy or those who are about to undergo surgery. • Close medical supervision is required when this drug is taken with guanethidine or Placidyl hypnotic. • This drug may cause changes in blood sugar levels. Diabetics should monitor their blood sugar more frequently when first taking this medication. • This drug interacts with alcohol, amphetamine, barbiturates, clonidine, epinephrine, oral anticoagulants, phenylephrine, and depressants; if you are currently taking any drugs of these types, consult your doctor about their use. If you are unsure of the type or contents of your medications, ask your doctor or pharmacist. • This drug may cause drowsiness; avoid tasks that require alertness. To prevent oversedation, avoid the use of alcohol or other drugs that have sedative properties. • Report any sudden mood changes to your doctor.

Comments: Take this medicine exactly as your doctor prescribes. Do not stop taking it without first checking with your doctor. • While taking this drug, do not take any nonprescription item for weight control, cough, cold, or sinus problems without first checking with your doctor. Be sure your doctor is aware of every medication you use, and do not stop or start any other drug without your doctor's approval. • The effects of therapy with this drug may not be apparent for two to four weeks. • Your doctor may adjust your dosage frequently during the first few months of therapy in order to find the best dose for you. • Notify your doctor if you develop signs of jaundice (yellow eyes or skin; dark urine). • Chew gum or suck on ice chips or a piece of hard candy to reduce mouth dryness • Avoid prolonged exposure to the sun while taking this drug, and wear protective clothing and a sunscreen when outdoors. • To avoid dizziness or light-headedness when you stand, contract and relax the muscles of your legs

CONSUMER GUIDE®

for a few moments before rising. Do this by pushing one foot against the floor while raising the other foot slightly, alternating feet so that you are "pumping" your legs in a pedaling motion. • Many people receive as much benefit from taking a single dose of this drug at bedtime as from taking multiple doses throughout the day. Talk to your doctor about this. • This drug is very similar in action to other antidepressants. If one of these antidepressant drugs is ineffective or is not well tolerated, your doctor may want you to try one of the others in order to find the best one for you.

Nor-Tet antibiotic (Vortech Pharmaceutical, Ltd.), see tetracycline hydrochloride antibiotic.

Nuprin anti-inflammatory (Bristol-Myers), see ibuprofen anti-inflammatory.

Nutracort topical steroid (Owen/Allercreme), see hydrocortisone topical steroid.

nystatin antifungal agent (various manufacturers), see Mycostatin antifungal agent.

Nystex antifungal agent (Savage Laboratories), see Mycostatin antifungal agent.

Octamide gastrointestinal stimulant (Adria Laboratories, Inc.), see Reglan gastrointestinal stimulant.

Ocusert Pilo-20 ophthalmic preparation (Alza Corporation), see Isopto Carpine ophthalmic preparation.

Ocusert Pilo-40 ophthalmic preparation (Alza Corporation), see Isopto Carpine ophthalmic preparation.

Omnipen antibiotic (Wyeth-Ayerst Laboratories), see ampicillin antibiotic.

Oragest S.R. antihistamine and decongestant (Major Pharmaceuticals), see Ornade Spansules antihistamine and decongestant.

oral contraceptives (birth control pills)

"Oral contraceptives" is a descriptive term.
Examples: Brevicon, Syntex (F.P.) Inc.; Demulen, Searle & Co.; Enovid, Searle & Co.; Gynex, Searle & Co.; Loestrin, Parke-Davis; Lo/Ovral, Wyeth-Ayerst Laboratories; Micronor, Ortho Pharmaceutical Corp.; Modicon, Ortho Pharmaceutical Corp.; Nordette, Wyeth-Ayerst Laboratories; Norinyl, Syntex (F.P.) Inc.; Norlestrin, Parke-Davis; Nor-Q.D., Syntex (F.P.) Inc.; Ortho-Novum, Ortho Pharmaceutical Corp.; Ovcon, Mead Johnson Nutritional; Ovral, Wyeth-Ayerst Laboratories; Ovrette, Wyeth-Ayerst Laboratories; Ovulen, Searle & Co.; Tri-Levlen, Berlex Laboratories, Inc.; Tri-Norinyl, Syntex (F.P.) Inc.; Triphasil, Wyeth-Ayerst Laboratories

Dosage Form: Tablets in packages. Some contain 20 or 21 tablets; others 28. When 28 are present, seven are blank or contain iron (see Comments).

Use: Birth control; control of painful menstruation (dysmenorrhea)

Minor Side Effects: Abdominal cramps; acne; backache; bloating; change in appetite; change in sexual desire; diarrhea; dizziness; fatigue; headache; hearing changes; itching; nasal congestion; nausea; nervousness; vaginal irritation; vomiting

Major Side Effects: Anemia; arthritis; birth defects; blood clots; breakthrough bleeding (spotting); cancer; cervical damage; cessation of menstruation; changes in menstrual flow; colitis; depression; elevated blood sugar; enlarged or tender breasts; eye damage; fluid retention; gallbladder disease; heart attack; high blood pressure; increase or decrease in hair growth; internal bleeding; jaundice; kidney damage; liver damage; lung damage; migraine; numbness or tingling; pain during menstruation; pancreatic changes; rash; reduced ability to conceive after drug is stopped; skin color changes; stroke; tumor growth; weight changes; yeast infection

Contraindications: This type of drug should not be used by women who smoke, by nursing women, or by women who have or have had breast cancer or certain types of heart disease, liver disease, blood disease, vaginal bleeding, blood clots, clotting disorders, strokes or mini-strokes, heart attack, or chest pain. Be sure your doctor knows if any of these conditions applies to you. • This drug should not be used by women who may have breast cancer or by women who have had liver tumors as a result of using drugs of this type. • Women who have certain other cancers or abnormal vaginal bleeding and those who may be pregnant should not take this drug.

Warnings: This type of drug has been known or suspected to cause cancer. If you have a family history of cancer, you should inform your doctor before taking oral contraceptives. • This type of drug should be used cautiously by women over age 30. • Oral contraceptives are known to cause an increased risk of heart attacks, stroke, liver disease, gallbladder disease, fluid retention, depression, clotting disorders, blood diseases, eye disease, cancer, birth defects, diabetes, high blood pressure, headache, bleeding disorders, and poor production of breast milk. • Caution should be observed while taking oral contraceptives if you have uterine tumors, mental depression, epilepsy, migraine, asthma, kidney disease, jaundice, or vitamin deficiency. Be sure your doctor knows if any of these conditions applies to you. • Oral contraceptives interact with oral anticoagulants, barbiturates, phenylbutazone, isoniazid, carbamazepine, primidone, chloramphenicol, phenytoin, ampicillin, tetracycline, rifampin, and steroids. Contact your doctor immediately if you are currently taking any drugs of these types. If you are unsure of the type or contents of your medications, ask your doctor or pharmacist. • Some women who have used oral contraceptives have had trouble becoming pregnant after they stopped using the drug. Most of these women had scanty or irregular menstrual periods before they started taking oral contraceptives. Possible subsequent difficulty in becoming pregnant is a matter that you should discuss with your doctor before using this drug. • You should have a complete physical, including a Pap smear, before you start taking oral contraceptives and then every year that you take them. • Oral contraceptives affect a wide variety of lab tests. Be sure your doctor knows you are taking oral contraceptives if you are being tested or examined for any reason. • Little is known about the long-term effects of the use of this type of drug on pituitary, ovarian, adrenal, liver, or uterine function or on the immune system. • Use of this drug may make it difficult to tell when menopause occurs.

Comments: Oral contraceptives currently are considered the most effective reversible method of birth control. The table on the following page shows various methods of birth control and their effectiveness.

Birth Control Method	Effectiveness*
Oral contraceptives	up to 3
Intrauterine device (IUD)	up to 6
Diaphragm (with cream or gel)	up to 20
Vaginal sponge	up to 20
Aerosol foam	up to 29
Condom	up to 36
Gel or cream	up to 36
Rhythm	up to 47
No contraception	up to 80

*Pregnancies per 100 woman years

Take an oral contraceptive at the same time every day—either with a meal or at bedtime—so that you get into the habit of taking the pills. Effectiveness depends on strict adherence to a dosing schedule. If you skip one day, take a tablet for the day you missed as soon as you think of it and another tablet at the regular time. If you miss two days, take two tablets each day for the next two days, then continue with your normal schedule. If you miss more than two days, contact your doctor and use supplemental contraceptive measures. • If you do not start to menstruate on schedule at the end of the pill cycle and you took all the pills as directed, begin the next cycle of pills at the prescribed time anyway. Many women taking oral contraceptives have irregular menstruation. Do not be alarmed, but consult your doctor. • Stop taking oral contraceptive tablets at least three months before you wish to become pregnant. Use another type of contraceptive during this three-month period. • Some oral contraceptive packets contain 28 tablets rather than the usual 20 or 21 tablets. The 28-tablet packets contain seven placebos (sugar pills) or iron tablets. The placebos help you remember to take a tablet each day even while you are menstruating, and the iron tablets help replace the iron that is lost in menstruation. • Nausea is common, especially during the first two or three months, but may be prevented by taking the tablets at bedtime. If nausea persists for more than three months, consult your doctor. • Although many brands of oral contraceptives are available, most differ in only minor ways, and you may have to try several brands before you find the product that is ideal for you. There are three categories of oral contraceptives that contain both estrogen and progestin: monophasic, biphasic, and triphasic. Monophasics contain a fixed dose of estrogen and progestin throughout the cycle. With the biphasics, the estrogen content remains the same while the progestin increases in the second half of the cycle. With the triphasics, the amount of both estrogen and progestin may vary throughout the cycle. The biphasics and triphasics are designed to more closely mimic the natural physiological process and thus limit side effects. Side effects are related to the potency of estrogen or progestin in the product. Your doctor may have you try several products to find the right balance of these two ingredients for you. • Some oral contraceptives contain progestin only (Micronor, Nor-QD, Ovrette). These products have a slightly higher failure rate than the estrogen/progestin combination products but have the advantage of fewer side effects, such as high blood pressure, headache, and swelling of feet and ankles. • With every prescription, your pharmacist will give you a booklet explaining birth control pills. Read this booklet carefully. It contains exact directions on how to use the medication correctly. • If you use oral contraceptives, you must not smoke cigarettes. • You should visit your doctor for a checkup at least once a year while you are taking oral contraceptives. • Women over 30 have an increased risk of adverse effects from use of oral contraceptives. • Spotting or breakthrough bleeding may occur during the first months of use of this drug. Call your physician if it continues past the second month. • Notify your doctor if you develop signs of jaundice (yellow eyes or skin; dark urine). • Use a supplemental method of birth control the first three weeks that you start taking oral contraceptives.

Oramide oral antidiabetic (Major Pharmaceuticals), see Orinase oral antidiabetic.

Oraminic Spancaps antihistamine and decongestant (Vortech Pharmaceutical, Ltd.), see Ornade Spansules antihistamine and decongestant.

Orasone steroid hormone (Reid-Rowell), see prednisone steroid hormone.

Oretic diuretic and antihypertensive (Abbott Laboratories), see hydrochlorothiazide diuretic and antihypertensive.

Oridol-C antitussive and expectorant (LuChem), see Tussi-Organidin antitussive and expectorant.

Orinase oral antidiabetic

Manufacturer: The Upjohn Company
Ingredient: tolbutamide
Equivalent Products: Oramide, Major Pharmaceuticals; tolbutamide, various manufacturers
Dosage Form: Tablet: 250 mg; 500 mg (both white)
Use: Treatment of diabetes mellitus not controlled by diet and exercise alone
Minor Side Effects: Cramps; diarrhea; dizziness; fatigue; headache; heartburn; loss of appetite; nausea; sensitivity to sunlight; stomach upset; vomiting; weakness
Major Side Effects: Blood disorders; breathing difficulties; bruising; dark urine; jaundice; light-colored stools; low blood sugar; muscle cramps; rash; ringing in the ears; seizures; sore throat; tingling in hands and feet
Contraindications: This drug should not be used to treat juvenile (insulin-dependent) or unstable diabetes. Diabetics who are subject to acidosis or ketosis and diabetics with a history of repeated diabetic comas should not use this drug. This drug should not be used be people with severe renal impairment or by those with an allergy to sulfonylureas. In the presence of fever, severe trauma, or infections, insulin should be used instead, at least during the acute stage of the problem. If any of these conditions applies to you, be sure your doctor knows before you begin taking this drug.
Warnings: Tolbutamide may not be safe for use during pregnancy. If you are or might become pregnant, be sure to tell your doctor before taking this drug. • Be sure you can recognize the symptoms of low blood sugar and know what to do if you begin to experience these symptoms. You will have to be especially careful during the transition from insulin to tolbutamide. • People with thyroid disease or kidney or liver damage and those who are malnourished must use this drug cautiously. Be sure your doctor knows if any of these conditions applies to you. • Thiazide diuretics (commonly used to treat high blood pressure) and beta-blocking drugs may interfere with control of your diabetes. If you are taking any drugs of either type, talk to your physician before you take this drug. If you are unsure of the type of your medications, ask your doctor or pharmacist. • Do not drink alcohol and do not take any other drugs while you are taking this drug unless your doctor tells you that you may. Be especially careful

with nonprescription cold remedies. • This drug interacts with anabolic steroids, anticoagulants, anticonvulsants, aspirin, chloramphenicol, guanethidine, propranolol, monoamine oxidase inhibitors, phenylbutazone, steroids, tetracycline; thiazide diuretics, and thyroid hormones; if you are currently taking any drugs of these types, consult your doctor about their use. If you are unsure of the type or contents of your medications, ask your doctor or pharmacist.

Comments: Take this drug at the same time every day. • Recent evidence indicates that not all generic forms of tolbutamide are equivalent. Ask your pharmacist for a product that is bioequivalent. • This drug makes you more sensitive to the sun. Avoid prolonged exposure to sunlight, and wear protective clothing and a sunscreen when outdoors. • This drug is not an oral form of insulin. • Studies have shown that a good diet and exercise program is extremely important in controlling diabetes. Oral antidiabetic drugs should only be used after diet and exercise alone have not proven adequate. However, these drugs allow diabetics more leeway in their lifestyles. Persons taking this drug should carefully watch their diet and exercise program and pay close attention to good personal hygiene. • Persons taking this drug should visit the doctor frequently during the first few weeks of therapy. They should check their urine for sugar and ketones at least three times a day. (Be sure that you know how to test your urine and that you know what the results mean.) They should also know how to recognize the first signs of low blood sugar. Signs of low blood sugar include chills; cold sweat; cool, pale skin; drowsiness; headache; nausea; nervousness; rapid pulse; tremors; weakness. If these symptoms develop, eat or drink something containing sugar and call your doctor. • Call your doctor if you develop an infection, fever, sore throat, unusual bleeding or bruising, yellow eyes or skin, excessive thirst or urination, or dark urine while taking this drug. • It may be advised that you carry a medical alert card or wear a medical alert bracelet indicating you are taking this medication. • There are other drugs that are similar to this one that vary slightly in activity (Diabinese, Glucotrol, Tolinase). Certain persons who do not benefit from one type of oral antidiabetic may benefit from another.

Ornade Spansules antihistamine and decongestant

Manufacturer: Smith Kline & French Laboratories
Ingredients: chlorpheniramine maleate; phenylpropanolamine hydrochloride
Equivalent Products: Allerest 12 Hour, Pharmacraft; Condrin-LA, Mallard, Inc.; Contac 12 Hour, SmithKline Consumer Products; Dehist, Forest Pharmaceuticals, Inc.; Drize, B.F. Ascher & Company, Inc.; Oragest S.R., Major Pharmaceuticals; Oraminic Spancaps, Vortech Pharmaceutical, Ltd.; Resaid S.R., Geneva Generics, Inc.; Rhinolar-EX 12, McGregor Pharmaceuticals; Ru-Tuss II, Boots Pharmaceuticals, Inc.; Triaminic-12, Sandoz Pharmaceuticals (see Comments)
Dosage Form: Sustained-release capsule: chlorpheniramine maleate, 12 mg and phenylpropanolamine hydrochloride, 75 mg (red/natural with red, white, and gray beads)
Uses: Symptomatic relief of upper respiratory tract congestion, hay fever, or other allergies
Minor Side Effects: Acne; blurred vision; confusion; constipation; diarrhea; dizziness; drowsiness; dry mouth; headache; heartburn; insomnia; irritability; loss of appetite; nasal congestion; nausea; restlessness; sedation; sun sensitivity; sweating; vomiting; weakness
Major Side Effects: Bruising; chest pain; convulsions; difficulty in urinating; high blood pressure; loss of coordination; low blood pressure; mood changes; palpitations; rash; severe abdominal pain; sore throat

Contraindications: This drug should not be taken by people who are allergic to any of its components, by people who are using monoamine oxidase inhibitors (ask your pharmacist if you are unsure), or by those who have asthma, certain types of heart disease, severe high blood pressure, obstructed bladder, obstructed intestine, or ulcer (certain types). Consult your doctor immediately if this drug has been prescribed for you and any of these conditions applies. • This drug should not be given to children under age six.

Warnings: This drug should be used cautiously by people who have glaucoma, heart or blood vessel disease, thyroid disease, diabetes, epilepsy, myasthenia gravis, hiatal hernia, or enlarged prostate and by women who are pregnant or nursing. Be sure your doctor knows if any of these conditions applies to you. • This drug may cause drowsiness; avoid tasks that require alertness. To prevent oversedation, avoid the use of alcohol or other drugs that have sedative properties.

Comments: Chew gum or suck on ice chips or a piece of hard candy to reduce mouth dryness. • Because this drug reduces sweating, avoid excessive work or exercise in hot weather and drink plenty of fluids. • This drug has sustained action; never increase your dose or take it more frequently than your doctor prescribes. A serious overdose could result. • This drug must be swallowed whole; do not crush or chew the capsule. • While taking this drug, do not take any nonprescription item for weight control, cough, cold, or sinus problems without first checking with your doctor. • This drug may be taken with food or milk to lessen stomach upset. • Triaminic-12, Allerest 12 Hour, and Contac 12 Hour tablets are available without a prescription. Compare prices and discuss this option with your doctor or pharmacist.

Orphengesic, Orphengesic Forte analgesics (various manufacturers), see Norgesic, Norgesic Forte analgesics.

Ortega Otic M preparation (Ortega Pharmaceutical Company), see Cortisporin Otic preparation.

Otocort otic preparation (Lemmon Company), see Cortisporin Otic preparation.

Otomycin-Hpn Otic preparation (Misemer Pharmaceuticals, Inc.), see Cortisporin Otic preparation.

Otoreid-HC otic preparation (Reid-Rowell), see Cortisporin Otic preparation.

O-V Statin antifungal agent (E. R. Squibb & Sons, Inc.), see Mycostatin antifungal agent.

oxazepam antianxiety and sedative (various manufacturers), see Serax antianxiety and sedative.

Oxycet analgesic (Halsey Drug Co., Inc.), see Percocet analgesic.

oxycodone HCl and acetaminophen analgesic (various manufacturers), see Percocet analgesic.

oxycodone hydrochloride, oxycodone terephthalate, and aspirin analgesic (various manufacturers), see Percodan analgesic.

Panasol steroid hormone (Seatrace Co.), see prednisone steroid hormone.

Panmycin antibiotic (The Upjohn Company), see tetracycline hydrochloride antibiotic.

Panwarfin anticoagulant (Abbott Laboratories), see Coumadin anticoagulant.

Papadeine analgesic (Vangard Laboratories), see acetaminophen with codeine analgesic.

PCE antibiotic (Abbott Laboratories), see erythromycin antibiotic.

Pediamycin antibiotic (Ross Laboratories), see erythromycin antibiotic.

Pediazole antibiotic

Manufacturer: Ross Laboratories
Ingredients: erythromycin ethylsuccinate; sulfisoxazole
Dosage Form: Oral Suspension (content per 5 ml teaspoon): erythromycin ethylsuccinate, 200 mg and sulfisoxazole, 600 mg
Use: Treatment of ear infections (predominantly those in children)
Minor Side Effects: Abdominal pain; diarrhea; dizziness; headache; increased sensitivity to sunlight; insomnia; loss of appetite; nausea; stomach upset; vomiting
Major Side Effects: Aching muscles or joints; allergic skin rash; bleeding or bruising; blood disorders; convulsions; depression; difficulty in swallowing; difficulty in urinating; fatigue; fever; hallucinations; hearing impairment; itching; jaundice; mouth sores; ringing in the ears; sore throat and fever; superinfection
Contraindications: This drug should not be used by persons who are allergic to either erythromycin or sulfa drugs, in infants less than two months old, by pregnant women at term, or by nursing women. Contact your doctor immediately if this drug has been prescribed for you and any of these conditions applies.
Warnings: This drug must be used cautiously by pregnant women and by persons with liver or kidney disease or a history of severe allergies or asthma. Make sure your doctor knows if any of these conditions applies to you. • If you develop a sore throat, fever, or yellowing of the skin or eyes while taking this drug, call your doctor immediately. • If a skin rash develops, discontinue taking the drug and contact your doctor. • Your doctor may want to test your blood periodically if you are taking this drug (or any sulfa drug) for an extended period of time. Prolonged use of this drug may allow organisms that are not susceptible to it to grow wildly. This is called a superinfection. • Do not use this drug unless your doctor has specifically told you to do so. • Avoid prolonged, unprotected exposure to sunlight, as this drug may make you more sensitive to the sun's effects.
Comments: Take this drug as prescribed. For best results, this drug should be taken at evenly spaced intervals around the clock. Continue taking it for the number of days indicated, even if the symptoms disappear within that time. • This medication must be stored in the refrigerator. Shake well before using. • Discard any unused portion after 14 days. • While taking this drug, it is recommended that you drink plenty of fluids each day.

Penapar VK antibiotic (Parke-Davis), see penicillin potassium phenoxymethyl (penicillin VK) antibiotic.

Penecort topical steroid (Herbert Laboratories), see hydrocortisone topical steroid.

penicillin G potassium antibiotic

Manufacturer: various manufacturers
Ingredient: penicillin G potassium
Equivalent Product: Pentids, E. R. Squibb & Sons, Inc.
Dosage Forms: Liquid; Tablet (various dosages and various colors)
Use: Treatment of a wide variety of bacterial infections
Minor Side Effects: Diarrhea; heartburn; nausea; vomiting
Major Side Effects: Bloating; breathing difficulties; chills; cough; fever; irritation of the mouth; muscle aches; rash; rectal and vaginal itching; severe diarrhea; sore throat; superinfection
Contraindication: This drug should not be taken by people who are allergic to any penicillin drug. Consult your doctor immediately if this drug has been prescribed for you and you have such an allergy.
Warnings: This drug should be used cautiously by people who have kidney disease, asthma, or other significant allergies. Be sure your doctor knows if you have any type of allergy. • This drug interacts with aspirin, probenecid, phenylbutazone, indomethacin, sulfinpyrazone, chloramphenicol, erythromycin, and tetracycline; if you are currently taking any drugs of these types, consult your doctor about their use. If you are unsure of the type or contents of your medications, ask your doctor or pharmacist. • This drug is readily destroyed by acids in the stomach; do not take this medication with fruit juice or carbonated beverages. It is best taken with water or milk. • Severe allergic reactions to this drug—indicated by breathing difficulties, rash, fever, and chills—have been reported but are rare when the drug is taken orally. If you experience any of these symptoms while taking this drug, contact your doctor. • Diabetics using Clinitest urine test may get a false high sugar reading while taking this drug. Change to Clinistix, Diastix, or Tes-Tape urine test to avoid this problem. • Prolonged use of this drug may allow organisms that are not susceptible to it to grow wildly. This is called a superinfection. • Do not use this drug unless your doctor has specifically told you to do so. Be sure to follow the directions carefully and report any unusual reactions to your doctor at once. • Complete blood cell counts and liver and kidney function tests should be done if you take this drug for a prolonged period. • This drug may affect the potency of oral contraceptives. Consult your doctor about using supplementary contraceptive measures while you are taking this drug.
Comments: This drug is very similar to penicillin potassium phenoxymethyl (see next profile) and can often be used interchangeably. Penicillin G potassium is less effective than penicillin potassium phenoxymethyl when taken with acidic fluids, such as fruit juice. • This drug should be taken for the full prescribed period, even if symptoms disappear within that time; stopping treatment early can lead to reinfection. • The liquid form of this drug should be stored in the refrigerator. This drug should not be frozen. Any unused portion should be discarded after 14 days. Shake well before using. • Take this drug on an empty stomach (one hour before or two hours after a meal) with a full glass of water. • It is best to take this drug at evenly spaced times throughout the day and night. Your doctor or pharmacist will help you set up a dosing schedule.

penicillin potassium phenoxymethyl
(penicillin VK) antibiotic

Manufacturer: various manufacturers

Ingredient: penicillin potassium phenoxymethyl

Equivalent Products: Beepen VK, Beecham Laboratories; Betapen-VK, Bristol Laboratories; Ledercillin VK, Lederle Laboratories; Penapar VK, Parke-Davis; Pen-V, Goldline Laboratories; Pen-Vee K, Wyeth-Ayerst Laboratories; Robicillin VK, A.H. Robins Company; Suspen, Circle Pharmaceutical, Inc.; V-Cillin K, Eli Lilly & Co.; Veetids, E. R. Squibb & Sons, Inc.

Dosage Forms: Liquid; Tablet (various dosages and various colors)

Use: Treatment of a wide variety of bacterial infections

Minor Side Effects: Diarrhea; heartburn; nausea; vomiting

Major Side Effects: Bloating; breathing difficulties; chills; cough; fever; irritation of the mouth; muscle aches; rash; rectal and vaginal itching; severe diarrhea; sore throat; superinfection

Contraindication: This drug should not be used by people allergic to any penicillin drug. Consult your doctor immediately if this drug has been prescribed for you and you have such an allergy.

Warnings: This drug should be used cautiously by people who have kidney disease or asthma or other significant allergies. Be sure your doctor knows if any of these conditions applies to you. • This drug interacts with chloramphenicol, probenecid, aspirin, phenylbutazone, indomethacin, sulfinpyrazone, erythromycin, and tetracycline; if you are currently taking any drugs of these types, consult your doctor about their use. If you are unsure of the type or contents of your medications, ask your doctor or pharmacist. • Severe allergic reactions to this drug — indicated by breathing difficulties, rash, fever and chills — have been reported but are rare when the drug is taken orally. Consult your doctor if you develop any of these symptoms while taking this drug. • Diabetics using Clinitest urine test may get a false high sugar reading while taking this drug. Change to Clinistix, Diastix, or Tes-Tape urine test to avoid this problem. • Prolonged use of this drug may allow organisms that are not susceptible to it to grow wildly. This is called a superinfection. • Do not use this drug unless your doctor has specifically told you to do so and do not take it more frequently than directed. Be sure to follow directions carefully and report any unusual reactions to your doctor at once. • This drug may affect the potency of oral contraceptives. Consult your doctor about using supplementary contraceptive measures while you are taking this drug.

Comments: "Penicillin V" is another name for this drug. • This drug has approximately the same antibacterial activity as the less expensive product penicillin G. However, this drug is more stable in the stomach and may be worth the extra cost. • This drug is similar in nature and action to amoxicillin and ampicillin. • This drug should be taken for the full prescribed course, even if symptoms disappear within that time; stopping treatment early can lead to reinfection. • Penicillin VK tablets should be stored at room temperature in a tightly closed container. • The liquid form of this drug should be stored in the refrigerator. This medication should never be frozen. Any unused portion should be discarded after 14 days. Shake well before use. • Take this drug on an empty stomach (one hour before or two hours after a meal). • It is best to take this drug at evenly spaced times throughout the day and night. Your doctor or pharmacist will help you set up a dosing schedule.

Pentids antibiotic (E. R. Squibb & Sons, Inc.), see penicillin G potassium antibiotic.

Pen-V antibiotic (Goldline Laboratories), see penicillin potassium phenoxymethyl (penicillin VK) antibiotic.

Pen-Vee K antibiotic (Wyeth-Ayerst Laboratories), see penicillin potassium phenoxymethyl (penicillin VK) antibiotic.

Pepcid antisecretory

Manufacturer: Merck Sharp & Dohme
Ingredient: famotidine
Dosage Forms: Oral suspension (content per 5 ml teaspoon): 40 mg. Tablet: 20 mg (beige); 40 mg (light brownish-orange)
Uses: Treatment of ulcers and hypersecretory conditions; prevention of recurrent ulcers
Minor Side Effects: Acne; altered sense of taste; constipation; decreased libido; diarrhea; dizziness; dry mouth; dry skin; fatigue; headache; muscle pain; nausea; somnolence; stomach upset
Major Side Effects: Anorexia; anxiety; blood disorders; breathing difficulties; depression; hair loss; palpitations; rash; tingling in the hands or feet; vomiting
Contraindication: This drug should not be taken by anyone who is allergic to it.
Warnings: This drug must be used with caution by pregnant or nursing women. Discuss the benefits and risks with your doctor. • This drug is not recommended for use in children. • Elderly persons and persons with kidney disease should use this drug cautiously; lower than normal doses may be required. • This drug has not been shown to interact with other medications; however, check with your doctor or pharmacist before taking any other medication in addition to this drug.
Comments: For best results with ulcers, this drug must be taken as directed for four to eight weeks, even if you feel better during that time. • This drug is usually taken twice a day or once daily at bedtime. • The oral suspension must be shaken well before use. • This drug is very similar in action to Zantac and Tagamet. Discuss these medications with your doctor in order to identify the best product for you.

Percocet analgesic

Manufacturer: Du Pont Pharmaceuticals, Inc.
Ingredients: acetaminophen; oxycodone hydrochloride
Equivalent Products: Oxycet, Halsey Drug Co., Inc.; oxycodone HCl and acetaminophen, various manufacturers; Roxicet, Roxane Laboratories, Inc.; Tylox, McNeil Pharmaceutical (see Comments)
Dosage Form: Tablet: acetaminophen, 325 mg and oxycodone hydrochloride, 5 mg (white)
Use: For relief of moderate to severe pain
Minor Side Effects: Anxiety; constipation, dizziness; drowsiness; euphoria; fatigue; light-headedness; loss of appetite; nausea; restlessness; sedation; sweating; vomiting; weakness
Major Side Effects: Breathing difficulties; dark urine; difficult or painful urination; hallucinations; jaundice; light-colored stools; palpitations; rash
Contraindication: This drug should not be used by persons allergic to either of its components. Consult your doctor immediately if this drug has been prescribed for you and you have such an allergy.
Warnings: This drug should be used cautiously by pregnant women, the elderly, children, persons with liver or kidney disease, persons with Addison's

disease, and in the presence of head injury or acute abdominal conditions. Be sure your doctor knows if any of these conditions applies to you. • This drug interacts with narcotic analgesics, tranquilizers, phenothiazines, sedatives, and hypnotics. If you are currently taking any drugs of these types, consult your doctor about their use. If you are unsure about the types or contents of your medications, ask your doctor or pharmacist. • Because this drug causes sedation, it should not be used with other sedative drugs or alcohol. • Avoid tasks requiring alertness, such as driving a car or operating machinery, while taking this drug. • This drug contains a narcotic, oxycodone HCl; therefore, it has the potential for abuse and must be used with caution. Tolerance may develop quickly. Do not increase your dose or take this drug more often than prescribed without first consulting your doctor. Products containing narcotics are usually not used for more than seven to ten days.

Comments: If stomach upset occurs, take this drug with food or milk. • Side effects of this drug may be somewhat relieved by lying down. • Notify your doctor if you develop signs of jaundice (yellow eyes or skin; dark urine). • While taking this medicine, be cautious of taking nonprescription medicines containing acetaminophen. • Percocet is similar to Percodan, the difference being that Percocet contains acetaminophen and Percodan contains aspirin. • For all intents and purposes, Tylox can be considered an equivalent to Percocet. Tylox contains acetaminophen, 500 mg; oxycodone HCl, 4.5 mg; and oxycodone terephthalate, 0.38 mg. • Roxicet is also available in liquid form, which contains the same amount (per 5 ml teaspoon) of acetaminophen and oxycodone as do the tablets.

Percodan analgesic

Manufacturer: Du Pont Pharmaceuticals, Inc.

Ingredients: aspirin; oxycodone hydrochloride; oxycodone terephthalate

Equivalent Products: Codoxy, Halsey Drug Co., Inc.; oxycodone hydrochloride, oxycodone terephthalate, and aspirin, various manufacturers; Roxiprin, Roxane Laboratories, Inc. (see Comments)

Dosage Form: Tablet: aspirin, 325 mg; oxycodone hydrochloride, 4.50 mg; oxycodone terephthalate, 0.38 mg (yellow)

Use: Relief of moderate to moderately severe pain

Minor Side Effects: Constipation; dizziness; drowsiness; dry mouth; euphoria; flushing; itching; light-headedness; loss of appetite; nausea; sedation; sweating; vomiting

Major Side Effects: Bloody stools; breathing difficulties; chest tightness; difficulty in urinating; jaundice; kidney disease; low blood sugar; odd movements; palpitations; rapid or slow heartbeat; rash; ringing in the ears; tremors; ulcer

Contraindication: This drug should not be taken by people who are allergic to any of its components. Consult your doctor immediately if this drug has been prescribed for you and you have such an allergy.

Warnings: This drug should be used cautiously by pregnant women, the elderly, children, and debilitated persons. It should be used cautiously by persons with anemia, colitis, lung disease, gallbladder disease, bleeding disorders, peptic ulcer, abdominal disease, head injuries, liver disease, kidney disease, thyroid disease, or prostate disease. Be sure your doctor knows if any of these conditions applies to you. • This drug must be used cautiously in conjunction with alcohol, methotrexate, 6-mercaptopurine, oral antidiabetics, phenytoin, oral anticoagulants, aspirin, or gout medications (probenecid, sulfinpyrazone). If you are unsure of the type or contents of your medications, ask your doctor or pharmacist. • This drug has the potential for abuse and must be used with caution. Tolerance may develop quickly; do not increase the dose of this drug without first consulting your doctor. • Products containing narcotics (e.g., oxycodone) are usually not used for more than seven to ten days. • This drug may cause drowsiness; avoid tasks requiring alertness, such as driving a car or operating machinery. To prevent oversedation, avoid the use of alcohol or other drugs that have sedative properties.

Comments: Take this drug with food or milk to lessen stomach upset. • While taking this medication, avoid the use of nonprescription medicines that contain aspirin. • Side effects caused by this drug may be somewhat relieved by lying down. • If your ears feel strange, if you hear buzzing or ringing, or if your stomach hurts, your dosage may need adjustment. Call your doctor. • Notify your doctor if you develop signs of jaundice (yellow eyes or skin; dark urine). • There are half-strength forms of this drug available. One is called Percodan-Demi and is also made by Du Pont Pharmaceuticals, Inc. (Only the oxycodone components are half strength.) There is also a generic form available.

Persantine antianginal and anticoagulant

Manufacturer: Boehringer Ingelheim
Ingredient: dipyridamole
Equivalent Products: dipyridamole, various manufacturers; Pyridamole, Major Pharmaceuticals
Dosage Form: Tablet: 25 mg; 50 mg; 75 mg (all are orange)
Uses: With Coumadin anticoagulant, for prevention of blood clot formation; may also be used to prevent angina (chest pain)
Minor Side Effects: Cramps; dizziness; fainting; fatigue; flushing; headache; nausea; weakness
Major Side Effects: Rash; worsening of chest pain (mainly at start of therapy)
Contraindications: None known
Warnings: This drug should be used cautiously by pregnant or nursing women and by patients with low blood pressure. This drug may cause allergic-type reactions, particularly in persons with aspirin hypersensitivity. Be sure your doctor knows if any of these conditions applies to you.
Comments: This drug is often used as a "blood thinner;" it prevents clots from forming and keeps blood flowing freely. While taking this drug, you will bleed longer than normal after a cut or scrape; be aware of this. Contact your doctor immediately if you sustain a severe cut or injury. • Your doctor may wish to perform periodic blood tests to determine the effectiveness of this drug. • This drug should be taken with a full glass of liquid on an empty stomach (one hour before or two hours after a meal) and only in the prescribed amount. • The effects of this drug may not become apparent for at least two months. • Do not suddenly stop taking this medication without consulting your doctor. • To avoid dizziness or light-headedness when you stand, contract and relax the muscles of your legs for a few moments before rising. Do this by pushing one foot against the floor while raising the other foot slightly, alternating feet so that you are "pumping" your legs. • Not all generic forms of this drug are identical. Consult your doctor or pharmacist about the use of a generic product.

Pertofrane antidepressant (Rorer Pharmaceuticals), see Norpramin antidepressant.

Phenameth with Codeine expectorant (Major Pharmaceuticals), see Phenergan, Phenergan with Codeine expectorants.

Phenaphen with Codeine analgesic (A. H. Robins Company), see acetaminophen with codeine analgesic.

Phenazodine analgesic (The Lannett Company, Inc.), see Pyridium analgesic.

phenazopyridine hydrochloride analgesic (various manufacturers), see Pyridium analgesic.

Phenergan, Phenergan with Codeine expectorants

Manufacturer: Wyeth-Ayerst Laboratories

Ingredients: promethazine hydrochloride; codeine phosphate (Phenergan with Codeine only); alcohol (syrup only)

Equivalent Products: Phenergan: promethazine hydrochloride, various manufacturers; Prothazine, Vortech Pharmaceutical, Ltd. Phenergan with Codeine: Phenameth with Codeine, Major Pharmaceuticals; promethazine hydrochloride with codeine, various manufacturers; Prometh with Codeine, Barre-National; Prothazine DC, Vortech Pharmaceutical, Ltd.

Dosage Forms: Phenergan: Liquid (content per 5 ml teaspoon): promethazine hydrochloride, 6.25 mg and alcohol, 7%. Tablet: promethazine hydrochloride, 12.5 mg (orange); 25 mg (white); 50 mg (pink). Phenergan with Codeine: Liquid (content per 5 ml teaspoon): codeine phosphate, 10 mg; promethazine hydrochloride, 6.25 mg; alcohol, 7%

Uses: Cough suppressant; relief of allergy symptoms; prevention and treatment of motion sickness and nausea and vomiting

Minor Side Effects: Blurred vision; confusion; constipation; diarrhea; dizziness; drowsiness; dry mouth, nose, and throat; headache; heartburn; insomnia; loss of appetite; nasal congestion; nausea; nervousness; rash; restlessness; sweating; trembling; vomiting; weakness

Major Side Effects: Breathing difficulties; convulsions; difficulty in urinating; disturbed coordination; excitation; jaundice; low blood pressure; muscle spasms; nightmares; palpitations; rash from exposure to sunlight; severe abdominal pain; sore throat

Contraindications: This drug should not be taken by nursing mothers, newborns, people who are allergic to any of its components, or those taking monoamine oxidase inhibitors (ask your pharmacist if you are unsure). Consult your doctor immediately if this drug has been prescribed for you and any of these conditions applies.

Warnings: This drug interacts with amphetamine, anticholinergics, levodopa, antacids, and trihexyphenidyl; if you are currently taking any drugs of these types, consult your doctor about their use. If you are unsure of the type or contents of your medications, ask your doctor or pharmacist. • This drug may cause drowsiness; avoid tasks that require alertness. To prevent oversedation, avoid the use of alcohol or other drugs that have sedative properties. • The codeine-containing form of this product has the potential for abuse and must be used with caution. It usually should not be taken for more than five days without some improvement of symptoms, nor for longer than ten days at a time if prescribed for use on a regular basis. Tolerance may develop quickly; do not increase the dosage without consulting your doctor. An overdose usually sedates an adult but may cause excitation leading to convulsions and death in a child. • This drug should be used cautiously by people who have glaucoma (certain types), asthma, high blood pressure, central nervous system disorders (such as seizures), colitis, gallbladder disease, liver disease, ulcers, blood vessel or heart disease, kidney disease, thyroid disease, bowel or bladder obstruction, prostate trouble, or diabetes. Be sure your doctor knows if any of these conditions applies to you. • This drug may affect the results of certain laboratory tests. Remind your doctor that you are taking this drug if you are scheduled for any tests.

Comments: If you need an expectorant, you need more moisture in your environment. The use of a vaporizer or humidifier may be beneficial. Consult your doctor. You should also drink nine to ten glasses of water daily. • Notify your doctor if you develop signs of jaundice (yellow eyes or skin; dark urine). • Chew gum or suck on ice chips or a piece of hard candy to reduce mouth dryness. • While taking this drug, do not take any nonprescription item for weight control, cough, cold, or sinus problems without first checking with your doctor. • This drug may make you more sensitive to the sun; avoid prolonged sun exposure.

Phenergan VC, Phenergan VC with Codeine expectorants

Manufacturer: Wyeth-Ayerst Laboratories

Ingredients: phenylephrine hydrochloride; promethazine hydrochloride; codeine phosphate (Phenergan VC with Codeine only); alcohol

Equivalent Products: Phenergan VC: Pherazine VC, Halsey Drug. Co., Inc.; promethazine hydrochloride VC, various manufacturers; Prometh VC Plain, Goldline Laboratories. Phenergan VC with Codeine: Mallergan VC with Codeine, W.E. Hauck, Inc.; Phenameth VC with Codeine, Major Pharmaceuticals; Pherazine VC with Codeine, Halsey Drug Co., Inc.; promethazine hydrochloride VC with codeine, various manufacturers; Prometh VC with Codeine, Barre-National

Dosage Form: Phenergan VC: Liquid (content per 5 ml teaspoon): phenylephrine hydrochloride, 5 mg; promethazine hydrochloride, 6.25 mg; alcohol, 7%. Phenergan VC with Codeine: Liquid (content per 5 ml teaspoon): codeine phosphate, 10 mg; phenylephrine hydrochloride, 5 mg; promethazine hydrochloride, 6.25 mg; alcohol, 7%

Uses: Relief of coughing, congestion, and other symptoms of allergies or the common cold

Minor Side Effects: Blurred vision; confusion; constipation; diarrhea; dizziness; drowsiness; dry mouth, nose, and throat; headache; heartburn; insomnia; loss of appetite; nasal congestion; nausea; nervousness; rash; restlessness; sweating; trembling; vomiting; weakness

Major Side Effects: Breathing difficulties; convulsions; difficulty in urinating; disturbed coordination; excitation; jaundice; low blood pressure; muscle spasms; nightmares; palpitations; rash from exposure to sunlight; severe abdominal pain; sore throat

Contraindications: This drug should not be taken by nursing mothers, by newborns, by people who are allergic to any of its components, and by those taking monoamine oxidase inhibitors. Consult your doctor immediately if this drug has been prescribed for you and any of these conditions applies.

Warnings: This drug interacts with amphetamine, anticholinergics, levodopa, guanethidine, antacids, and trihexyphenidyl; if you are currently taking any drugs of these types, consult your doctor about their use. If you are unsure of the type or contents of your medications, ask your doctor or pharmacist. • This drug may cause drowsiness; avoid tasks that require alertness. • To prevent oversedation, avoid the use of alcohol or other drugs that have sedative properties. • The codeine-containing form of this product has the potential for abuse and must be used with caution. It usually should not be taken for more than five days without improvement of symptoms, nor for longer than ten days at a time if prescribed for use on a regular basis. Tolerance may develop quickly; do not increase the dosage without consulting your doctor. An overdose usually sedates an adult but may cause excitation leading to convulsions and death in a child. • This drug should be used cautiously by people who have glaucoma (certain types), asthma, high blood pressure, seizure disorders, colitis, gallbladder disease, liver disease, ulcers, blood vessel or heart disease, kidney disease, thyroid disease, bowel or bladder obstruction, prostate trouble, or diabetes. Be sure your doctor knows if any of these conditions applies to you. • This drug may effect the results of certain laboratory tests. Remind your doctor that you are taking this drug if you are scheduled for any tests.

Comments: If you need an expectorant, you need more moisture in your environment. The use of a vaporizer or humidifier may be beneficial; consult your doctor. You should also drink nine to ten glasses of water daily. • Notify your doctor if you develop signs of jaundice (yellow eyes or skin; dark urine). • Chew gum or suck on ice chips or a piece of hard candy to reduce mouth dryness. • While taking this drug, do not take any nonprescription item for weight control, cough, cold, or sinus problems without first checking with your doctor. • This drug may make you more sensitive to the sun; avoid prolonged sun exposure and use a sunscreen

phenobarbital sedative and hypnotic

Manufacturer: various manufacturers
Ingredient: phenobarbital
Equivalent Products: Barbita, Vortech Pharmaceutical, Ltd.; Solfoton, Poythress Laboratories, Inc.
Dosage Forms: Capsule; Liquid; Tablet (various dosages and various colors)
Uses: Control of convulsions; relief of anxiety or tension; sleeping aid
Minor Side Effects: Diarrhea; dizziness; drowsiness; headache; muscle pain; nausea; stomach upset; vomiting
Major Side Effects: Breathing difficulties or other allergic reactions; bruising; chest tightness; confusion; depression; excitation; loss of coordination; low blood pressure; skin rash; slow heart rate; slurred speech
Contraindications: This drug should not be used by people who are allergic to it, by those who have porphyria or respiratory disease, or by those with a history of drug abuse. Consult your doctor immediately if this drug has been prescribed for you and any of these conditions applies.
Warnings: This drug should be used cautiously by people who have liver or kidney disease or certain lung diseases, by women who are pregnant or nursing, and by children. Be sure your doctor knows if any of these conditions applies to you. • This drug interacts with alcohol, central nervous system depressants, griseofulvin, oral contraceptives, cyclophosphamide, digitalis, rifampin, chloramphenicol, theophylline, aminophylline, oral anticoagulants, phenytoin, steroids, sulfonamides, tetracycline, and antidepressants; if you are currently taking any drugs of these types, consult your doctor about their use. If you are unsure of the type or contents of your medications, ask your doctor or pharmacist. • This drug may cause drowsiness; avoid tasks that require alertness. • To prevent oversedation and serious adverse reactions, avoid the use of alcohol or other drugs that have sedative properties while taking this drug. • This drug has the potential for abuse and must be used with caution. Tolerance may develop quickly; do not increase the dose without first consulting your doctor. • Do not stop taking this drug without first consulting your doctor. If you have been taking the drug for a long time, the dose should be reduced gradually. • Children may respond to this drug differently than adults; they may become excited, irritable, and aggressive. • Periodic laboratory tests may be necessary if you are taking this drug for prolonged periods.
Comments: Phenobarbital is an effective sedative and hypnotic, and it is rel-

atively inexpensive. ● Notify your doctor if you develop fever, mouth sores, sore throat, or unusual bleeding or bruising while taking this drug.

Phentox Compound decongestant and antihistamine (My-K Labs), see Naldecon decongestant and antihistamine.

phenytoin sodium anticonvulsant (various manufacturers), see Dilantin anticonvulsant.

Pherazine VC, Pherazine VC with Codeine expectorants (Halsey Drug Co., Inc.), see Phenergan VC, Phenergan VC with Codeine expectorants.

Phyllocontin bronchodilator (The Purdue Frederick Company), see aminophylline bronchodilator.

Pilocar ophthalmic preparation (Iolab), see Isopto Carpine ophthalmic preparation.

pilocarpine hydrochloride ophthalmic preparation (various manufacturers), see Isopto Carpine ophthalmic preparation.

Pilopine HS ophthalmic preparation (Alcon Laboratories, Inc.), see Isopto Carpine ophthalmic preparation.

Polycillin antibiotic (Bristol Laboratories), see ampicillin antibiotic.

Polymox antibiotic (Bristol Laboratories), see amoxicillin antibiotic.

Polytabs-F vitamin and fluoride supplement (Major Pharmaceuticals), see Poly-Vi-Flor vitamin and fluoride supplement.

Poly-Vi-Flor vitamin and fluoride supplement

Manufacturer: Mead Johnson Nutritional
Ingredients: vitamins A, D, E, C; folic acid (tablet only); thiamin; riboflavin; niacin; vitamins B_6, B_{12}; fluoride
Equivalent Products: Florvite, Everett Laboratories, Inc.; Polytabs-F, Major Pharmaceuticals; Poly-Vitamins with Fluoride, various manufacturers; Polyvite with Fluoride Drops, Geneva Generics, Inc.; Vi-Daylin/F, Ross Laboratories (see Comments)
Dosage Forms: Chewable tablet: vitamin A, 2500 I.U.; vitamin D, 400 I.U.; vitamin E, 15 mg; vitamin C, 60 mg; folic acid, 0.3 mg; thiamin, 1.05 mg; riboflavin, 1.2 mg; niacin, 13.5 mg; vitamin B_6, 1.05 mg; vitamin B_{12}, 4.5 mcg; fluoride, 1.0 mg, 0.25 mg, and 1 mg. Drops (content per ml): vitamin A, 1500 I.U.; vitamin D, 400 I.U.; vitamin E, 4.1 mg; vitamin C, 35 mg; thiamin, 0.5 mg; riboflavin, 0.6 mg; niacin, 8 mg; vitamin B_6, 0.4 mg; vitamin B_{12}, 2 mcg; fluoride, 0.5 mg and 0.25 mg

Uses: Protection against tooth decay and vitamin deficiencies in children

Minor Side Effects: Rash (rare); stomach upset

Major Side Effects: Allergic reactions

Contraindications: This product should not be used when fluoride content of drinking water is 0.7 parts per million or more. The drops form should not be used by infants from birth to two years of age in areas where the drinking water contains 0.3 parts per million or more of fluoride. If you are unsure of the fluoride content of your drinking water, ask your doctor or call your County Health Department. • This product should not be used in the presence of frank dental fluorosis.

Warnings: The recommended dose should not be exceeded or other fluoride-containing drugs given concurrently, since prolonged, excessive fluoride intake may cause dental fluorosis in children. • This drug should be used cautiously by those with heart disease, kidney disease, bone disease, or thyroid disease. • Keep this product out of the reach of children.

Comments: This product should never be referred to as candy or "candy-flavored vitamins." Your child may take you literally and swallow too many. • Mead Johnson Nutritional also manufactures a similar product, Tri-Vi-Flor vitamin and fluoride supplement, which contains only vitamins A, C, and D, and sodium fluoride. • The chewable tablets and drops discussed here are very similar to each other, but they do not contain exactly the same kinds and amounts of vitamins. Both of these products are available without fluoride as well. They are called Poly-Vi-Sol and Tri-Vi-Sol. Poly-Vi-Flor is also available with iron and may be prescribed if your doctor determines that extra iron is necessary. Numerous multiple vitamin products are available. Discuss the differences with your doctor or pharmacist, and purchase the one that best suits your needs. • Vitamins are used to supplement the diet. Discuss proper diet with your doctor to ensure that you and your family are eating balanced meals. • The drops are best suited for infants and the chewable tablets for young children.

Poly-Vi-Sol vitamin supplement (Mead Johnson Nutritional), see Poly-Vi-Flor vitamin and fluoride supplement (comments).

Poly-Vitamins with Fluoride vitamin and fluoride supplement (various manufacturers), see Poly-Vi-Flor vitamin and fluoride supplement.

Polyvite with Fluoride Drops vitamin and fluoride supplement (Geneva Generics, Inc.), see Poly-Vi-Flor vitamin and fluoride supplement.

Potachlor potassium chloride replacement (My-K Labs), see potassium chloride replacement.

Potage potassium chloride replacement (Lemmon Company), see potassium chloride replacement.

Potasalan potassium chloride replacement (The Lannett Company, Inc.), see potassium chloride replacement.

potassium chloride replacement

Manufacturer: various manufacturers
Ingredient: potassium chloride
Equivalent Products: Cena-K, Century Pharmaceuticals, Inc.; Kaochlor, Adria Laboratories, Inc.; Kaon, Adria Laboratories, Inc.; Kato, ICN Pharmaceuticals, Inc.; Kay Ciel, Forest Pharmaceuticals, Inc.; Kaylixir, The Lannett Company, Inc.; K-G, Geneva Generics, Inc.; K-Lor, Abbott Laboratories; Klor-Con, Upsher-Smith Laboratories, Inc.; Klor-Con/EF, Upsher-Smith Laboratories, Inc.; Klorvess, Sandoz Pharmaceuticals; Klotrix, Mead Johnson Nutritional; K-Lyte, Mead Johnson Nutritional; K-Lyte/Cl, Mead Johnson Nutritional; K-Lyte DS, Mead Johnson Nutritional; Kolyum, Pennwalt Pharmaceutical Division; K-Tab, Abbott Laboratories; Micro-K, A. H. Robins Company; My-K Elixir, My-K Labs; Potachlor, My-K Labs; Potage, Lemmon Company; Potasalan, The Lannett Company, Inc.; Rum-K, Fleming & Co.; Slow-K, Ciba Pharmaceutical Company; Ten-K, Ciba Pharmaceutical Company
Dosage Forms: Controlled-release capsule; Controlled-release tablet; Effervescent tablet; Liquid; Powder (various dosages and various colors)
Use: Prevention or treatment of potassium deficiency, especially that caused by diuretics
Minor Side Effects: Diarrhea; nausea; stomach pains; vomiting
Major Side Effects: Breathing difficulties; confusion; dark, tarry stools; numbness or tingling in arms or legs; palpitations; ulcer
Contraindications: This drug should not be used by people who have severe kidney disease, high blood levels of potassium, or Addison's disease. This drug should not be used by those allergic to it. Consult your doctor immediately if any of these conditions applies to you.
Warnings: This drug should be used cautiously by people who have heart disease (certain types), intestinal blockage, peptic ulcer, or acute dehydration. Be sure your doctor knows if any of these conditions applies to you. • This drug interacts with amiloride, captopril, spironolactone, and triamterene; if you are currently taking any drugs of these types, consult your doctor about their use. If you are unsure of the type or contents of your medications, ask your doctor or pharmacist. • Follow your doctor's dosage instructions exactly and do not stop taking this medication without first consulting your doctor. • Supplements of potassium should be administered with caution, since the amount of potassium deficiency may be difficult to determine accurately; too much potassium can also be dangerous. Potassium intoxication, however, rarely occurs in patients with normal kidney function. • This drug should be taken cautiously by digitalized patients, and such patients should be monitored by ECG for heart problems. • If you develop severe nausea and vomiting, black stools, abdominal pain, or unusual weakness while taking this drug, call your doctor.
Comments: This drug should be taken with food. • The liquid and powder forms of this drug may be added to one-half or one full glass of cold water, then swallowed. The effervescent tablet form of this drug must be completely dissolved in a full glass of water before being swallowed. Do not crush or chew the slow-release tablets; this form of the drug must be swallowed whole. • Ask your doctor about using a salt substitute in addition to, or instead of, potassium chloride. • Potassium supplements usually have a low rate of patient compliance. People usually take them infrequently, or they stop taking them altogether. If a potassium product is prescribed for you, be sure to take the medication exactly as directed and do not stop taking it without first consulting your doctor. • Some of these products are sugar-free. • There are many forms of this drug available. Discuss the various forms with your doctor or pharmacist to find the one that best suits you. • Ask your doctor whether you should include potassium-rich foods in your diet. Foods rich in potassium include meat, bananas, raisins,

dates, prunes, avocados, broccoli, watermelon, brussels sprouts, lentils, and spinach.

Prednicen-M steroid hormone (Central Pharmaceuticals, Inc.), see prednisone steroid hormone.

prednisone steroid hormone

Manufacturer: various manufacturers
Ingredient: prednisone
Equivalent Products: Deltasone, The Upjohn Company; Liquid Pred, Muro Pharmaceutical, Inc.; Meticorten, Schering Corp.; Orasone, Reid-Rowell; Panasol, Seatrace Co.; Prednicen-M, Central Pharmaceuticals, Inc.; Sterapred, Mayrand, Inc.
Dosage Forms: Oral Solution; Syrup (content per 5 ml teaspoon): 5 mg. Tablet: 1 mg; 2.5 mg; 5 mg; 10 mg; 20 mg; 25 mg; 50 mg (various colors)
Uses: Treatment of endocrine or rheumatic disorders; asthma; blood diseases; certain cancers; eye disorders; gastrointestinal disturbances such as ulcerative colitis; respiratory diseases; inflammations such as arthritis, dermatitis, and poison ivy
Minor Side Effects: Dizziness; headache; increased hair growth; increased susceptibility to infection; increased sweating; indigestion; insomnia; menstrual irregularities; muscle weakness; nervousness; reddening of the skin on the face; restlessness; thin skin; weight gain
Major Side Effects: Abdominal enlargement; blurred vision; bone loss; bruising; cataracts; convulsions; diabetes; euphoria; fluid retention; fracture; glaucoma; growth impairment in children; heart failure; high blood pressure; impaired healing of wounds; mood changes; mouth sores; muscle wasting; nightmares; peptic ulcer; potassium loss; salt retention; weakness
Contraindications: This drug should not be taken by people who are allergic to it or by those who have systemic fungal infections. Consult your doctor if this drug has been prescribed for you and either of these conditions applies.
Warnings: If you use this drug for more than a week and are subjected to stress such as serious infection, injury, or surgery, you may need to receive higher dosages. • This drug may mask signs of infection or cause new infections to develop. • This drug may cause glaucoma or cataracts, high blood pressure, high blood sugar, fluid retention, and potassium loss. • This drug has not been proven safe for use during pregnancy. • While you are taking this drug you should not be vaccinated or immunized. • This drug should be used cautiously by people who have had tuberculosis and by those who have thyroid disease, liver disease, severe ulcerative colitis, diabetes, seizures, a history of ulcers, kidney disease, high blood pressure, a bone disease, or myasthenia gravis. Be sure your doctor knows if any of these conditions applies to you. • If you have been taking this drug for more than a week, do not stop taking it suddenly. Your doctor will gradually reduce your dose. Never increase the dose or take the drug for a longer time than prescribed without consulting your doctor. • Report mood swings or depression to your doctor. • Growth of children may be affected by this drug. • This drug interacts with aspirin, barbiturates, diuretics, rifampin, cyclophosphamide, estrogens, indomethacin, oral anticoagulants, antidiabetics, and phenytoin; if you are currently taking any drugs of these types, consult your doctor about their use. If you are unsure of the type or contents of your medications, ask your doctor or pharmacist. • Blood pressure, body weight, and vision should be checked at regular intervals. Stomach X rays are advised for persons with suspected or known peptic ulcers who take this drug for a prolonged period.

Comments: This drug is often taken on a decreasing-dosage schedule (four times a day for several days, then three times a day, etc.). • Often, taking the entire daily dose at one time (about 8:00 A.M.) gives the best results. • To help avoid potassium loss while using this drug, take your dose with a glass of fresh or frozen orange juice, or eat a banana each day. The use of a salt substitute also helps prevent potassium loss. Do not change your diet, however, without consulting your doctor. Too much potassium may also be dangerous. • If you are using this drug chronically, you should wear or carry a notice that you are taking a steroid. • To prevent stomach upset, take this drug with food or a snack. • Take this drug exactly as directed. Do not take extra doses or skip a dose without first consulting your doctor. For long-term treatment, taking the drug every other day is permitted. Ask your doctor about alternate-day dosing.

Premarin estrogen hormone

Manufacturer: Wyeth-Ayerst Laboratories
Ingredients: conjugated estrogens
Equivalent Products: conjugated estrogens, various manufacturers; Progens, Major Pharmaceuticals
Dosage Forms: Tablet: 0.3 mg (green); 0.625 mg (maroon); 0.9 mg (white); 1.25 mg (yellow); 2.5 mg (purple). Vaginal Cream (per gram): 0.625 mg
Uses: Estrogen replacement therapy; symptoms of menopause; treatment of prostatic cancer in men, uterine bleeding, and some cases of breast cancer; and prevention of osteoporosis
Minor Side Effects: Bleeding; bloating; change in sexual desire; cramps; depression; diarrhea; dizziness; headache; increased sensitivity to sunlight; loss of appetite; nausea; swelling of ankles and feet; vomiting
Major Side Effects: Allergic rash; breathing difficulties; cervical damage; change in menstrual patterns; chest pain; cystitis; diabetes; eye damage; fibroid growth; fluid retention; fungal infections; gallbladder disease; high blood pressure; jaundice; loss of coordination; migraine; pain in calves; severe headache; skin color changes; slurred speech; vision changes; weight gain or loss
Contraindications: This drug should not be used by pregnant women, by people who have blood clotting disorders or a history of such disorders due to estrogen use, or by those who have certain cancers or vaginal bleeding. In most cases, this drug should not be used by people who have breast cancer. Consult your doctor immediately if this drug has been prescribed for you and any of these conditions applies.
Warnings: Studies have shown that prolonged use of estrogens increases the risk of endometrial cancer. Your pharmacist has a brochure that describes the benefits and risks involved with estrogen therapy. Your pharmacist is required by law to give you a copy each time you have your prescription filled. Read this material carefully. • This drug should be used cautiously by people who have asthma, diabetes, epilepsy, gallbladder disease, heart disease, high blood levels of calcium, high blood pressure, kidney disease, liver disease, migraine, porphyria, uterine fibroid tumors, or a history of depression and by nursing women. Be sure your doctor knows if any of these conditions applies to you. • This drug may retard bone growth and therefore should be used cautiously by young patients who have not yet completed puberty. • This drug interacts with oral anticoagulants, barbiturates, rifampin, ampicillin, anticonvulsants, and steroids; if you are currently taking any drugs of these types, consult your doctor about their use. If you are unsure of the type or contents of your medications, ask your doctor or pharmacist. • This drug may alter the body's tolerance to glucose. Diabetics should monitor urine sugar or blood glucose and report any changes to their doctors. • Notify your doctor immediately if you experience abnormal vaginal bleeding, breast lumps, pains in the calves or

chest, sudden shortness of breath, coughing up of blood, severe headaches, dizziness, faintness, changes in vision or skin color, or dark urine. • This drug may affect a number of laboratory tests; remind your doctor that you are taking it if you are scheduled for any tests. • You should have a complete physical examination at least once a year while you are on this medication.

Comments: This drug is usually taken for 21 days followed by a seven-day rest. • Compliance is mandatory with this drug. Take it exactly as prescribed. • This drug is probably effective in preventing estrogen-deficiency osteoporosis when used in conjunction with calcium and exercise. • Special applicators are available with the vaginal cream to ensure proper dosing. Insert the cream high into the vagina unless otherwise directed.

Prenatal 1 mg + Iron vitamin-mineral supplement (Everett Laboratories, Inc.), see Stuartnatal 1+1 vitamin-mineral supplement.

Prenatal-1 vitamin-mineral supplement (Major Pharmaceuticals), see Stuartnatal 1+1 vitamin-mineral supplement.

Principen antibiotic (E. R. Squibb & Sons, Inc.), see ampicillin antibiotic.

procainamide hydrochloride antiarrhythmic (various manufacturers), see Pronestyl antiarrhythmic.

Procamide SR antiarrhythmic (Reid-Rowell), see Pronestyl antiarrhythmic.

Procan SR antiarrhythmic (Parke-Davis), see Pronestyl antiarrhythmic.

Procardia antianginal

Manufacturer: Pfizer Laboratories Division
Ingredient: nifedipine
Equivalent Product: Adalat, Miles Pharmaceutical
Dosage Form: Capsule: 10 mg (orange); 20 mg (orange and light brown)
Use: Treatment of various types of angina (chest pain)
Minor Side Effects: Bloating; blurred vision; cough; dizziness; flushing; gas; giddiness; headache; heartburn; heat sensation; loss of balance; muscle cramps; nasal congestion; nausea; nervousness; sleep disturbances; sweating; tremors; weakness
Major Side Effects: Breathing difficulties; chills; confusion; fainting; fever; impotence; low blood pressure; mood changes; rapid and pounding heart rate; sore throat; swelling of ankles, feet, or lower legs
Contraindication: This drug should not be used by people who are allergic to it. Consult your doctor immediately if this drug has been prescribed for you and you have such an allergy.
Warnings: This drug should be used cautiously by people who have low blood pressure or heart disease (certain types) and by pregnant or nursing women. Be sure your doctor knows if any of these conditions applies to you. • This drug may interact with beta blockers, digoxin, phenytoin, quinidine, warfarin, calcium supplements, and digitalis. If you are taking antihypertensive medication, the dose may have to be adjusted. If you are currently taking any of these drug types, consult your doctor about their use. If you are unsure of the

type or contents of your medications, ask your doctor or pharmacist. • This drug may make you dizzy, especially during the first few days of therapy; avoid activities that require alertness, and limit your consumption of alcohol, which exaggerates this effect.

Comments: Your doctor may want to see you regularly while you are taking this drug to check your response and to conduct liver function tests. • Learn how to monitor your pulse and blood pressure; discuss this with your doctor. • It may take several days before the effects of this drug are noticed. Compliance is necessary to prevent chest pain. This drug will not stop an attack of chest pain that is already in progress. • Swallow the capsule whole without breaking or chewing it unless otherwise instructed by your physician. • Do not suddenly stop taking this drug, unless you consult with your doctor first. Your dosage may have to be decreased gradually. • Protect this drug from light and moisture. • If you feel dizzy or light-headed, sit or lie down for a while; get up slowly from a sitting or reclining position, and be careful on stairs. • Contact your doctor if this drug causes severe or persistent dizziness, constipation, nausea, shortness of breath, swelling of hands and feet, or irregular heartbeat.

prochlorperazine phenothiazine (various manufacturers), see Compazine phenothiazine.

Progens estrogen hormone (Major Pharmaceuticals), see Premarin estrogen hormone.

Proloid thyroid hormone (Parke-Davis), see thyroid hormone.

promethazine hydrochloride expectorant plain (various manufacturers), see Phenergan, Phenergan with Codeine expectorants.

promethazine hydrochloride VC expectorant (various manufacturers), see Phenergan VC, Phenergan VC with Codeine expectorants.

promethazine hydrochloride VC with codeine expectorant (various manufacturers), see Phenergan VC, Phenergan VC with Codeine expectorants.

promethazine hydrochloride with codeine expectorant (various manufacturers), see Phenergan, Phenergan with Codeine expectorants.

Prometh VC Plain, Prometh VC with Codeine expectorants (Barre-National), see Phenergan VC, Phenergan VC with Codeine expectorants.

Prometh with Codeine expectorant (Barre-National), see Phenergan, Phenergan with Codeine expectorants.

Promine antiarrhythmic (Major Pharmaceuticals), see Pronestyl antiarrhythmic.

Pronestyl antiarrhythmic

Manufacturer: Princeton Pharmaceutical Products
Ingredient: procainamide hydrochloride
Equivalent Products: procainamide hydrochloride, various manufacturers; Procamide SR, Reid-Rowell; Procan SR, Parke-Davis; Promine, Major Pharmaceuticals; Rhythmin, Sidmark Co.
Dosage Forms: Capsule: 250 mg (yellow); 375 mg (white/orange); 500 mg (yellow/orange). Sustained-release tablet: 500 mg (greenish yellow). Tablet: 250 mg (yellow); 375 mg (orange); 500 mg (red); see Comments
Use: Treatment of some heart arrhythmias
Minor Side Effects: Bitter taste in the mouth; diarrhea; dizziness; dry mouth; headache; itching; loss of appetite; nausea; stomach upset; vomiting
Major Side Effects: Bruising; chest pains; chills; confusion; depression; fatigue; fever; giddiness; hallucinations; low blood pressure; pain in the joints; palpitations; psychosis; rash; sore throat; weakness
Contraindications: This drug should not be taken by people who are allergic to it or to some local anesthetics. The drug should not be taken by people who have myasthenia gravis or certain types of heart disease. Consult your doctor immediately if this drug has been prescribed for you and any of these conditions applies.
Warnings: People who have liver or kidney disease or certain types of heart disease should use this drug with caution. Be sure your doctor knows if any of these conditions applies to you. • Notify your doctor if you experience soreness around the mouth, throat, or gums; unexplained fever; a head cold or respiratory infection; or joint pain or stiffness.
Comments: This drug may interact with other heart drugs, diuretics, lidocaine, and cimetidine. If you are taking any drugs of these types, ask your doctor about their use. If you are unsure about the type or contents of your medications, ask your doctor or pharmacist. • Alcohol consumption may affect the way the body handles this drug. Use caution if you consume alcohol while taking this drug. While taking this drug, do not take any nonprescription item for weight control, cough, cold or sinus problems without first checking with your doctor. • Follow your doctor's dosage instructions carefully; it is especially important that this drug be taken on schedule. It should be taken at evenly spaced intervals around the clock. Do not take extra doses and do not skip a dose without first consulting your doctor. • It is best to take this drug on an empty stomach (one hour before or two hours after meals). However, if this drug causes stomach upset, it may be taken with food or milk. • Chew gum or suck on ice chips or a piece of hard candy to reduce mouth dryness. • Do not crush or chew any of the dosage forms of this drug; it must be swallowed whole. • Sustained-release tablets require less frequent dosing than the regular tablets. Sustained-release tablets should not be used for initial therapy but can be substituted once the dosage is stabilized. Consult your doctor about the use of this dosage form. • Some of products that are equivalent to Pronestyl are also available in 250 mg, 750 mg, and 1000 mg sustained-release capsules. • Do not be alarmed if you notice an empty tablet in your bowel movements. This is the core of the tablet, which is made of wax. Since it is not digestible, it is excreted from the body. • Your doctor may want to check your blood levels of this drug periodically. Blood levels indicate the effectiveness of the dosage.

Propacet 100 analgesic (Lemmon Company), see Darvocet-N analgesic.

propoxyphene hydrochloride compound analgesic (various manufacturers), see Darvon Compound-65 analgesic.

propoxyphene napsylate and acetaminophen analgesic (various manufacturers), see Darvocet-N analgesic.

propranolol and hydrochlorothiazide diuretic and antihypertensive (various manufacturers), see Inderide diuretic and antihypertensive.

propranolol beta blocker

Manufacturer: various manufacturers

Ingredient: propranolol hydrochloride

Equivalent Products: Inderal, Wyeth-Ayerst Laboratories; Ipran, Major Pharmaceuticals

Dosage Forms: Sustained-release capsule: 80 mg; 120 mg; 160 mg. Tablet: 10 mg; 20 mg; 40 mg; 60 mg; 80 mg; 90 mg (see Comments)

Uses: Treatment of angina pectoris, certain heart arrhythmias, and thyroid disorders; prevention of heart attacks, high blood pressure, and migraine headaches

Minor Side Effects: Abdominal cramps; blurred vision; constipation; dry mouth; fatigue; gas; insomnia; light-headedness; loss of appetite; nausea; sweating; vomiting; weakness

Major Side Effects: Breathing difficulties; bruises; cold hands and feet; decreased sexual ability; depression; diarrhea; difficulty in urinating; dizziness; fever; hair loss; hallucinations; heart failure; nightmares; rash; ringing in the ears; shortness of breath; slow pulse; slurred speech; sore throat; tingling in fingers; visual disturbances

Contraindications: This drug should not be used by persons with bronchial asthma, severe hay fever, or certain types of heart problems. Be sure your doctor knows if any of these conditions applies to you. • This drug should not be used with monoamine oxidase inhibitors or during the two-week withdrawal period from such drugs. If you are currently taking any drugs of this type, consult your doctor about their use. If you are unsure of the type or contents of your medications, ask your doctor or pharmacist.

Warnings: This drug should be used with caution by persons with certain respiratory problems, diabetes, certain types of heart problems, liver and kidney diseases, hypoglycemia, or thyroid disease. Be sure your doctor knows if any of these conditions applies to you. • Diabetics taking this medication should watch for signs of altered blood glucose levels. • This drug should be used cautiously by pregnant women. • This drug should be used with care during anesthesia. If possible, this drug should be withdrawn 48 hours prior to major surgery. • This drug should be used cautiously when insulin, digoxin, reserpine, cimetidine, theophylline, or aminophylline are taken. • Do not suddenly stop taking this drug unless directed to do so by your doctor. Your doctor will reduce your dosage gradually or substitute another drug if this medication is no longer to be used.

Comments: Your doctor may want you to take your pulse and blood pressure every day while you take this medication. Discuss this with your doctor. • Be sure to take your medication doses at the same time each day. It is best to take it with food. • While taking this drug, do not take any nonprescription item for weight control, cough, cold, or sinus problems without first checking with your doctor; such medications may contain ingredients that can increase blood pressure. • Notify your doctor if breathing difficulties, dizziness, or diarrhea develops. • This drug is of value in preventing further heart attacks among patients who have already suffered a heart attack. • This drug may make you more sensitive to the cold; dress warmly. • The sustained-release capsule form of this drug is available under the name Inderal LA, which requires less frequent dosing. Consult your doctor about its use.

Prothazine DC expectorant (Vortech Pharmaceutical, Ltd.), see Phenergan, Phenergan with Codeine expectorants.

Prothazine expectorant (Vortech Pharmaceutical, Ltd.), see Phenergan, Phenergan with Codeine expectorants.

Protostat antimicrobial and antiparasitic (Ortho Pharmaceutical Corp.), see Flagyl antimicrobial and antiparasitic.

Proval analgesic (Reid-Rowell), see acetaminophen with codeine analgesic.

Proventil bronchodilator (Schering Corp.), see Ventolin bronchodilator.

Provera progesterone hormone

Manufacturer: The Upjohn Company
Ingredient: medroxyprogesterone acetate
Equivalent Products: Amen, Carnrick Laboratories, Inc.; Curretab, Reid-Provident Laboratories, Inc.
Dosage Form: Tablet: 2.5 mg (orange); 5 mg (white); 10 mg (white)
Uses: Treatment of abnormal menstrual bleeding, difficult menstruation, or lack of menstruation
Minor Side Effects: Acne; dizziness; hair growth; headache; nausea; sensitivity to the sun; vomiting
Major Side Effects: Breast tenderness; birth defects (if used during pregnancy); cervical damage; change in menstrual patterns; depression; fainting; fluid retention; hair loss; itching; jaundice; rash; spotting or breakthrough or unusual vaginal bleeding; weight gain or loss
Contraindications: This drug should not be taken by people who have cancer of the breast or genitals, clotting disorders or a history of clotting disorders, vaginal bleeding of unknown cause, or liver disease; by those who are pregnant, especially during the first trimester; or by those who have had a stroke. The drug should not be used by anyone with a history of missed abortion (retention of a dead fetus in the uterus for a number of weeks). This drug should not be used if you are allergic to it. Consult your doctor immediately if this drug has been prescribed for you and any of these conditions applies. • This drug should not be used as a test to determine pregnancy.
Warnings: This drug should be used cautiously by nursing women and by people who have porphyria, gallbladder disease, epilepsy, migraine, asthma, heart or kidney disease, depression, or diabetes. Be sure your doctor knows if any of these conditions applies to you. • Watch for early signs of clotting disorders, loss of vision, or headache; report any such signs to your doctor immediately. • Notify your doctor if any unusual vaginal bleeding occurs. • If you take this drug and later discover that you are pregnant, consult your doctor immediately. • This drug should not be used in conjunction with oral anticoagulants, barbiturates, or steroids; if you are currently taking any drugs of these types, consult your doctor about their use. If you are unsure about the type or contents of your medications, ask your doctor or pharmacist. • Before you begin to take this drug, you should have a complete physical examination,

including a Pap smear. • Very little is known about the long-term effects of using this drug. Consider your decision to use it carefully. • This drug may mask the signs of menopause. • This drug may affect the results of many laboratory tests and other medical examinations. Be sure your doctor knows you are taking this drug if you are being tested for any medical condition.

Comments: Progesterone-type drugs have been included in birth control pills. It is thought that most of the adverse effects of the pill are due to the estrogen component rather than the progesterone, but this has not been proven. For a more complete listing of the adverse effects associated with these hormones, see the profile on oral contraceptives. • Your pharmacist has a brochure that describes this drug. Your pharmacist is required by law to give you a copy each time you have your prescription filled. Read this material carefully. • Notify your doctor if you develop signs of jaundice (yellow eyes or skin; dark urine).

Pyridamole antianginal and anticoagulant (Major Pharmaceuticals), see Persantine antianginal.

Pyridiate analgesic (various manufacturers), see Pyridium analgesic.

Pyridium analgesic

Manufacturer: Parke-Davis
Ingredient: phenazopyridine hydrochloride
Equivalent Products: Azo-Standard, Webcon Drug Co.; Baridium, Pfeiffer; Di-Azo, Kay Pharmacal Co., Inc.; Geridium, Goldline Laboratories; Phenazodine, The Lannett Company, Inc.; phenazopyridine hydrochloride, various manufacturers; Pyridiate, various manufacturers; Urodine, various manufacturers; Urogesic, Edwards Pharmacal (see Comments)
Dosage Form: Tablet: 100 mg; 200 mg (both are maroon)
Use: Symptomatic relief of the burning and pain of urinary tract disorders
Minor Side Effects: Change in urine color; dizziness; headache; indigestion; nausea; stomach cramps; vomiting
Major Side Effects: Anemia; jaundice; rash
Contraindications: This drug should not be taken by people who are allergic to phenazopyridine hydrochloride or by those who have severe kidney disease. Consult your doctor immediately if this drug has been prescribed for you and either of these conditions applies.
Warnings: This drug should be used with caution by pregnant women and by elderly persons. • This drug will cause your urine to become orange-red in color. Do not be alarmed by this side effect. The urine will return to its normal color soon after the drug has been discontinued. • This drug should not be used for pain other than that associated with the urinary tract. • Diabetics may get a false reading for sugar or ketones while using this drug. • This drug may interfere with certain urine and blood laboratory tests. • This drug is often used in combination with an antibiotic to treat urinary tract infections. Treatment with this drug should not exceed two days. Studies indicate that this drug, taken in conjunction with an antibiotic, is no more effective if taken for more than two days.
Comments: Take this drug with at least a full glass of water. Drink at least eight to ten glasses of water daily. This drug is best when taken after meals. • Notify your doctor if you develop signs of jaundice (yellow eyes or skin; dark urine). • Azo-Standard, Baridium, and Di-Azo are available without prescription in 100 mg strength tablets. Compare prices, and ask your doctor or pharmacist about using the nonprescription brands. • Parke-Davis also makes Pyridium

Plus tablets; each tablet contains phenazopyridine hydrochloride, 150 mg; hyoscyamine hydrobromide, 0.3 mg; and butabarbital, 15 mg. Due to the antispasmodic and sedative ingredients, it may be more effective than Pyridium for some persons. Pyridium Plus is available by prescription only.

Pyridium Plus analgesic (Parke-Davis), see Pyridium analgesic (comments).

Quibron-T bronchodilator (Bristol Laboratories), see theophylline bronchodilator.

Quinidex Extentabs antiarrhythmic (A. H. Robins Company), see quinidine sulfate antiarrhythmic.

quinidine sulfate antiarrhythmic

Manufacturer: various manufacturers
Ingredient: quinidine sulfate
Equivalent Products: Cin-Quin, Reid-Rowell; Quinidex Extentabs, A. H. Robins Company; Quinora, Key Pharmaceuticals, Inc. (see Comments)
Dosage Forms: Capsule: 200 mg; 300 mg. Sustained-release tablet: 300 mg. Tablet: 100 mg; 200 mg; 300 mg (various colors)
Use: Treatment of certain types of heart arrhythmias
Minor Side Effects: Abdominal pain; bitter taste in mouth; confusion; cramping; diarrhea; flushing; loss of appetite; nausea; restlessness; vomiting
Major Side Effects: Anemia; bleeding; blurred vision; breathing difficulties; bruising; dizziness; fainting; fever; headache; jaundice; light-headedness; palpitations; ringing in the ears; sore throat
Contraindications: This drug should not be used by people who are allergic to it or by those who have had a blood disease caused by previous quinidine therapy. Consult your doctor immediately if this drug has been prescribed for you and either of these conditions applies.
Warnings: This drug should be used cautiously by people who are also taking digitalis; by those who have liver or kidney disease, low blood pressure, low blood levels of potassium, myasthenia gravis, thyroid disease, or certain types of heart disease; and by pregnant women. Be sure your doctor knows if any of these conditions applies to you. • The amount of potassium in your blood affects the activity of quinidine. Your doctor will want to check your blood potassium levels occasionally while you take quinidine. • This drug interacts with acetazolamide, anticholinergics, antacids, anticonvulsants, diuretics, oral anticoagulants, sodium bicarbonate, and potassium. If you are currently taking any drugs of these types, consult your doctor about their use. If you are unsure of the type or contents of your medications, ask your doctor or pharmacist. • If you take this drug for prolonged periods, your doctor may perform blood tests to monitor its effectiveness. • If you develop ringing or thumping in your ears, light-headedness, or blurred vision, contact your doctor immediately; these may be symptoms of drug toxicity.
Comments: Although many quinidine sulfate products are on the market, they are not all bioequivalent; that is, they may not all be absorbed into the bloodstream at the same rate or have the same overall pharmacologic activity. To make sure you are receiving an identically functioning product, don't change brands of this drug without consulting your doctor or pharmacist • If you are being treated for a heart arrhythmia, do not take any nonprescription item for weight control, cough, cold, or sinus problems without first checking with your

doctor. • Take this medication with food or milk to help avoid stomach upset. • Take this drug exactly as directed. Do not take extra doses or skip a dose without first consulting your doctor. Do not stop taking it unless your doctor advises you to do so. • Notify your doctor if you develop signs of jaundice (yellow eyes or skin; dark urine). • The sustained-release tablet form of this drug must be swallowed whole; do not crush or chew.

Quinora antiarrhythmic (Key Pharmaceuticals, Inc.), see quinidine sulfate antiarrhythmic.

Razepam sedative and hypnotic (Major Pharmaceuticals), see Restoril sedative and hypnotic.

Reclomide gastrointestinal stimulant (Major Pharmaceuticals), see Reglan gastrointestinal stimulant.

Rectacort steroid-hormone-containing anorectal product (Century Pharmaceuticals, Inc.), see Anusol-HC steroid-hormone-containing anorectal product.

Reglan gastrointestinal stimulant

Manufacturer: A. H. Robins Company
Ingredient: metoclopramide
Equivalent Products: Clopra, Quantum Pharmics; Maxolon, Beecham Laboratories; metoclopramide, various manufacturers; Octamide, Adria Laboratories, Inc.; Reclomide, Major Pharmaceuticals
Dosage Forms: Syrup (content per 5 ml teaspoon): 5 mg. Tablet: 10 mg (pink)
Uses: Relief of the symptoms associated with diabetic gastric stasis or gastric reflux; prevention of nausea and vomiting
Minor Side Effects: Diarrhea; dizziness; drowsiness; fatigue; headache; insomnia; nausea; restlessness
Major Side Effects: Anxiety; depression; involuntary movements of the face, mouth, jaw, and tongue; uncoordinated movements
Contraindications: This drug should not be used by persons with pheochromocytoma or epilepsy or in the presence of gastrointestinal bleeding, obstruction, or perforation. Reglan should not be prescribed for persons who are allergic to it. Consult your doctor if this drug has been prescribed for you and any of these conditions applies.
Warnings: This drug should be used cautiously by children and by nursing mothers. • This drug should be used with extreme caution during pregnancy. Talk to your doctor about the use of this medication if you are pregnant. • Diabetics who require insulin should use this drug cautiously, as the dosage or timing of the insulin may need adjustment. Discuss this with your doctor. • This drug may cause motor restlessness, uncoordinated movements, or fine tremors of the tongue. Contact your doctor immediately if you notice any of these symptoms. • Because this drug may cause drowsiness, avoid tasks that require alertness for a few hours after taking each dose. • This drug interacts with narcotic analgesics, anticholinergics, alcohol, sedatives, hypnotics, and tranquilizers. If you are currently taking any drugs of these types, consult your doctor about their use. If you are unsure about the types or contents of your medications, ask your doctor or pharmacist. • Persons with previously detected breast cancer should be monitored closely while using this drug. An increase in

breast cancer has been found in laboratory rats who were given large doses of this drug for a prolonged period. These findings have not been duplicated in humans.

Comments: This medication is usually taken 30 minutes before each meal. For maximum benefit, take this drug exactly as prescribed. Do not take extra doses or skip doses without first consulting your doctor. • Because this drug causes stimulation of the gastrointestinal tract, talk to your doctor about the effect this may have on any other medications you are taking. For some drugs, the timing of doses may need to be adjusted. • If you experience involuntary movements of the face, hands, legs, or eyes, call your doctor.

Relaxadon sedative and anticholinergic (Geneva Generics, Inc.), see Donnatal sedative and anticholinergic.

Reposans-10 antianxiety (Wesley Pharmacal Co.), see Librium antianxiety.

Resaid S.R. antihistamine and decongestant (Geneva Generics, Inc.), see Ornade Spansules antihistamine and decongestant.

Respbid bronchodilator (Boehringer Ingelheim), see theophylline bronchodilator.

Restoril sedative and hypnotic

Manufacturer: Sandoz Pharmaceuticals
Ingredient: temazepam
Equivalent Products: Razepam, Major Pharmaceuticals; Temaz, Quantum Pharmics; temazepam, various manufacturers
Dosage Form: Capsule: 15 mg (maroon/pink); 30 mg (maroon/blue)
Use: Short-term relief of insomnia
Minor Side Effects: Constipation; decreased sex drive; diarrhea; dizziness; drowsiness; dry mouth; heartburn; lethargy; loss of appetite; relaxed feeling
Major Side Effects: Blurred vision; breathing disorders; confusion; depression; euphoria; hallucinations; palpitations; tremors; weakness
Contraindications: This drug should not be used by persons allergic to it or by pregnant women. Consult your doctor immediately if this drug has been prescribed for you and either of these conditions applies.
Warnings: This drug should be used with caution by depressed people; nursing mothers; persons under the age of 18; and people with liver or kidney diseases, narrow-angle glaucoma, or psychosis. Be sure your doctor knows if any of these conditions applies to you. • Because this drug has the potential for abuse, it must be used with caution, especially by those with a history of drug dependence. Tolerance may develop quickly; do not increase the dose or take this drug more often than prescribed without first consulting your doctor. If you have been taking this drug for a long time, do not stop taking it suddenly unless directed to do so by your doctor. Your doctor may gradually reduce your dosage. • When this drug is combined with other sedative drugs or alcohol, serious adverse reactions may develop. Avoid the use of alcohol, other sedatives, or central nervous system depressants. If you are currently taking any drugs of these types, consult your doctor about their use. If you are unsure of the type or contents of your medications, ask your doctor or pharmacist. • This drug causes drowsiness; avoid tasks that require alertness. • The elderly are more sensitive to this drug, so smaller doses are often prescribed for them.

Comments: After you stop taking this drug, your sleep may be disturbed for a few nights. • Take this drug one-half to one hour before bedtime unless otherwise prescribed. • This drug is similar in action to Dalmane but has a shorter duration of action. Restoril is believed to cause less sluggishness and lethargy in the morning than Dalmane does.

Retin-A acne preparation

Manufacturer: Ortho Pharmaceutical Corp.
Ingredient: tretinoin (retinoic acid; vitamin A acid)
Dosage Forms: Cream: 0.025%; 0.05%; 0.1%. Gel: 0.025%; 0.01%. Liquid: 0.05%
Use: Topical application in treatment of acne vulgaris
Minor Side Effects: Localized rash; stinging
Major Side Effects: Blistering or crusting of the skin; heightened susceptibility to sunlight; peeling; temporary change in skin color
Contraindication: This drug should not be used by people who are allergic to it. Consult your doctor immediately if this drug has been prescribed for you and you have such an allergy.
Warnings: This drug should not be used in conjunction with other acne preparations, particularly peeling agents containing sulfur, resorcinol, benzoyl peroxide, or salicylic acid. • While using this drug, exposure to sunlight (or sunlamps), wind, and/or cold should be minimized or totally avoided to prevent skin irritation. If you are sunburned, wait for the sunburn to heal before using this product. • This drug should be used with extreme caution by persons suffering from eczema. • Medicated or abrasive soaps, cosmetics that have a strong drying effect, and locally applied products containing high amounts of alcohol, spices, or lime should be used with caution because of a possible negative interaction with the drug. • Applying this product more often than recommended will not hasten improvement of the condition and is likely to cause further irritation.
Comments: This drug should be kept away from the eyes, the mouth, the angles of the nose, and the mucous membranes. • A temporary feeling of warmth or a slight stinging may be noted following application of this drug. This effect is normal and not dangerous. • The liquid form of this drug may be applied with a fingertip, gauze pad, or cotton swab. If gauze or cotton is used, do not oversaturate so that the liquid runs onto areas that are not intended for treatment. • During the early weeks of using this drug, there may be an apparent increase in skin lesions. This is usually not a reason to discontinue its use; however, your doctor may wish to modify the concentration of the drug. Therapeutic effects may be noted within two to three weeks although more than six weeks may be required before definite benefits are seen. • There are claims that Retin-A can help prevent premature aging of the skin and help eliminate wrinkles. This drug is not approved for such a purpose. More studies are needed to evaluate these claims. You may want to discuss this with your doctor.

Rhinolar-EX 12 antihistamine and decongestant (McGregor Pharmaceuticals), see Ornade Spansules antihistamine and decongestant.

Rhythmin antiarrhythmic (Sidmark Co.), see Pronestyl antiarrhythmic.

Ritalin central nervous system stimulant

Manufacturer: Ciba Pharmaceutical Company

Ingredient: methylphenidate hydrochloride

Equivalent Product: methylphenidate hydrochloride, various manufacturers

Dosage Forms: Sustained-release tablet: 20 mg (white). Tablet: 5 mg (yellow); 10 mg (green); 20 mg (yellow) (see Comments)

Uses: Treatment of hyperactivity in children; treatment of narcolepsy; relief of mild depression

Minor Side Effects: Abdominal pain; dizziness; drowsiness; dry mouth; headache; insomnia; loss of appetite; nausea; nervousness; vomiting; weakness

Major Side Effects: Bruising; chest pain; fever; hair loss; heart irregularities; high or low blood pressure; hives; joint pain; mood changes; palpitations; psychosis; rash; seizures; sore throat; uncoordinated movements. In children: abdominal pain; impairment of growth; weight loss

Contraindications: This drug should not be taken by persons with marked anxiety, tension, or agitation, since it may aggravate these symptoms. This drug should not be taken by people who are allergic to it or by people with glaucoma. Consult your doctor immediately if this drug has been prescribed for you and any of these conditions applies.

Warnings: This drug is not recommended for use by children under six years of age, since suppression of growth has been reported with long-term use. The long term effects of this drug on children have not been well established. Your doctor may want to stop the medication periodically to determine effectiveness. Treatment is usually discontinued after puberty. • This drug should be used cautiously by persons with severe depression, epilepsy, high blood pressure, or eye disease. Be sure your doctor knows if any of these conditions applies to you. • This drug should not be used for the prevention or treatment of normal fatigue. • This drug should be used with caution by pregnant women and women of childbearing age. • This drug should be used cautiously by people with a history of drug dependence or alcoholism. Do not increase the dose of this drug without consulting your doctor. Chronic abuse of this drug can lead to tolerance and psychological dependence. • Do not stop taking this drug without consulting your doctor. • Periodic blood tests are recommended for patients on long-term therapy with this drug. • This drug interacts with acetazolamide, guanethidine, monoamine oxidase inhibitors, sodium bicarbonate, antidepressants, anticoagulants, anticonvulsants, and phenylbutazone. If you are currently taking any drugs of these types, consult your doctor about their use. If you are unsure of the type or contents of your medications, ask your doctor or pharmacist.

Comments: To avoid sleeplessness, this drug should not be taken later than 6:00 P.M. • While taking this drug, do not take any nonprescription item for weight control, cough, cold, or sinus problems without first checking with your doctor. • Avoid foods rich in tyramine, such as aged cheeses, chicken livers, and chocolate; ask your doctor for a list of such foods. • This drug may mask symptoms of fatigue and pose serious danger; never take this drug as a stimulant to keep you awake. • If your child's teacher tells you that your child is hyperkinetic (hyperactive), take the child to a physician for a thorough diagnosis. • If a hyperkinetic child needs to take a dose of this drug at noontime, make arrangements with the school nurse. • The sustained-release tablets, called Ritalin SR, must be swallowed whole; do not crush or chew them.

Robicillin VK antibiotic (A. H. Robins Company), see penicillin potassium phenoxymethyl (penicillin VK) antibiotic.

Robimycin antibiotic (A. H. Robins Company), see erythromycin antibiotic.

Robitet antibiotic (A.H. Robins Company), see tetracycline hydrochloride antibiotic.

Ronase oral antidiabetic (Reid-Rowell), see Tolinase oral antidiabetic.

Roxicet analgesic (Roxane Laboratories, Inc.), see Percocet analgesic.

Roxiprin analgesic (Roxane Laboratories, Inc.), see Percodan analgesic.

R-Tannate antihistamine and decongestant (various manufacturers), see Rynatan antihistamine and decongestant.

Rufen anti-inflammatory (Boots Pharmaceuticals, Inc.), see ibuprofen anti-inflammatory.

Rum-K potassium chloride replacement (Fleming & Co.), see potassium chloride replacement.

Ru-Tuss II antihistamine and decongestant (Boots Pharmaceuticals, Inc.), see Ornade Spansules antihistamine and decongestant.

Ru-Vert-M antinauseant (Reid-Provident Laboratories, Inc.), see Antivert antinauseant.

Rymed-TR decongestant and expectorant (Edwards Pharmacal), see Entex LA decongestant and expectorant.

Rynatan antihistamine and decongestant

Manufacturer: Wallace Laboratories
Ingredients: phenylephrine tannate; chlorpheniramine tannate; pyrilamine tannate
Equivalent Product: R-Tannate, various manufacturers; see Comments
Dosage Forms: Pediatric syrup (content per 5 ml teaspoon): phenylephrine tannate, 5 mg; chlorpheniramine tannate, 2 mg; pyrilamine tannate, 12.5 mg. Tablet: phenylephrine tannate, 25 mg; chlorpheniramine tannate, 8 mg; pyrilamine tannate, 25 mg (buff)
Uses: Symptomatic relief of upper respiratory tract congestion, hay fever, or allergic conditions
Minor Side Effects: Dizziness; drowsiness; dry mouth; headache; nausea; sedation; stomach upset
Major Side Effects: Change in blood pressure; chest pain; palpitations; weakness
Contraindications: This drug should not be used by persons who are allergic to any of its ingredients, by newborns, by nursing mothers, or by persons

taking monoamine oxidase inhibitors. Consult your doctor if this drug has been prescribed for you and any of these conditions applies.

Warnings: This drug must be used cautiously by persons with high blood pressure, certain heart diseases, thyroid disease, diabetes, narrow-angle glaucoma, or enlarged prostate. Be sure your doctor knows if any of these conditions applies to you. • This drug should be used with extreme caution during pregnancy; discuss the benefits and risks with your doctor. • This drug causes drowsiness; avoid tasks requiring alertness. To prevent oversedation, avoid the use of alcohol, sedatives, tranquilizers, or other central nervous system depressant agents. If you are unsure about the type or contents of your medications, ask your doctor or pharmacist.

Comments: Side effects of this drug are usually mild and transient. During the first few days, you may experience light-headedness. If it continues or becomes more pronounced, contact your doctor. • Antihistamines are more likely to cause dizziness, sedation, and blood pressure changes in elderly persons. In children, antihistamines may cause excitation or mild stimulation. This drug should be used cautiously by the elderly and in children under two years of age. • Chew gum or suck on ice chips or a piece of hard candy to relieve mouth dryness. • Drink plenty of fluids while taking this drug to aid in breaking up congestion. • Because this drug reduces sweating, avoid excessive work and exercise in hot weather. • Do not take this drug more frequently than prescribed. • This drug may be taken with food to prevent stomach upset. • If you have high blood pressure, do not take any nonprescription item for weight control, cough, cold, or sinus problems without first checking with your doctor or pharmacist. • There are many drugs of this type on the market that vary slightly in ingredients and amounts. Some are available without a prescription. Your doctor or pharmacist can help select an antihistamine and decongestant medication best for you.

Scabene pediculicide and scabicide (Stiefel Laboratories, Inc.), see Kwell pediculicide and scabicide.

Seldane antihistamine

Manufacturer: Merrell Dow Pharmaceuticals, Inc.
Ingredient: terfenadine
Dosage Form: Tablet: 60 mg (white)
Use: Relief of allergy symptoms
Minor Side Effects: Alteration of sexual desire; blurred vision; chills; confusion; constipation; depression; diarrhea; dizziness; drowsiness; dry mouth, nose, and throat; euphoria; excitation; headache; increased frequency of urination; insomnia; loss of appetite; muscle pain; nasal stuffiness; nausea; nightmares; sedation; sun sensitivity; sweating; vomiting; weight gain
Major Side Effects: Breathing difficulties; difficulty in urinating; menstrual disorders; palpitations; rash; ringing in the ears; tingling of hands and feet; thinning of hair; tremors
Contraindications: This drug should not be taken by people who are allergic to it, by persons taking monoamine oxidase inhibitors, or by nursing mothers. Consult your doctor immediately if any of these conditions applies to you. • This drug is not recommended for use in infants or children under 12 years of age. • This drug should not be used to treat asthma or lower respiratory tract symptoms.
Warnings: This drug must be used cautiously by persons with glaucoma (certain types), ulcers (certain types), thyroid disease, certain urinary difficulties, enlarged prostate, or heart disease (certain types). Be sure your doctor

knows if any of these conditions applies to you. • Elderly persons may be more likely than others to experience side effects, especially sedation, and should use this drug with caution. • Because this drug may cause drowsiness, avoid tasks requiring alertness. • The sedative effects of this drug are enhanced by alcohol and other central nervous system depressants. If you are currently taking drugs of these types, consult your doctor about their use. If you are unsure about the type or contents of your medications, ask your doctor or pharmacist.

Comments: Chew gum or suck on ice chips or a piece of hard candy to relieve mouth dryness. • If stomach upset occurs, try taking each dose with food or milk. • While taking this medication, do not take any nonprescription item for weight control, cough, cold, or sinus problems without first consulting your doctor or pharmacist. • This drug has effects similar to Benadryl antihistamine but is less sedating and therefore may be a better alternative for persons requiring antihistamine use during the day. Discuss this with your doctor. • This drug may make you more sensitive to the effects of the sun. Wear protective clothing and use a sunscreen when outdoors.

Septra and Septra DS antibacterials (Burroughs Wellcome Co.), see Bactrim and Bactrim DS antibacterials.

Serax antianxiety and sedative

Manufacturer: Wyeth-Ayerst Laboratories
Ingredient: oxazepam
Equivalent Products: oxazepam, various manufacturers; Zaxopam, Quantum Pharmics
Dosage Forms: Capsule: 10 mg (pink/white); 15 mg (red/white); 30 mg (maroon/white). Tablet: 15 mg (yellow)
Uses: Relief of anxiety, nervousness, tension; relief of muscle spasms; withdrawal from alcohol addiction
Minor Side Effects: Confusion; constipation; depression; diarrhea; dizziness; drooling; drowsiness; dry mouth; fatigue; headache; heartburn; nausea; sweating
Major Side Effects: Blurred vision; breathing difficulties; decreased or increased sexual drive; euphoria; excitement; fainting; fever; fluid retention; hallucinations; jaundice; menstrual irregularities; palpitations; rash; slurred speech; sore throat; tremors; uncoordinated movements
Contraindications: This drug should not be used by persons allergic to it or by those with acute narrow-angle glaucoma. Consult your doctor immediately if this drug has been prescribed for you and either of these conditions applies. This drug should not be used to treat psychotic disorders.
Warnings: This drug should be used cautiously by pregnant women; people with a history of drug abuse; people with lung disease, epilepsy, porphyria, liver or kidney disease, or myasthenia gravis; and people for whom a drop in blood pressure may lead to heart problems. Be sure your doctor knows if any of these conditions applies to you. • Do not stop taking this drug suddenly without consulting your doctor. If you have been taking this drug for a long period, your dosage should be reduced gradually according to your doctor's directions. • This drug may cause drowsiness; avoid tasks that require alertness. • This drug is not recommended for children under six years of age and should be used with caution in children between six and twelve years of age. • Persons taking this drug for prolonged periods should have periodic liver function tests and blood counts. • This drug should not be taken with other sedatives, alcohol, or central nervous system depressants. This drug should be used cautious-

ly in conjunction with cimetidine or phenytoin. If you are currently taking any drugs of these types, consult your doctor about their use. If you are unsure of the type or contents of your medications, ask your doctor or pharmacist. • This drug has the potential for abuse and must be used with caution. Tolerance may develop quickly; do not increase the dose of this drug without first consulting your doctor.

Comments: This drug currently is used by many people to relieve nervousness. It is effective for this purpose, but it is important to try to remove the cause of the anxiety as well. • Chew gum or suck on ice chips or a piece of hard candy to reduce mouth dryness. • To lessen stomach upset, take this drug with food or a full glass of water. • Notify your doctor if you develop signs of jaundice (yellow eyes or skin; dark urine).

Sinemet antiparkinson drug

Manufacturer: Merck Sharp & Dohme
Ingredients: carbidopa; levodopa
Dosage Form: Tablet: Sinemet-10/100: carbidopa, 10 mg and levodopa, 100 mg (dark blue); Sinemet-25/100: carbidopa, 25 mg and levodopa, 100 mg (yellow); Sinemet-25/250: carbidopa, 25 mg and levodopa, 250 mg (light blue)
Use: Treatment of symptoms of Parkinson's disease
Minor Side Effects: Abdominal pain; agitation; anxiety; bitter taste in the mouth; confusion; constipation; diarrhea; discoloration or darkening of the urine; dizziness; dry mouth; excessive salivation; faintness; fatigue; fluid retention; flushing; headache; hiccups; hot flashes; increased sexual interest; insomnia; loss of appetite; low blood pressure; nausea; offensive body odor; sweating; vision changes; vomiting; weakness
Major Side Effects: Aggressive behavior; anemia; blood clots; blood disorders; burning of the tongue; convulsions; delusions; depression; difficulty in swallowing; difficulty in urinating; double vision; euphoria; gastrointestinal bleeding; grinding of teeth; hallucinations; high blood pressure; involuntary movements; irregular heartbeats; jaw stiffness; loss of balance; loss of hair; mental changes; nightmares; numbness; palpitations; persistent erection; skin rash; suicidal tendencies; tremors; ulcer; weight gain or loss
Contraindications: Monoamine oxidase inhibitors and this drug should not be taken together. You must stop taking such drugs at least two weeks prior to starting therapy with this drug. Be sure your doctor knows about all the medications you take. • This drug should not be taken by people with narrow-angle glaucoma or hypersensitivity to either of the drug's ingredients. This drug should not be taken by people with certain cancers or skin diseases. Consult your doctor immediately if any of these conditions applies to you.
Warnings: This drug should be used with caution by people with heart, lung, kidney, liver, or glandular diseases; epilepsy; diabetes; low blood pressure; asthma; or ulcers. Be sure your doctor knows if any of these conditions applies to you. • Pregnant women, nursing mothers, and children should use this drug with caution. Consult your doctor if you experience a drastic mood change or if you notice any involuntary movements of the hands or tongue. • Periodic evaluations of liver, blood, heart, and kidney function are recommended during extended therapy with this drug. • This drug should be taken with caution by people who are taking drugs to treat high blood pressure. When this drug is started, dosage adjustment of the antihypertensive drug may be required. • This drug interacts with hypoglycemics, monoamine oxidase inhibitors, antipsychotics, phenytoin, papaverine, adrenergics, and antidepressants. If you are currently taking any drugs of these types, consult your doctor about their use. If you are unsure about the type or contents of your medications, ask your doctor or pharmacist. • When this drug is administered to patients currently taking

levodopa (L-dopa), the levodopa must be discontinued at least eight hours before. • This drug may cause dizziness or drowsiness; avoid tasks that require alertness.

Comments: Persons taking levodopa products are told to avoid taking vitamin B_6 (pyridoxine) products and to avoid eating foods rich in this vitamin. This precaution is not necessary with Sinemet antiparkinson drug. • This drug causes beneficial effects in Parkinson's disease similar to levodopa. Because of its ingredient, carbidopa, lower doses of levodopa contained in the tablet give better results than if the levodopa were taken alone. • If dizziness or light-headedness occurs when you stand, contract and relax the muscles of your legs for a few moments before rising. Do this by pushing one foot against the floor while raising the other foot slightly, alternating feet so that you are "pumping" your legs in a pedaling motion. • Take this drug with food or milk to lessen stomach upset. • It may take several weeks before the full effect of this drug is evident. Compliance with therapy will ensure maximum effectiveness.

Sinequan antidepressant and antianxiety

Manufacturer: Roerig
Ingredient: doxepin hydrochloride
Equivalent Products: Adapin, Pennwalt Pharmaceutical Division; Doxepin HCl, various manufacturers
Dosage Forms: Capsule: 10 mg (red/pink); 25 mg (blue/pink); 50 mg (light pink/pink); 75 mg (light brown); 100 mg (blue/light pink); 150 mg (blue). Oral concentrate liquid (content per ml): 10 mg
Use: Relief of depression and anxiety
Minor Side Effects: Agitation; anxiety; blurred vision; confusion; constipation; cramps; diarrhea; dizziness; drowsiness; dry mouth; fatigue; flushing; headache; increased sensitivity to light; indigestion; insomnia; loss of appetite; nausea; peculiar tastes; restlessness; stomach upset; sweating; vomiting; weakness
Major Side Effects: Chills; convulsions; difficulty in urinating; enlarged or painful breasts (in both sexes); fluid retention; hair loss; hallucinations; high or low blood pressure; impotence; jaundice; mental disorders; mood changes; nervousness; nightmares; numbness in fingers or toes; palpitations; psychosis; rash; ringing in the ears; sleep disorders; sore throat; tendency to bleed or bruise; testicular swelling; tremors; uncoordinated movements or balance problems; weight loss or gain
Contraindications: This drug should not be used by people who are allergic to it. Consult your doctor immediately if this drug has been prescribed for you and you have such an allergy. • This drug should not be used by persons, particularly older patients, who have glaucoma or urinary retention. Be sure your doctor knows if either of these conditions applies to you.
Warnings: The dosage of this drug should be carefully adjusted in elderly patients, those with other illnesses, and those taking other medications. • This drug should be used cautiously by pregnant women, nursing mothers, and children under 12. • This drug interacts with alcohol and other sedatives, monoamine oxidase inhibitors, amphetamines, epinephrine, methylphenidate, and phenylephrine. If you are currently taking any drugs of these types, consult your doctor about their use. If you are unsure of the type or contents of your medications, ask your doctor or pharmacist. • This drug may cause drowsiness; avoid tasks requiring alertness. To prevent oversedation, avoid the use of alcohol or other drugs with sedative properties. • Report eye pain, sore throat, fever, unusual bruising or bleeding, or any sudden mood swings to your doctor.
Comments: The effects of this drug may not be apparent for at least two weeks. Your doctor may adjust your dose frequently during the first few weeks

of therapy in order to find the best dose for you. • Minor side effects such as dizziness, light-headedness, and blurred vision tend to disappear as therapy continues. If they persist and become a problem, consult your physician. • While taking this drug, do not take any nonprescription item for weight control, cough, cold, or sinus problems without first checking with your doctor. Do not stop or start any other drug without notifying your doctor or pharmacist. • Chew gum or suck on ice chips or a piece of hard candy to reduce mouth dryness. • Take this drug with food or milk to lessen stomach upset. • This drug causes increased sensitivity to the sun; use a sunscreen and avoid long exposure to the sun. • Notify your doctor if you develop signs of jaundice (yellow eyes or skin; dark urine). • Immediately before you take the oral concentrate form, you should dilute it in about a half-glassful of water, juice (not grape), or milk. Do not mix your dose until just before you take it. Do not use carbonated beverages to dilute this drug. • To avoid dizziness or light-headedness when you stand, contract and relax the muscles of your legs for a few moments before rising. Do this by pushing one foot against the floor while raising the other foot slightly, alternating feet so that you are "pumping" your legs in a pedaling motion. • There are many antidepressant drugs available. If this drug is ineffective or not well tolerated, your doctor may want you to try another antidepressant.

Slo-bid bronchodilator (Rorer Pharmaceuticals), see theophylline bronchodilator.

Slo-Phyllin bronchodilator (Rorer Pharmaceuticals), see theophylline bronchodilator.

Slow-K potassium chloride replacement (Ciba Pharmaceutical Company), see potassium chloride replacement.

SMZ-TMP antibacterial (various manufacturers), see Bactrim and Bactrim DS antibacterials.

Sofarin anticoagulant (Lemmon Company), see Coumadin anticoagulant.

Solfoton sedative and hypnotic (Poythress Laboratories, Inc.), see phenobarbital sedative and hypnotic.

Somophyllin bronchodilator (Fisons Corporation), see aminophylline bronchodilator.

Somophyllin-DF bronchodilator (Fisons Corporation), see aminophylline bronchodilator.

Somophyllin-T bronchodilator (Fisons Corporation), see theophylline bronchodilator.

Sorbitrate antianginal (ICI Pharma), see Isordil antianginal.

Spaslin sedative and anticholinergic (Blaine Co., Inc.), see Donnatal sedative and anticholinergic.

Spasmolin sedative and anticholinergic (various manufacturers), see Donnatal sedative and anticholinergic.

Spasmophen sedative and anticholinergic (The Lannett Company, Inc.), see Donnatal sedative and anticholinergic.

Spasquid sedative and anticholinergic (Geneva Generics, Inc.), see Donnatal sedative and anticholinergic.

Spironazide diuretic and antihypertensive (Henry Schein, Inc.), see Aldactazide diuretic and antihypertensive.

spironolactone diuretic and antihypertensive (various manufacturers), see Aldactone diuretic and antihypertensive.

spironolactone with hydrochlorothiazide diuretic and antihypertensive (various manufacturers), see Aldactazide diuretic and antihypertensive.

Spirozide diuretic and antihypertensive (Rugby Laboratories), see Aldactazide diuretic and antihypertensive.

S-P-T thyroid hormone (Fleming & Co.), see thyroid hormone.

Stelazine antipsychotic

Manufacturer: Smith Kline & French Laboratories
Ingredient: trifluoperazine hydrochloride
Equivalent Products: Suprazine, Major Pharmaceuticals; trifluoperazine, various manufacturers
Dosage Forms: Liquid concentrate (content per ml): 10 mg. Tablet: 1 mg; 2 mg; 5 mg; 10 mg (all are blue)
Uses: Management of certain psychotic disorders; relief of excessive anxiety or tension
Minor Side Effects: Blurred vision; change in urine color; constipation; decreased sweating; diarrhea; dizziness; drooling; drowsiness; dry mouth; fatigue; headache; impotence; insomnia; jitteriness; loss of appetite; menstrual irregularities; milk production; nausea; photosensitivity; restlessness; tremors; weakness
Major Side Effects: Arthritis; blood disorders; breast enlargement (in both sexes); breathing difficulties; convulsions; difficulty in swallowing; difficulty in urinating; eye changes; fluid retention; heart attack; involuntary movements of the mouth, face, neck, and tongue; liver damage; low blood pressure; muscle spasm; rash; skin darkening
Contraindications: This drug should not be taken by persons who have drug-induced depression, blood disease, severe high or low blood pressure, bone-marrow depression, Parkinson's disease, or liver damage. This drug should not be used by children under the age of two. Consult your doctor immediately if this drug has been prescribed for you and any of these conditions applies.
Warnings: This drug should be used with caution by patients who are allergic to phenothiazine. Consult your doctor immediately if this drug has been prescribed for you and you have such an allergy. • This drug may cause drowsiness; avoid tasks that require alertness. To prevent oversedation, avoid the use

of alcohol or other drugs with sedative properties. • This drug should be used cautiously by pregnant women and by people with heart or blood vessel disease, diabetes, epilepsy, brain damage, kidney disease, peptic ulcer, breast cancer, or enlarged prostate. Be sure your doctor knows if any of these conditions applies to you. • Use of this drug may cause blood diseases, jaundice, liver damage, or motor restlessness. • Notify your doctor immediately if you notice visual disturbances. • This drug interacts with other depressant drugs, antacids, alcohol, and anticholinergics. If you are currently taking any drugs of these types, consult your doctor about their use. If you are unsure of the type or contents of your medications, ask your doctor or pharmacist. • If you take this drug for a prolonged time, it may be desirable for you to stop taking it for awhile in order to see if you still need it. However, do not stop taking this drug without talking to your doctor first. You may have to reduce your dosage gradually. • This drug may interfere with certain laboratory tests. Remind your doctor that you are taking this drug before undergoing any tests.

Comments: The effects of therapy with this drug may not be apparent for at least two weeks. • This drug has sustained action; never take it more frequently than your doctor prescribes. A serious overdose may result. • While taking this drug, do not take any nonprescription item for weight control, cough, cold, or sinus problems without first checking with your doctor. • Chew gum or suck on ice chips or a piece of hard candy to reduce mouth dryness. • The liquid concentrate form of this drug should be added to 60 ml ($\frac{1}{4}$ cup) or more of water, milk, juice, coffee, tea, or carbonated beverages or to pulpy foods (applesauce, etc.) just prior to administration. • To avoid dizziness or lightheadedness when you stand, contract and relax the muscles of your legs for a few moments before rising. Do this by pushing one foot against the floor while raising the other foot slightly, alternating feet so that you are "pumping" your legs in a pedaling motion. • If you notice fine tremors of your tongue, call your doctor. • Some of the side effects of this drug can be prevented by taking an antiparkinson drug. Discuss this with your doctor. • Antacids may prevent the absorption of this drug. Don't take them at the same time that you take this drug. • This drug may make you more sensitive to sunlight. Avoid prolonged exposure to the sun, and wear protective clothing and a sunscreen when outdoors. • Take extra precautions if you are using this medication during hot weather. It may increase your risk of heat stroke. Avoid strenuous activity during hot weather and drink plenty of fluids. • Notify your doctor if you develop signs of jaundice (yellow eyes or skin; dark urine).

Sterapred steroid hormone (Mayrand, Inc.), see prednisone steroid hormone.

Stuartnatal 1+1 vitamin-mineral supplement

Manufacturer: Stuart Pharmaceuticals
Ingredients: calcium; copper; iron; vitamins A, D, E, B_1, B_2, B_3, B_6, B_{12}, C; folic acid; zinc
Equivalent Products: Prenatal 1mg + Iron, Everett Laboratories, Inc.; Prenatal-1, Major Pharmaceuticals
Dosage Form: Tablet: calcium, 200 mg; iron, 65 mg; vitamin A, 4,000 I.U.; vitamin D, 400 I.U.; vitamin E, 11 mg; vitamin B_1, 1.5 mg; vitamin B_2, 3 mg; vitamin B_3, 20 mg; vitamin B_6, 10 mg; vitamin B_{12}, 12 mcg; vitamin C, 90 mg; folic acid, 1.0 mg; copper, 2 mg; zinc, 25 mg (yellow)
Use: Vitamin-mineral supplement for use during pregnancy and nursing
Minor Side Effects: Constipation; diarrhea; nausea; stomach upset; vomiting

Major Side Effects: None

Contraindication: This drug should not be used by anyone who is allergic to any of its ingredients. Contact your doctor if you have such an allergy.

Warning: Because this product may mask symptoms of pernicious anemia, it should be used only under a doctor's supervision.

Comments: If this drug upsets your stomach, take it with food or milk. • You may wish to continue taking this product for a few weeks after delivery, especially if you are nursing your baby. • While not all prenatal vitamin-mineral formulations are identical to this product, some are similar. Ask your doctor if you can use a less expensive version, then discuss various products with your pharmacist. • Because of its iron content, this product may cause constipation, diarrhea, nausea, or stomach pain. These symptoms usually disappear or become less severe after two or three days. Taking your dose with food or milk may help minimize these side effects. If they persist, ask your pharmacist to recommend another product. • Black stools are a normal consequence of iron therapy; do not be alarmed.

sulfamethoxazole and trimethoprim antibacterial (various manufacturers), see Bactrim and Bactrim DS antibacterials.

Sulfatrim and Sulfatrim DS antibacterials (various manufacturers), see Bactrim and Bactrim DS antibacterials.

Sumycin antibiotic (E.R. Squibb & Sons, Inc.), see tetracycline hydrochloride antibiotic.

Suprazine antipsychotic (Major Pharmaceuticals), see Stelazine antipsychotic.

Susano sedative and anticholinergic (Halsey Drug Co., Inc.), see Donnatal sedative and anticholinergic.

Suspen antibiotic (Circle Pharmaceutical, Inc.), see penicillin potassium phenoxymethyl (penicillin VK) antibiotic.

Sustaire bronchodilator (Pfipharmecs Division), see theophylline bronchodilator.

Symadine antiviral and antiparkinson (Reid-Rowell), see Symmetrel antiviral and antiparkinson.

Symmetrel antiviral and antiparkinson

Manufacturer: Du Pont Pharmaceuticals, Inc.

Ingredient: amantadine hydrochloride

Equivalent Products: amantadine HCl, Rugby Laboratories; Symadine, Reid-Rowell

Dosage Forms: Capsule: 100 mg (red). Syrup (content per 5 ml teaspoon): 50 mg

Uses: Symptomatic treatment of Parkinson's disease; prevention and treatment of respiratory illness due to flu

Minor Side Effects: Blurred vision; constipation; dry mouth; fatigue; headache; irritability; light-headedness; loss of appetite; nausea; slurred speech; vomiting; weakness

Major Side Effects: Blood disorders; changes in vision; depression; difficulty in urinating; heart failure; psychiatric disorders; rash; shortness of breath

Contraindication: This drug should not be used by persons who are allergic to it. Consult your doctor immediately if this drug has been prescribed for you and you have such an allergy.

Warnings: This drug must be used with caution by persons with seizure disorders, heart failure, kidney disease, liver disease, or psychiatric disorders and by pregnant or nursing women. Be sure your doctor knows if any of these conditions applies to you. • This drug is not recommended for use in children less than one year of age. • If you are taking this drug for Parkinson's disease, do not suddenly stop taking it without consulting your doctor; stopping treatment early can lead to a worsening of symptoms. • This drug may become ineffective after long periods of use. If this occurs, your doctor may have you stop taking the drug for a short period. When you start taking the drug again, it should be effective. If you must take this drug for a prolonged period, discuss this type of therapy with your doctor. • This drug interacts with central nervous system stimulants, anticholinergics, and levodopa. If you are currently taking any drugs of these types, consult your doctor about their use. If you are unsure of the types or contents of your medications, consult your doctor or pharmacist. • This drug may cause drowsiness; avoid tasks that require alertness.

Comments: This drug is used for prevention of respiratory tract illness due to influenza A virus in persons with a high risk of contracting it, such as persons with chronic medical problems. If this drug is being used for prevention of respiratory illness, begin therapy as soon as possible after contact has been made with a person having the influenza virus. Therapy should be continued for at least ten days. • To prevent dizziness and light-headedness when you stand, contract and relax the muscles of your legs for a few minutes before rising. Do this by pushing one foot against the floor while raising the other foot slightly. Alternate feet so that you are "pumping" your legs in a pedaling motion. While taking this drug, limit your consumption of alcoholic beverages in order to minimize dizziness. • Notify your doctor if you experience shortness of breath, difficulty in urinating, mood changes, or swelling of the extremities while taking this drug.

Synacort topical steroid (Syntex Laboratories, Inc.), see hydrocortisone topical steroid.

Synalar topical steroid hormone

Manufacturer: Syntex Laboratories, Inc.

Ingredient: fluocinolone acetonide

Equivalent Products: fluocinolone acetonide, various manufacturers; Fluonid, Herbert Laboratories; Flurosyn, Rugby Laboratories; Synemol, Syntex Laboratories, Inc.

Dosage Forms: Cream: 0.01%; 0.025%; 0.2%%. Ointment: 0.025%. Topical solution: 0.01%

Use: Relief of skin inflammation associated with such conditions as dermatitis, eczema, and poison ivy

Minor Side Effects: Blistering; burning sensation; dryness; increased hair growth; irritation; itching; rash

Major Side Effects: Loss of skin color; secondary infection; skin wasting

Contraindications: This drug should not be used by people who are allergic to it. Consult your doctor immediately if this drug has been prescribed for you and you have such an allergy. • This drug should not be used on infants less than two years old. • This drug should not be used in the presence of infection or severe circulatory system disease or in the ear if the eardrum is perforated.

Warnings: If irritation develops when using this drug, immediately discontinue its use and notify your doctor. • If extensive areas are treated or if an occlusive bandage is used, there will be increased systemic absorption of this drug; suitable precautions should be taken, particularly in children and infants. If this medication is applied to the diaper area of an infant, tight-fitting diapers or plastic pants should not be used. • This drug should be used with caution by pregnant women. • This drug is not meant for use in the eyes.

Comments: If the affected area is extremely dry or scaling, the skin may be moistened before applying the medication by soaking in water or by applying water with a clean cloth. The ointment form is probably better for dry skin. The solution form is best for hairy areas. • A mild, temporary stinging may be apparent after the medicine is applied. • Do not use this drug with an occlusive wrap unless directed to do so by your doctor. If it is necessary for you to use this drug under a wrap, follow your doctor's instructions exactly; do not leave the wrap in place longer than specified. • Use this drug only as prescribed. Do not use more often or for a longer period than your doctor ordered. • Use this drug only for the condition for which it was prescribed. • Applying this drug to burns or infections may delay healing.

Synemol topical steroid hormone (Syntex Laboratories, Inc.), see Synalar topical steroid hormone.

Synthroid thyroid hormone

Manufacturer: Flint Laboratories
Ingredient: levothyroxine sodium
Equivalent Products: Levothroid, Rorer Pharmaceuticals; levothyroxine sodium, Lederle Laboratories; Synthrox, Vortech Pharmaceutical, Ltd.; Syroxine, Major Pharmaceuticals
Dosage Form: Tablet: 0.025 mg (orange); 0.05 mg (white); 0.075 mg (violet); 0.1 mg (yellow); 0.125 mg (brown); 0.15 mg (blue); 0.2 mg (pink); 0.3 mg (green); see Comments
Use: Thyroid replacement therapy
Minor Side Effects: Diarrhea; headache; irritability; vomiting
Major Side Effects: In overdose: Chest pain; diarrhea; fever; heat intolerance; insomnia; leg cramps; menstrual irregularities; nervousness; palpitations; shortness of breath; sweating; trembling; weight loss
Contraindications: Although there are no absolute contraindications to this drug, special care should be taken if it is used by persons who have recently had a heart attack and those with defective adrenal glands or an overactive thyroid gland. Be sure your doctor knows if any of these conditions applies to you.
Warnings: This drug should be used cautiously by people who have heart disease, high blood pressure, kidney disease, or diabetes. Be sure your doctor knows if any of these conditions applies to you. • This drug interacts with cholestyramine, digitalis, oral anticoagulants, oral antidiabetics, oral contraceptives, epinephrine, and phenytoin; if you are currently taking any drugs of these types, consult your doctor about their use. If you are unsure of the type or contents of your medications, ask your doctor or pharmacist. • While taking this drug, do not take any nonprescription item for weight control, cough, cold, or sinus problems without first checking with your doctor. • If you are taking digitalis in addition to this drug, watch carefully for symptoms of increased digitalis effects (e.g., nausea, blurred vision, palpitations), and notify your doctor immediately if they occur. • Be sure to follow your doctor's dosage instructions exactly. Most side effects from this drug can be controlled by dosage adjustment; consult your doctor if you experience side effects. • This drug should not be

used to treat obesity. Using this drug in conjunction with appetite suppressants is particularly dangerous.

Comments: For most patients, generic thyroid hormone tablets (see the profile on thyroid hormone) will work as well as this drug and may be less expensive. Check with your doctor. Not all levothyroxine products are true equivalents. Do not switch brands without consulting your doctor or pharmacist; a dosage adjustment may be necessary. • Do not stop taking this drug without first consulting your doctor. Compliance with the prescribed therapy is essential. Get into the habit of taking this drug at the same time every day. • Levothroid is also available in a 0.175 mg tablet.

Synthrox thyroid hormone (Vortech Pharmaceutical, Ltd.), see Synthroid thyroid hormone.

Syroxine thyroid hormone (Major Pharmaceuticals), see Synthroid thyroid hormone.

Tagamet antisecretory

Manufacturer: Smith Kline & French Laboratories
Ingredients: cimetidine; alcohol (in liquid form only)
Dosage Forms: Liquid (content per 5 ml teaspoon): 300 mg; alcohol, 2.8%. Tablet: 200 mg; 300 mg; 400 mg; 800 mg; (all are light green)
Uses: Treatment of duodenal and gastric ulcer; long-term treatment of excessive gastric acid secretion; prevention of recurrent ulcers
Minor Side Effects: Diarrhea; dizziness; drowsiness; headache; muscle pain
Major Side Effects: Breast enlargement (when taken in extremely high doses over a prolonged period); confusion; easy bruising; fever; hair loss; impotence (when taken in extremely high doses over a prolonged period); jaundice; palpitations; rash; sore throat; weakness
Contraindication: This drug should not be taken by anyone who is allergic to it. Consult your doctor if this drug has been prescribed for you and you have such an allergy.
Warnings: This drug should be used with caution by pregnant women or women who may become pregnant and by nursing mothers. • This drug is not recommended for use by children under 16 years of age unless your doctor feels the benefits outweigh any potential risks. • This drug should be used with caution by people with liver or kidney disease, or organic brain syndrome. Be sure your doctor knows if any of these conditions applies to you. • This drug may interact with theophylline, aminophylline, phenytoin, beta blockers, anticoagulants, and certain tranquilizers. If you are currently taking any drugs of these types, consult your doctor about their use. If you are unsure about the type or contents of your medications, ask your doctor or pharmacist. Taking this drug at bedtime may reduce the potential for drug interaction.
Comments: Although this drug is classified as a histamine blocker, its major action on histamine in the body is in the stomach and intestine, unlike other antihistamines, which act primarily on the skin. • This drug should not be crushed or chewed because cimetidine has a bitter taste and an unpleasant odor. • Antacid therapy may be continued while taking this drug, but the two drugs should not be taken at the same time. For maximum benefit, stagger the doses of antacid and Tagamet by at least two hours. • This drug is usually taken throughout the day. It should be taken with, or immediately following, a meal. • When used as a preventive, the medication may be taken as a single dose at bedtime. • Take this drug for the prescribed period, even if you feel better, to ensure adequate results. • This drug may cause changes in blood cells;

therefore, periodic blood tests may be requested by your doctor if you take this medication for prolonged periods. • This drug is similar but not equivalent in action to Zantac and Pepcid. Talk to your doctor about these drugs to see if they may be less expensive alternatives. • If you become dizzy or sleepy or if you develop a rash or diarrhea while taking this medication, call your doctor. • Notify your doctor if you develop signs of jaundice (yellow eyes or skin; dark urine).

Talacen Caplets analgesic (Winthrop-Breon Laboratories), see Talwin Nx analgesic (comments).

Talwin Compound analgesic (Winthrop-Breon Laboratories), see Talwin Nx analgesic (comments).

Talwin Nx analgesic

Manufacturer: Winthrop-Breon Laboratories
Ingredients: pentazocine hydrochloride; naloxone hydrochloride
Dosage Form: Tablet: pentazocine hydrochloride, 50 mg and naloxone hydrochloride, 0.5 mg (yellow)
Use: Relief of moderate to severe pain
Minor Side Effects: Change in sense of taste; constipation; diarrhea; dizziness; drowsiness; dry mouth; flushing; headache; indigestion; insomnia; lightheadedness; loss of appetite; nausea; vomiting
Major Side Effects: Blurred vision; breathing difficulties; chest tightness; difficulty in urinating; disorientation; euphoria; hallucinations; loss of hearing; mood changes; nightmares; ringing in the ears; tingling in the hands and feet
Contraindications: This drug should not be used by people who are allergic to it or to narcotic analgesics. Consult your doctor immediately if this drug has been prescribed for you and you have such an allergy.
Warnings: This drug should be used with caution by pregnant and nursing women; by people who have been taking narcotics; by people with head injuries, enlarged prostate, peptic ulcer, severe respiratory problems, severe bronchial asthma, liver or kidney disease, or epilepsy; by those about to undergo gallbladder surgery; by those who have suffered a heart attack; and by those with a history of drug abuse. Be sure your doctor knows if any of these conditions applies to you. • This drug is not recommended for use by children under 12. • This drug has the potential for abuse. Tolerance may develop quickly; do not increase the dose of this drug without first consulting your doctor. • This medication is for oral use only. Naloxone is added to prevent misuse; it may cause fatal reactions if injected. • Do not stop taking this drug suddenly without consulting your doctor. • This drug has, on rare occasions, produced hallucinations (usually visual), disorientation, and confusion in some patients. These side effects have cleared spontaneously in a few hours. • Use of this drug may cause drowsiness; avoid tasks that require alertness such as driving or operating machinery. To prevent oversedation, avoid the use of alcohol or other drugs that have sedative properties while taking this drug. • This drug interacts with alcohol, narcotics, phenothiazines, antidepressants, and monoamine oxidase inhibitors. If you are currently taking any drugs of these types, consult your doctor about their use. If you are unsure of the type or contents of your medications, ask your doctor or pharmacist. • If a rash develops or if you become confused or disoriented while taking this drug, call your doctor.
Comments: Winthrop-Breon Laboratories also markets Talwin Compound caplets, which contain pentazocine hydrochloride, 12.5 mg and aspirin, 325 mg; and Talacen Caplets, which contain pentazocine hydrochloride, 25 mg and acetaminophen, 650 mg. Both are combination pain relievers.

CONSUMER GUIDE®

Tavist-D antihistamine and decongestant

Manufacturer: Sandoz Pharmaceuticals
Ingredients: phenylpropanolamine hydrochloride; clemastine fumarate
Dosage Form: Sustained-release tablet: phenylpropanolamine hydrochloride, 75 mg and clemastine fumarate, 1.34 mg (white)
Use: Relief of hay fever and allergy symptoms, such as sneezing, runny nose, teary eyes, and nasal congestion
Minor Side Effects: Blurred vision; chills; confusion; constipation; diarrhea; dizziness; drowsiness; dry mouth, throat, and nose; euphoria; fatigue; headache; irritability; loss of appetite; nasal congestion; nausea; nervousness; restlessness; ringing or buzzing in the ears; sedation; stomach upset; sun sensitivity; sweating; tremors; weakness; wheezing
Major Side Effects: Convulsions; difficulty in urinating; high blood pressure; loss of coordination; low blood pressure; menstrual changes; palpitations; rash; sore throat and fever; tightness in the chest; tingling in the hands and feet
Contraindications: This drug should not be taken by people who are allergic to either of its components, persons taking monoamine oxidase inhibitors, nursing mothers, or persons with severe high blood pressure or coronary artery disease. Consult your doctor immediately if any of these conditions applies to you. • This drug is not recommended for use in children under 12 years of age. • This drug should not be used to treat asthma or to treat lower respiratory tract symptoms.
Warnings: This drug must be used cautiously by persons with glaucoma (certain types), ulcers (certain types), thyroid disease, diabetes, certain urinary difficulties, enlarged prostate, and certain heart diseases. Be sure your doctor knows if any of these conditions applies to you. • Elderly persons may be more likely than others to experience side effects, especially sedation, and should use this drug with caution. • Because this drug may cause drowsiness, avoid tasks requiring alertness. • The sedative effects of this drug are enhanced by alcohol and other central nervous system depressants. If you are currently taking any drugs of these types, consult your doctor about their use. If you are unsure about the type or contents of your medications, ask your doctor or pharmacist.
Comments: Chew gum or suck on ice chips or a piece of hard candy to reduce mouth dryness. • If stomach upset occurs, try taking each dose with food or milk. • While taking this drug, do not take any nonprescription medication for weight control, cough, cold, or sinus problems without first consulting your doctor or pharmacist. • These tablets must be swallowed whole. Do not crush or chew them, as the sustained action will be lost and side effects will be increased. • Take this medication as prescribed; never take it more frequently or increase your dose unless instructed to do so by your doctor; a serious overdose may result. • Because this medication reduces sweating, avoid excessive work or exercise in hot weather and drink plenty of fluids.

Tebamide antinauseant (G&W Laboratories, Inc.), see Tigan antinauseant.

Tega decongestant and expectorant (Ortega Pharmaceutical Company), see Entex LA decongestant and expectorant.

Tegretol anticonvulsant

Manufacturer: Geigy Pharmaceuticals
Ingredient: carbamazepine

Equivalent Products: carbamazepine, Rugby Laboratories; Epitol, Lemmon Company

Dosage Forms: Chewable tablet: 100 mg (red/pink). Oral suspension (content per 5 ml teaspoon): 100 mg. Tablet: 200 mg (white)

Uses: Treatment of seizure disorders; relief of neuralgia pain

Minor Side Effects: Agitation; blurred vision; confusion; constipation; diarrhea; dizziness; drowsiness; dry mouth; eye discomfort; fainting; headache; loss of appetite; muscle or joint pain; nausea; restlessness; sensitivity to sunlight; sweating; vomiting; weakness

Major Side Effects: Abdominal pain; breathing difficulties; bruising; chills; dark urine; depression; difficulty in urinating; fever; hair loss; hallucinations; impotence; jaundice; loss of balance; mouth sores; nightmares; numbness or tingling; pale stools; rapid and pounding heart rate; ringing in the ears; sore throat; skin rash; swelling of hands or feet; twitching

Contraindications: This drug should not be used by people who are allergic to it or to tricyclic antidepressants. This drug should not be taken by anyone who has bone marrow depression or who has taken a monoamine oxidase inhibitor within the past two weeks. Consult your doctor immediately if this drug has been prescribed for you and any of these conditions applies.

Warnings: This drug should be used cautiously by pregnant or nursing women and by people who have glaucoma, blood disorders, kidney or liver disease, or heart disease. Be sure your doctor knows if any of these conditions applies to you. • This drug interacts with oral anticoagulants, digitalis, erythromycin, tetracycline, troleandomycin, oral contraceptives, painkillers, tranquilizers, and other anticonvulsants. If you are currently taking any drugs of these types, consult your doctor about their use. If you are unsure of the type or contents of your medications, ask your doctor or pharmacist. Do not use any other medicines without first checking with your doctor or pharmacist.

Comments: It is important that all doses of this medication are taken on time. • If this drug causes stomach upset, take it with food. • This drug increases your sensitivity to sunlight; limit your exposure to the sun, wear protective clothing and sunglasses, and use an effective sunscreen. • Chew gum or suck on ice chips or a piece of hard candy to reduce mouth dryness. • This drug may cause dizziness or drowsiness; avoid tasks that require alertness. • While taking this drug, your doctor will want to see you regularly for blood tests, liver and kidney function tests, and eye examinations. • Notify your doctor if you develop a sore throat, mouth sores, fever, chills, unusual bruising, pale stools, dark urine, yellow eyes or skin, or edema (swelling) while taking this medication. • Do not stop taking this drug suddenly and do not increase the dosage without your doctor's approval. • It is recommended that persons taking this medication carry a medical alert card or wear a medical alert bracelet.

temazepam sedative and hypnotic (various manufacturers), see Restoril sedative and hypnotic.

Temaz sedative and hypnotic (Quantum Pharmics), see Restoril sedative and hypnotic.

Ten-K potassium chloride replacement (Geigy Pharmaceuticals), see potassium chloride replacement.

Tenoretic diuretic and antihypertensive

Manufacturer: ICI Pharma
Ingredients: atenolol; chlorthalidone

Dosage Form: Tablet: Tenoretic 50: atenolol, 50 mg and chlorthalidone, 25 mg; Tenoretic 100: atenolol, 100 mg and chlorthalidone, 25 mg (both white)

Use: Treatment of high blood pressure

Minor Side Effects: Cold extremities; constipation; cramps; diarrhea; dizziness; dreaming; drowsiness; fatigue; headache; heartburn; increased sensitivity to sunlight; lethargy; light-headedness; loss of appetite; nausea; restlessness

Major Side Effects: Blood disorders; breathing difficulties; confusion; depression; fever; jaundice; leg pain; muscle spasm; skin rash; sore throat; trembling; weak pulse; wheezing

Contraindications: This drug should not be used by persons with certain heart diseases, persons with anuria (inability to urinate), or persons with an allergy to sulfa drugs. Consult your doctor immediately if this drug has been prescribed for you and any of these conditions applies.

Warnings: This drug should be used with caution by pregnant or nursing women and by persons with kidney disease, liver disease, diabetes, gout, allergies, or asthma. Be sure your doctor knows if any of these conditions applies to you. • This drug may cause gout and low blood levels of potassium; it may also trigger the appearance of diabetes that has been latent. Periodic blood tests are advisable if you are taking this drug for prolonged periods. • Use of this drug may affect thyroid tests. If you are scheduled to have such tests, remind your doctor that you are taking this drug. • This drug may add to the actions of other blood pressure drugs. If you are taking any such medications, a dosage adjustment may be necessary. • This drug also interacts with digitalis, indomethacin, lithium, oral antidiabetics, steroids, and curare. Persons taking this drug and digitalis should watch carefully for signs of increased digitalis effects (e.g., nausea, blurred vision, palpitations), and notify their doctors immediately if symptoms occur. If you are currently taking any drugs of these types, consult your doctor about their use. If you are unsure of the types or contents of your medications, ask your doctor or pharmacist.

Comments: This drug causes frequent urination. Expect this effect; it should not alarm you. • Notify your doctor if you develop signs of jaundice (yellow eyes or skin; dark urine). • This drug can cause potassium loss. Signs of such loss include dry mouth, thirst, weakness, muscle pain or cramps, nausea, and vomiting. If you experience such symptoms, call your doctor. To help avoid potassium loss, take this drug with a glass of fresh or frozen orange juice. You may also eat a banana each day. The use of a salt substitute helps prevent potassium loss. Do not change your diet, however, without consulting your doctor. Too much potassium may also be dangerous. • Learn how to monitor your pulse and blood pressure while taking this drug; discuss this with your doctor. • Try not to take this drug at bedtime. This drug is best taken as a single dose in the morning with food. • This drug must be taken exactly as directed. Do not take extra doses or skip a dose without first consulting your doctor. • While taking this drug, as with many drugs that lower blood pressure, you should limit your consumption of alcoholic beverages in order to prevent dizziness or light-headedness. To avoid dizziness or light-headedness when you stand, contract and relax the muscles of your legs for a few moments before rising. Do this by pushing one foot against the floor while raising the other foot slightly, alternating feet so that you are "pumping" your legs in a pedaling motion. • If you have high blood pressure, do not take any nonprescription item for weight control, cough, cold, or sinus problems without first checking with your doctor. Such medications may contain ingredients that can increase blood pressure. • A doctor probably should not prescribe this drug or other "fixed dose" products as the first choice in treatment of high blood pressure. The patient should be treated first with each of the component drugs individually. If the response is adequate to the doses contained in this product, then this fixed dose product can be substituted. Combination products offer the advantage of increased convenience to the patient.

Tenormin beta blocker

Manufacturer: ICI Pharma
Ingredient: atenolol
Dosage Form: Tablet: 50 mg; 100 mg (white)
Uses: Treatment of high blood pressure and chest pain
Minor Side Effects: Abdominal pain; bloating; blurred vision; constipation; drowsiness; dry eyes, mouth, or skin; gas or heartburn; headache; insomnia; loss of appetite; nasal congestion; nausea; slowed heart rate; sweating; vivid dreams; vomiting
Major Side Effects: Bleeding or bruising; confusion; decreased sexual ability; depression; diarrhea; difficulty in urinating; dizziness; earache; fever; hair loss; hallucinations; mouth sores; night cough; nightmares; numbness and tingling in the fingers and toes; rash; ringing in the ears; shortness of breath; swelling in the hands or feet.
Contraindications: This drug should not be used by people who are allergic to atenolol or any other beta blocker. This drug may interact with monoamine oxidase inhibitors. Consult your doctor if you are taking any drugs of this type. If you are unsure about the type or contents of your medications, ask your doctor or pharmacist. • This drug should not be used by persons who have certain types of heart disease (bradycardia, severe heart failure, shock).
Warnings: This drug should be used with caution by persons with certain respiratory problems, diabetes, certain heart problems, liver or kidney diseases, hypoglycemia, or certain types of thyroid disease. Be sure your doctor knows if any of these conditions applies to you. • This drug should be used cautiously by pregnant women and by women of childbearing age. • This drug should be used with care during anesthesia and by patients undergoing major surgery. If possible, this drug should be withdrawn 48 hours prior to surgery. • This drug should be used cautiously when reserpine, cimetidine, theophylline, aminophylline, phenytoin, or digoxin is taken. • This drug is a potent medication; do not stop taking it abruptly, unless your doctor directs you to do so. Chest pain—even heart attacks—can occur if this medicine is stopped suddenly. • Diabetics should be aware that this drug may mask signs of hypoglycemia, such as changes in heart rate and blood pressure. If you are diabetic, you will need to monitor your blood glucose level more closely, especially when first taking this drug.
Comments: Your doctor may want you to take your pulse and blood pressure every day while you are taking this medication. Learn what your normal values are and what they should be; discuss this with your doctor. • Be sure to take your medication at the same time each day. • While taking this drug, do not take any nonprescription items for weight control, cough, cold, or sinus problems without first checking with your doctor or pharmacist; such items may contain ingredients that can increase blood pressure. • Notify your doctor if dizziness, diarrhea, depression, breathing difficulties, sore throat, or unusual bruising develops. • This drug may cause you to become more sensitive to the cold; dress warmly. • There are many beta blockers available. Your doctor may have you try different ones if this drug is ineffective.

Tetracap antibiotic (Circle Pharmaceutical, Inc.), see tetracycline hydrochloride antibiotic.

tetracycline hydrochloride antibiotic

Manufacturer: various manufacturers
Ingredient: tetracycline hydrochloride

Equivalent Products: Achromycin V, Lederle Laboratories; Cyclopar, Parke-Davis; Nor-Tet, Vortech Pharmaceutical, Ltd.; Panmycin, The Upjohn Company; Robitet, A. H. Robins Company; Sumycin, E. R. Squibb & Sons, Inc.; Tetracap, Circle Pharmaceutical, Inc.; Tetracyn, Pfipharmecs Division; Tetralan-250 and Tetralan-500, The Lannett Company, Inc.; Tetram, Dunhall Pharmaceuticals, Inc.

Dosage Forms: Capsule; Liquid; Tablet (various strengths and colors)

Uses: Treatment of acne and a wide variety of bacterial infections

Minor Side Effects: Diarrhea; increased sensitivity to sunlight; loss of appetite; nausea; stomach cramps and upset; vomiting

Major Side Effects: Anemia; black tongue; breathing difficulties; mouth irritation; rash; rectal and vaginal itching; sore throat; superinfection

Contraindication: This drug should not be taken by people who are allergic to any tetracycline drug. Consult your doctor immediately if this drug has been prescribed for you and you have such an allergy.

Warnings: This drug may cause permanent discoloration of the teeth if used during tooth development; therefore, it should be used cautiously by pregnant or nursing women and in infants and children under nine years of age. This drug should be used cautiously by people who have liver or kidney disease, or diabetes. Be sure your doctor knows if any of these conditions applies to you. • This drug interacts with antacids, barbiturates, carbamazepine, lithium, diuretics, digoxin, oral contraceptives, penicillin, and phenytoin; if you are currently taking any drugs of these types, consult your doctor about their use. If you are unsure of the type or contents of your medications, ask your doctor or pharmacist. • Milk, other dairy products, and antacids interfere with the body's absorption of this drug, so separate taking this drug and any dairy product or antacid by at least two hours. Do not take this drug at the same time as any iron preparation; their use should be separated by at least two hours. • This drug may cause you to be especially sensitive to the sun, so avoid exposure to sunlight as much as possible. • This drug may affect syphilis tests; if you are being treated for this disease, make sure that your doctor knows you are taking this drug. • If you are taking an anticoagulant in addition to this drug, remind your doctor. • Prolonged use of this drug may allow organisms that are not susceptible to it to grow wildly. Do not use this drug unless your doctor has specifically told you to do so. Be sure to follow the directions carefully and report any unusual reactions to your doctor at once. • Complete blood cell counts and liver and kidney function tests should be done if you take this drug for a prolonged period.

Comments: Ideally, you should take this drug on an empty stomach (one hour before or two hours after a meal). If this drug causes stomach upset, you may take it with food. Take it with at least eight ounces of water. • This drug should be taken for as long as prescribed, even if symptoms disappear within that time. Stopping treatment too soon can lead to reinfection. • This drug is most effective when taken at evenly spaced intervals throughout the day and night. Ask your doctor or pharmacist for help in planning a medication schedule. • The liquid form of this drug must be shaken before use. • Any unused medication should be discarded. Make sure your prescription is marked with the drug's expiration date. Do not use tetracycline after that date, as it can cause serious liver damage. • Tetracycline is also available in a topical solution that is used to treat acne.

Tetracyn antibiotic (Pfipharmecs Division), see tetracycline hydrochloride antibiotic.

Tetralan-250 and Tetralan-500 antibiotics (The Lannett Company, Inc.), see tetracycline hydrochloride antibiotic.

Tetram antibiotic (Dunhall Pharmaceuticals, Inc.), see tetracycline hydrochloride antibiotic.

T-Gen antinauseant (Goldline Laboratories), see Tigan antinauseant.

Thalitone diuretic and antihypertensive (Boehringer Ingelheim), see Hygroton diuretic and antihypertensive.

Theo-24 bronchodilator (Searle & Co.), see theophylline bronchodilator.

Theobid bronchodilator (Glaxo, Inc.), see theophylline bronchodilator.

Theoclear bronchodilator (Central Pharmaceuticals, Inc.), see theophylline bronchodilator.

Theo-Dur bronchodilator (Key Pharmaceuticals, Inc.), see theophylline bronchodilator.

Theolair bronchodilator (Riker Laboratories, Inc.), see theophylline bronchodilator.

Theon bronchodilator (Bock Pharmacal Company), see theophylline bronchodilator.

theophylline bronchodilator

Manufacturer: various manufacturers
Ingredient: theophylline, anhydrous
Equivalent Products: Accurbron, Merrell Dow Pharmaceuticals, Inc.; Aerolate, Fleming & Co.; Aquaphyllin, Ferndale Laboratories, Inc.; Asmalix, Century Pharmaceuticals, Inc.; Bronkodyl, Winthrop-Breon Laboratories; Constant-T, Geigy Pharmaceuticals; Elixicon, Berlex Laboratories, Inc.; Elixomin, Cenci; Elixophyllin, Forest Pharmaceuticals, Inc.; Lanophyllin, The Lannett Company, Inc.; Lixolin, Mallard, Inc.; Lodrane, Poythress Laboratories, Inc.; Quibron-T, Bristol Laboratories; Respbid, Boehringer Ingelheim; Slo-bid, Rorer Pharmaceuticals; Slo-Phyllin, Rorer Pharmaceuticals; Somophyllin-T, Fisons Corporation; Sustaire, Pfipharmecs Division; Theo-24, Searle & Co.; Theobid, Glaxo, Inc.; Theoclear, Central Pharmaceuticals, Inc.; Theo-Dur, Key Pharmaceuticals, Inc.; Theolair, Riker Laboratories, Inc.; Theon, Bock Pharmacal Company; Theospan, Laser, Inc.; Theostat, Laser, Inc.; Theo-Time, Major Pharmaceuticals; Theovent, Schering Corp.; Uniphyl, The Purdue Frederick Company
Dosage Forms: Capsule; Liquid; Tablet; Time-release capsule; Time-release tablet (various strengths) (see Comments)
Use: Symptomatic relief and prevention of bronchial asthma and bronchospasm
Minor Side Effects: Dizziness; flushing; gastrointestinal disturbances (diarrhea, nausea, stomach pain, vomiting); headache; heartburn; increased urination; insomnia; irritability; loss of appetite; low blood pressure; nervousness; paleness

Major Side Effects: Black, tarry stools; breathing difficulties; confusion; convulsions; high blood sugar; muscle twitches; palpitations; rash; ulcer; weakness

Contraindication: This drug should not be taken by people who are allergic to it. Consult your doctor immediately if you have such an allergy.

Warnings: This drug should be used cautiously by newborns, pregnant women, and the elderly and by people who have peptic ulcer, liver disease, chronic obstructive lung disease, certain types of heart disease, kidney disease, low or high blood pressure, or thyroid disease. Be sure your doctor knows if any of these conditions applies to you. • This drug should be used with caution in conjunction with furosemide, reserpine, chlordiazepoxide, cimetidine, oral anticoagulants, phenobarbital, certain antibiotics, disulfiram, ephedrine, lithium carbonate, propranolol, or other xanthines; if you are currently taking any drugs of these types, consult your doctor about their use. If you are unsure of the type or contents of your medication, ask your doctor or pharmacist. • This drug may interfere with certain blood and urine laboratory tests. Remind your doctor you are taking this drug before undergoing tests. • Before receiving an influenza vaccine, tell your doctor you are taking this drug.

Comments: While taking this drug, do not use any nonprescription item for asthma without first checking with your doctor. • Avoid drinking alcohol, coffee, tea, cola drinks, cocoa, or other beverages that contain caffeine. Caffeine produces side effects that are similar to those of this drug. • This drug may aggravate an ulcer; call your doctor if you experience stomach pain, vomiting, or restlessness. • While taking this drug, drink at least eight glasses of water daily. • Be sure to take your dose at exactly the right time. It is best to take this drug on an empty stomach one hour before or two hours after a meal (unless otherwise prescribed). • If taking this drug causes you minor gastrointestinal distress, use a nonprescription antacid product for relief. • The time-release forms must be swallowed whole; do not chew or crush them. If you are unable to swallow the capsule, you may mix its contents with jelly or applesauce and swallow the mixture without chewing. • Your doctor may want to check your blood levels of this drug in order to ensure its effectiveness. Ask your doctor to explain what the blood level means. Learn to keep track of your blood levels. • Cigarette smoking may affect this drug's action. Be sure your doctor knows you smoke. Also, do not suddenly stop smoking without informing your doctor. • Do not switch brands without checking with your doctor or pharmacist, as your dosage may need to be adjusted. There are many theophylline products that are similar but are not true "generic" substitutes. Consult with your doctor or pharmacist about the use of an inexpensive product.

Theospan bronchodilator (Laser, Inc.), see theophylline bronchodilator.

Theostat bronchodilator (Laser, Inc.), see theophylline bronchodilator.

Theo-Time bronchodilator (Major Pharmaceuticals), see theophylline bronchodilator.

Theovent bronchodilator (Schering Corp.), see theophylline bronchodilator.

thioridazine antipsychotic (various manufacturers), see Mellaril antipsychotic.

thiothixene antipsychotic (various manufacturers), see Navane antipsychotic.

Thiuretic diuretic and antihypertensive (Warner Chilcott Laboratories), see hydrochlorothiazide diuretic and antihypertensive.

Thyrar thyroid hormone (USV [P.R.] Development Corp.), see thyroid hormone.

thyroid hormone

Manufacturer: various manufacturers
Ingredient: thyroid
Equivalent Products: Armour Thyroid, Rorer Pharmaceuticals; Proloid, Parke-Davis; S-P-T, Fleming & Co.; Thyrar, USV [P.R.] Development Corp. (see Comments)
Dosage Forms: Capsule; Enteric-coated tablet; Tablet (various dosages and various colors)
Use: Thyroid-hormone replacement therapy
Minor Side Effects: Diarrhea; headache; irritability; vomiting
Major Side Effects: In overdose: Chest pain; fever; heat intolerance; insomnia; leg cramps; menstrual irregularities; nervousness; palpitations; shortness of breath; sweating; trembling; weight loss
Contraindications: This drug should not be used to treat obesity, especially in conjunction with amphetamine-type diet pills; such therapy is dangerous. • This drug should not be used by people with an overactive thyroid gland or by those whose adrenal glands are malfunctioning. Be sure your doctor knows if either of these conditions applies to you. • In most cases, this drug should not be used by people with heart disease. However, if the thyroid disease was a contributing or causative factor in the heart condition, this drug can be tried cautiously.
Warnings: This drug should be used cautiously by people who have cardiovascular disease, high blood pressure, kidney disease, or diabetes. Be sure your doctor knows if any of these conditions applies to you. • This drug interacts with cholestyramine, epinephrine, digitalis, phenytoin, oral contraceptives, oral anticoagulants, and antidiabetics; if you are currently taking any drugs of these types, consult your doctor about their use. If you are unsure of the type or contents of your medications, ask your doctor or pharmacist. • While taking this drug, do not take any nonprescription item for weight control, cough, cold, or sinus problems without first checking with your doctor. • If you are taking digitalis in addition to this drug, watch carefully for symptoms of increased digitalis effects (e.g., nausea, blurred vision, palpitations), and notify your doctor immediately if they occur.
Comments: Compliance with prescribed therapy is essential with this drug. Be sure to follow your doctor's dosage instructions exactly. Get into the habit of taking the drug at the same time each day. • Most side effects from this drug can be controlled by dosage adjustment; consult your doctor if you experience side effects. • Do not stop taking this drug without consulting your doctor. • Although many thyroid products are on the market, they are not all bioequivalent; that is, they may not all be absorbed into the bloodstream at the same rate or have the same overall pharmacologic activity. To make sure you are receiving an identically functioning product, don't change brands of this drug without consulting your doctor or pharmacist.

Tigan antinauseant

Manufacturer: Beecham Laboratories
Ingredient: trimethobenzamide hydrochloride
Equivalent Products: Tebamide, G&W Laboratories, Inc.; T-Gen, Goldline Laboratories; trimethobenzamide, various manufacturers
Dosage Forms: Capsule: 100 mg (blue/white); 250 mg (blue). Pediatric suppository: 100 mg. Suppository: 200 mg
Use: Control of nausea and vomiting
Minor Side Effects: Diarrhea; dizziness; drowsiness; headache; muscle cramps
Major Side Effects: Back pain; blood disorders; blurred vision; coma; convulsions; depression; disorientation; jaundice; mouth sores; rash; tremors; unusual hand or face movements; vomiting
Contraindications: This drug should not be taken by people who are allergic to it. Consult your doctor immediately if this drug has been prescribed for you and you have such an allergy. • The suppository form of this drug should not be given to newborn infants.
Warnings: This drug should be used with extreme caution in children for the treatment of vomiting. This drug is not recommended for treatment of uncomplicated vomiting in children; its use should be limited to prolonged vomiting of known cause. • Since this drug may cause drowsiness, patients should not operate motor vehicles or dangerous machinery until their individual responses to the drug have been determined. To avoid excessive sedation, avoid taking alcohol and other depressive drugs while taking this drug. If you are unsure of the type or contents of your medications, ask your doctor or pharmacist. • This drug should be used cautiously by pregnant or nursing women. • This drug should be used with caution by patients (especially children and the elderly or debilitated) who have acute fever, encephalitis, viral infection, intestinal infection, gastroenteritis, dehydration, or electrolyte imbalance. Be sure your doctor knows if any of these conditions applies to you. • This drug may render diagnosis more difficult in such conditions as appendicitis and may obscure signs of toxicity due to overdose of other drugs. • This drug should be discontinued at the first sign of sensitivity to it.

Timoptic ophthalmic preparation

Manufacturer: Merck Sharp & Dohme
Ingredient: timolol maleate
Dosage Form: Drop (content per ml): 0.25%; 0.5%
Uses: Treatment of some types of chronic glaucoma and ocular hypertension
Minor Side Effects: Mild eye irritation; temporary blurred vision
Major Side Effects: Major side effects are rare when this product is used correctly. However, rare occurrences of anxiety, bronchospasm, confusion, depression, dizziness, drowsiness, generalized rash, indigestion, loss of appetite, nausea, weakness, and slight reduction of the resting heart rate have been observed in some users of this drug.
Contraindication: This drug should not be used by people who are allergic to it. Consult your doctor immediately if this drug has been prescribed for you and you have such an allergy.
Warnings: This drug should be used with caution by people with bronchial asthma, myasthenia gravis, heart disease, or narrow-angle glaucoma. Be sure your doctor knows if any of these conditions applies to you. • This drug is not recommended for use by children. • This drug should be used cautiously by pregnant women. If you are pregnant, be sure your doctor knows about your

condition before you take this drug. • People taking beta blockers should use this drug with caution. If you are presently taking any drugs of this type, consult your doctor about their use. If you are unsure of the type or contents of your medications, ask your doctor or pharmacist.

Comments: This product is also available in a white plastic ophthalmic dispenser with a controlled-drop tip, called an Ocumeter. Your pharmacist can give you details. • Be careful about the contamination of drops used for the eyes. Wash your hands before administering eye drops. Do not touch the dropper to the eye. Do not wash or wipe the dropper before replacing it in the bottle. Close the bottle tightly to keep out moisture. See the chapter Administering Medication Correctly for instructions on using eye drops. • This product may sting at first, but this is normal and usually goes away after continued use. Like other eye drops, this product may cause some temporary clouding or blurring of vision. This symptom will go away quickly. • Unlike other drugs used to treat glaucoma, this agent needs to be administered only once or twice a day. • If you are using more than one type of eye product, wait at least five minutes between administrations of different medications.

Tipramine antidepressant (Major Pharmaceuticals), see Tofranil antidepressant.

Tobrex ophthalmic antibiotic

Manufacturer: Alcon Laboratories, Inc.
Ingredient: tobramycin
Dosage Forms: Ointment (per gram); Solution (per ml): tobramycin, 0.3%
Use: Treatment of eye infections
Minor Side Effects: Mild irritation; redness; stinging; tearing; temporary blurred vision
Major Side Effects: Eyelid swelling; itching
Contraindications: This drug should not be used by persons allergic to tobramycin or aminoglycoside antibiotics. Consult your doctor immediately if this drug has been prescribed for you and you have such an allergy.
Warnings: Use this drug exactly as prescribed for as long as prescribed, even if symptoms disappear within that time. Stopping therapy early can lead to reinfection. Prolonged use may allow organisms that are not susceptible to it to grow wildly, resulting in another infection. • Use this drug only for the condition for which it was prescribed. • This drug must be used cautiously by pregnant women. Nursing mothers who must take this drug should stop nursing. • This drug must be used cautiously in the presence of an injured cornea.
Comments: Upon instillation of this drug, there may be mild and temporary burning and stinging. Vision may also be blurred for a short time. If the effects continue or worsen, contact your doctor. • Symptoms should improve within a few days. If they persist or worsen, contact your doctor. • Be careful when administering eye medications. Wash your hands before using. To avoid contamination of the medication, do not touch the ointment tube to your eye. See the chapter Administering Medication Correctly for detailed instructions on proper use of eye medications.

Tofranil antidepressant

Manufacturer: Geigy Pharmaceuticals
Ingredient: imipramine hydrochloride
Equivalent Products: imipramine hydrochloride, various manufacturers; Janimine, Abbott Laboratories; Tipramine, Major Pharmaceuticals

Dosage Form: Tablet: 10 mg; 25 mg; 50 mg (all are coral); see Comments

Uses: Control of bed-wetting; relief of depression

Minor Side Effects: Agitation; anxiety; black tongue; blurred vision; confusion; constipation; cramps; diarrhea; dizziness; drowsiness; dry mouth; fatigue; flushing; headache; heartburn; increased sensitivity to light; insomnia; loss of appetite; nausea; peculiar tastes in the mouth; restlessness; stomach upset; sweating; urine color change; vomiting; weakness

Major Side Effects: Bleeding; convulsions; difficulty in urinating; enlarged or painful breasts (in both sexes); fainting; fever; fluid retention; hair loss; hallucinations; heart attack; high or low blood pressure; impotence; jaundice; loss of balance; mood changes; mouth sores; nervousness; nightmares; numbness in fingers or toes; palpitations; psychosis; rash; ringing in the ears; sleep disorders; sore throat; stroke; testicular swelling; tremors; uncoordinated movements; weight loss or gain

Contraindications: This drug should not be taken by people who are allergic to it or by anyone who has recently had a heart attack. This drug should not be taken by people who are using monoamine oxidase inhibitors (ask your pharmacist if you are unsure). Consult your doctor immediately if this drug has been prescribed for you and any of these conditions applies.

Warnings: This drug should be used cautiously by the elderly and by people who have glaucoma, high blood pressure, enlarged prostate, porphyria, intestinal blockage, heart disease, epilepsy, thyroid disease, liver or kidney disease, or a history of urinary retention problems. Pregnant or nursing women, people who receive electroshock therapy, and those who use drugs that lower blood pressure should also use this drug cautiously. Be sure your doctor knows if any of these conditions applies to you. • This drug must be used cautiously by children. • Notify your doctor if you experience abrupt changes in mood or if you have a sore throat with fever. • If you are going to have any type of surgery, be sure your doctor knows that you are taking this drug; the drug should be discontinued before surgery. (Consult your doctor before stopping the drug.) • This drug interacts with alcohol, amphetamines, barbiturates, central nervous system depressants, clonidine, anticholinergics, epinephrine, guanethidine, methylphenidate hydrochloride, monoamine oxidase inhibitors, oral anticoagulants, and phenylephrine; if you are currently taking any drugs of these types, consult your doctor about their use. If you are unsure of the type or contents of your medications, ask your doctor or pharmacist. • Do not stop taking this drug suddenly without consulting your doctor. It may be necessary to reduce your dosage gradually.

Comments: The effects of therapy with this drug may not be apparent for at least two weeks. Your doctor may adjust your dosage frequently during the first few months of therapy in order to find the best dose for you. • Take this medication exactly as prescribed. • If this drug is being used to control bed-wetting, it should be taken one hour before bedtime. • Chew gum or suck on ice chips or a piece of hard candy to reduce mouth dryness. • Many people receive as much benefit from taking a single dose of this drug at bedtime as from taking multiple doses throughout the day. Talk to your doctor about this dosage plan. • Tofranil antidepressant is also available in capsules that contain larger doses of the drug than the tablets. The capsule form, called Tofranil-PM, should not be used by children because the greater potency increases the risk of overdose. • While taking this drug, do not take any nonprescription item for weight control, cough, cold, or sinus problems without first checking with your doctor. • This drug may cause drowsiness; avoid tasks that require alertness. To prevent oversedation, avoid the use of alcohol or other drugs that have sedative properties. • This drug may cause you to be especially sensitive to the sun, so avoid exposure to sunlight as much as possible. • To avoid dizziness or light-headedness when you stand, contract and relax the muscles of your legs for a few moments before rising. Do this by pushing one foot against the floor while raising the other foot slightly, alternating feet so that you are "pumping" your legs in a pedaling motion. • This drug may be taken with food to lessen stomach upset. • This drug is similar in action to other antidepressants. If this drug is ineffective or not well tolerated, your doctor may have you try another in order to find the best drug for you.

Tofranil-PM antidepressant (Geigy Pharmaceuticals), see Tofranil antidepressant (comments).

Tolamide oral antidiabetic (Major Pharmaceuticals), see Tolinase oral antidiabetic.

tolazamide oral antidiabetic (various manufacturers), see Tolinase oral antidiabetic.

tolbutamide oral antidiabetic (various manufacturers), see Orinase oral antidiabetic.

Tolectin anti-inflammatory

Manufacturer: McNeil Pharmaceuticals
Ingredient: tolmetin sodium
Dosage Forms: Capsule: 400 mg (orange). Tablet: 200 mg (white)
Use: Relief of pain and swelling due to arthritis
Minor Side Effects: Bloating; blurred vision; constipation; diarrhea; dizziness; drowsiness; gas; headache; heartburn; insomnia; itching; nausea; nervousness; stomach upset; vomiting; weakness
Major Side Effects: Blood in stools; breathing difficulties; chest pain; depression; difficulty in urinating; fluid retention; high blood pressure; rash; ringing in the ears; sore throat; ulcers; visual disturbances; weight gain
Contraindications: This drug should not be taken by people who are allergic to it or to aspirin or similar drugs. Consult your doctor immediately if this drug has been prescribed for you and you have such an allergy.
Warnings: This drug should be used with extreme caution by patients with upper gastrointestinal tract disease, peptic ulcer, heart disease, high blood pressure, kidney disease, or bleeding diseases. Be sure your doctor knows if any of these conditions applies to you. • Persons taking this drug for prolonged periods should have regular eye examinations. • Use of this drug by pregnant women, nursing mothers, and children under two years of age is not recommended. • Persons using this drug should have periodic urine tests performed. • This drug should be used cautiously in conjunction with aspirin, diuretics, oral anticoagulants, oral antidiabetics, phenytoin, and probenecid. If you are currently taking any drugs of these types, consult your doctor. If you are unsure of the type or contents of your medications, ask your doctor or pharmacist.
Comments: In numerous tests, this drug has been shown to be as effective as aspirin in the treatment of arthritis, but aspirin is still the drug of choice for the disease. This drug is often prescribed when aspirin proves ineffective. • If you are allergic to aspirin, you may not be able to use this drug. • Do not take aspirin or alcohol while taking this drug without first consulting your doctor. • This drug may cause drowsiness; avoid tasks that require alertness, such as driving and operating machinery. • You should note improvement of your condition soon after you start using this drug; however, full benefit may not be obtained for one to two weeks. It is important not to stop taking this drug even

though symptoms have diminished or disappeared. • This drug is not a substitute for rest, physical therapy, or other measures recommended by your doctor to treat your condition. • If this drug upsets your stomach, take it with food or an antacid other than sodium bicarbonate. • Notify your doctor if skin rash, itching, black tarry stools, swelling of the hands or feet, or persistent headache occurs. • This drug is similar in action to other anti-inflammatory agents, such as Indocin, Naprosyn, and ibuprofen. If one of these drugs is not well tolerated, your doctor may have you try the others in order to find the drug that is best for you.

Tolinase oral antidiabetic

Manufacturer: The Upjohn Company
Ingredient: tolazamide
Equivalent Products: Ronase, Reid-Rowell; Tolamide, Major Pharmaceuticals; tolazamide, various manufacturers
Dosage Form: Tablet: 100 mg; 250 mg; 500 mg (all are white)
Use: Treatment of diabetes mellitus not controlled by diet and exercise alone
Minor Side Effects: Cramps; diarrhea; dizziness; fatigue; gas; headache; heartburn; loss of appetite; nausea; rash; stomach upset; sun sensitivity; vomiting; weakness
Major Side Effects: Blood disorders; breathing difficulties; bruising; convulsions; dark urine; jaundice; light-colored stools; low blood sugar; ringing in the ears; sore throat; tingling in the hands or feet; visual disturbances
Contraindications: This drug should not be taken by diabetic patients who have infections, are undergoing surgery or severe trauma, or have ketosis, acidosis, or a history of repeated bouts of ketoacidosis or coma. This drug is not indicated for persons with insulin-dependent or "brittle" diabetes. This drug should not be taken by people with liver disease, kidney disease, endocrine disease, uremia, or an allergy to sulfonylureas. Be sure your doctor knows if any of these conditions applies to you. • This drug should be used cautiously by pregnant women. Discuss this with your doctor.
Warnings: Be sure you receive full instructions on how to take this drug and how to control your diabetes. Know how to prevent low blood sugar and recognize its symptoms, as well as what to do if such a complication occurs. You cannot neglect your dietary restrictions or disregard instructions about weight, exercise, hygiene, and avoidance of infection. Be sure you know how and when to test your urine and what the results mean. You must be particularly careful during the transition from insulin to this oral antidiabetic. • This drug should be taken with caution when thiazide-type diuretics are also being taken, since such combinations can aggravate diabetes mellitus. • This drug should be used cautiously by persons who are malnourished, debilitated, or of advanced age and by those who suffer from alcoholism or adrenal or pituitary gland problems. Be sure your doctor knows if any of these conditions applies to you. • This drug interacts with alcohol, anabolic steroids, anticoagulants, aspirin, chloramphenicol, guanethidine, monoamine oxidase inhibitors, phenylbutazone, probenecid, propranolol, steroids, sulfonamides, tetracycline, thiazide diuretics, and thyroid hormone. If you are currently taking any drugs of these types, consult your doctor about their use. If you are unsure of the type or contents of your medications, ask your doctor or pharmacist.
Comments: Studies have shown that a good diet and exercise program is extremely important in controlling diabetes. Persons taking this drug should carefully watch their diet and exercise program. • Oral antidiabetic drugs are not effective in treating diabetes in children under age 12. • Take your dose of this drug at the same time each day. • Ask your doctor how to recognize the first signs of low blood sugar and how and when to test for glucose and ketones

in the urine. Signs of low blood sugar include cold sweat; chills; drowsiness; cool, pale skin; headache; nausea; rapid pulse; tremors; and weakness. If these signs develop, eat or drink something containing sugar and call your doctor immediately. • During the first few weeks of therapy with this drug, visit your doctor frequently. • You will have to be switched to insulin therapy if complications (e.g., ketoacidosis, severe trauma, severe infection, diarrhea, nausea, or vomiting) or the need for major surgery develops. • Do not use alcohol while taking this drug. Avoid any other drugs unless your doctor tells you to take them. Be especially careful of nonprescription cold remedies. • Notify your doctor if you develop signs of jaundice (yellow eyes or skin; dark urine). • You may sunburn easily while taking this product. Avoid prolonged exposure to the sun and wear a protective sunscreen. • It is advised that you carry a medical alert card or wear a medical alert bracelet indicating that you are taking this drug. • There are other drugs similar to this one that vary slightly in activity (see Glucotrol, Diabinese, Orinase). Certain persons who do not benefit from one type of oral antidiabetic may benefit from another.

Totacillin antibiotic (Beecham Laboratories), see ampicillin antibiotic.

Trandate antihypertensive (Allen & Hanburys), see Normodyne antihypertensive.

Transderm-Nitro transdermal antianginal (Ciba Pharmaceutical Company), see nitroglycerin transdermal antianginal.

Tranxene antianxiety and anticonvulsant

Manufacturer: Abbott Laboratories
Ingredient: clorazepate dipotassium
Equivalent Product: Gen-Xene, Alra Laboratories, Inc.
Dosage Forms: Sustained-action tablet: 11.25 mg (blue); 22.5 mg (tan). Tablet: 3.75 mg (blue); 7.5 mg (peach); 15 mg (lavender)
Uses: Relief of anxiety, nervousness, tension and symptoms of withdrawal from alcohol addiction
Minor Side Effects: Confusion; constipation; diarrhea; dizziness; drooling; drowsiness; dry mouth; fatigue; headache; heartburn; insomnia; irritability; loss of appetite; nausea; nervousness; sweating; vomiting
Major Side Effects: Blurred vision; breathing difficulties; depression; difficulty in swallowing; difficulty in urinating; double vision; fever; hallucinations; jaundice; low blood pressure; menstrual irregularities; palpitations; rash; slow heartbeat; slurred speech; sore throat; tremors
Contraindications: This drug should not be taken by people who are allergic to it or by those who have acute narrow-angle glaucoma. Consult your doctor immediately if this drug has been prescribed for you and either condition applies.
Warnings: This drug is not recommended for use by people who are severely depressed, those who have severe mental illness, or those under the age of nine. This drug should be used cautiously by people with a history of drug dependence; by pregnant or nursing women; by the elderly or debilitated; and by people with impaired liver or kidney function, lung disease, epilepsy, porphyria, or myasthenia gravis. Be sure your doctor knows if any of these conditions applies to you. • This drug may cause drowsiness, especially during the first few days of therapy; avoid tasks that require alertness, such as driving a car or operating machinery. • This drug should not be taken with alcohol or

other central nervous system depressants; serious adverse reactions may develop. This drug should be used cautiously in conjunction with cimetidine, phenytoin, or oral anticoagulants. If you are currently taking any drugs of these types, consult your doctor about their use. If you are unsure about the type or contents of your medications, ask your doctor or pharmacist. • This drug has the potential for abuse and must be used with caution. Tolerance may develop quickly; do not increase the dose without first consulting your doctor. • Do not stop taking this drug suddenly without first consulting your doctor. If you have been taking this drug regularly, your dosage will have to be reduced gradually according to your doctor's directions. • If you take this drug for long periods, you may need to have periodic blood counts and liver function tests.

Comments: This drug currently is used by many people to relieve nervousness. It is effective for this purpose, but it is important to try to remove the cause of the anxiety as well. • Chew gum or suck on ice chips or a piece of hard candy to reduce mouth dryness. • Never take the sustained-action tablets more frequently than your doctor prescribes; a serious overdose may result. • Take this medication with food or a full glass of water to lessen stomach upset. Do not take it with an antacid, which may retard absorption of the drug. Space dosing of this drug and an antacid by 30 minutes. • Notify your doctor if you develop signs of jaundice (yellow eyes or skin; dark urine).

trazodone HCI antidepressant (various manufacturers), see Desyrel antidepressant.

Trendar anti-inflammatory (Whitehall Laboratories, Inc.), see ibuprofen anti-inflammatory.

Trental hemorrheologic (blood flow promoter)

Manufacturer: Hoechst-Roussel Pharmaceutical, Inc.
Ingredient: pentoxifylline
Dosage Form: Sustained-release tablet: 400 mg (pink)
Use: Promotes blood flow in the treatment of certain blood vessel diseases
Minor Side Effects: Anxiety; bad taste in mouth; bloating; blurred vision; brittle fingernails; confusion; constipation; diarrhea; dizziness; drowsiness; dry mouth; earache; gas; headache; loss of appetite; nasal congestion; nausea; sore throat; stomach upset; thirst; tremor; weakness; weight change
Major Side Effects: Bleeding or bruising; blood disorders; breathing difficulties; chest pain; faintness; fluid retention; flushing; hallucinations; jaundice; low blood pressure; palpitations; rash; sleeping disorders; swollen neck glands
Contraindications: This drug should not be used by persons allergic to it or to caffeine, theophylline, or theobromine. Consult your doctor immediately if this drug has been prescribed for you and you have such an allergy. • This drug is not recommended for use by children under 18 years of age or by nursing mothers.
Warnings: This drug must be used cautiously by pregnant women and persons with coronary artery disease. Consult your doctor if either of these conditions applies to you. • This drug may interact with antihypertensive medications. This medication should be used cautiously by persons taking warfarin, aspirin, or salicylates. If you are currently taking any drugs of these types, consult your doctor about their use. If you are unsure about the type or contents of your medications, ask your doctor or pharmacist.
Comments: This drug is taken with food unless otherwise prescribed. • The tablets are sustained release and must be swallowed whole; do not crush or

chew them. • It may take two to four weeks before the effects of this drug are evident. Therapy is usually continued for at least eight weeks. • Side effects should subside with continued treatment. If they persist or become bothersome, contact your physician. An alteration in dosage may alleviate side effects. Do not, however, stop taking this drug or change the dose without your doctor's advice. • Notify your doctor if you develop signs of jaundice (yellow eyes or skin; dark urine). • Be cautious about taking nonprescription medicines containing aspirin.

Trialodine antidepressant (Quantum Pharmics), see Desyrel antidepressant.

triamcinolone and nystatin topical steroid hormone and anti-infective (various manufacturers), see Mycolog II topical steroid hormone and anti-infective.

Triaminic-12 antihistamine and decongestant (Sandoz Pharmaceuticals), see Ornade Spansules antihistamine and decongestant.

triamterene diuretic and antihypertensive (various manufacturers), see Dyazide diuretic and antihypertensive.

Triavil phenothiazine and antidepressant

Manufacturer: Merck Sharp & Dohme
Ingredients: amitriptyline hydrochloride; perphenazine
Equivalent Product: Etrafon, Schering Corp.
Dosage Form: Tablet: Triavil 2-10: amitriptyline hydrochloride, 10 mg and perphenazine, 2 mg (blue); Triavil 2-25: amitriptyline hydrochloride, 25 mg and perphenazine, 2 mg (orange); Triavil 4-10: amitriptyline hydrochloride, 10 mg and perphenazine, 4 mg (salmon); Triavil 4-25: amitriptyline hydrochloride, 25 mg and perphenazine, 4 mg (yellow); Triavil 4-50: amitriptyline hydrochloride, 50 mg and perphenazine, 4 mg (orange)
Uses: Relief of anxiety or depression
Minor Side Effects: Blurred vision; change in urine color; confusion; constipation; decreased sweating; diarrhea; dizziness; drooling; drowsiness; dry mouth; excitement; fatigue; headache; heartburn; increased salivation; jitteriness; loss of appetite; menstrual irregularities; nasal congestion; nausea; peculiar taste in the mouth; restlessness; skin darkening; sun sensitivity; vomiting; weakness
Major Side Effects: Aching or numbness in arms or legs; chest pain; convulsions; difficulty in urinating; enlarged or painful breasts (in both sexes); eye pain; fainting; fluid retention; hair loss; high or low blood pressure; high or low blood sugar; imbalance; impotence; insomnia; involuntary movements of the face, mouth, jaw, and tongue; jaundice; mouth sores; muscle stiffness; nervousness; nightmares; palpitations; rash; ringing in the ears; sore throat; stroke; swelling of the testicles; tremors; weight gain or loss
Contraindications: This drug should not be taken by persons with drug-induced depression, recent heart attack, or blood disease. This drug should not be taken by people who are allergic to either of its components or by those taking monoamine oxidase inhibitors. Consult your doctor immediately if this drug has been prescribed for you and any of these conditions applies.

Warnings: This drug should be used with caution by persons with thyroid disease, certain types of glaucoma, impaired liver function, certain types of heart disease, epilepsy, difficulty in urinating, intestinal blockage, high or low blood pressure, diabetes, brain disease, Parkinson's disease, peptic ulcer, enlarged prostate, breast cancer, or asthma or other respiratory disorders. Be sure your doctor knows if any of these conditions applies to you. • This drug may cause drowsiness; avoid tasks requiring alertness, such as driving or operating machinery. To prevent oversedation, avoid the use of alcohol or other drugs with sedative properties. • This drug is not recommended for use by pregnant women or by children. • Use of this drug may cause mood changes and a rise in body temperature. Call your doctor if you experience either. • This drug should be used with caution by persons undergoing elective surgery or electroshock therapy. • This drug has been shown to result in both elevation and lowering of blood sugar levels. Diabetics should monitor their urine sugar and blood glucose closely while taking this drug, and report any abnormalities to their doctors. • This drug should not be taken with alcohol, amphetamine, barbiturates, epinephrine, guanethidine, monoamine oxidase inhibitors, oral anticoagulants, phenylephrine, antacids, ethchlorvynol, anticholinergics, central nervous system depressants, or clonidine. If you are currently taking any drugs of these types, consult your doctor about their use. If you are unsure of the type or contents of your medications, ask your doctor or pharmacist. • Take this drug exactly as directed; an overdose could be fatal. • This drug may interfere with certain laboratory tests. Remind your doctor you are taking this drug before undergoing any tests.

Comments: The effects of this drug may not be apparent for at least two weeks. • While taking this drug, avoid using alcohol and do not start or stop taking any other drug, including nonprescription items, without consulting your doctor. • Chew gum or suck on ice chips or a piece of hard candy to reduce mouth dryness. • This drug may make you more sensitive to sunlight; avoid prolonged exposure and wear protective clothing and a sunscreen when outdoors. • To avoid dizziness or light-headedness when you stand, contract and relax the muscles of your legs for a few moments before rising. Do this by pushing one foot against the floor while raising the other foot slightly, alternating feet so that you are "pumping" your legs in a pedaling motion. • If you notice fine tremors of your tongue, call your doctor. • Antacids may prevent the absorption of this drug. Don't take them at the same time as you take this drug; space them by at least two hours. • If this drug causes stomach upset, you may take it with food or milk.

trifluoperazine antipsychotic (various manufacturers), see Stelazine antipsychotic.

trimethobenzamide antinauseant (various manufacturers), see Tigan antinauseant.

Trimox antibiotic (E. R. Squibb & Sons, Inc.), see amoxicillin antibiotic.

Trinalin antihistamine and decongestant

Manufacturer: Schering Corp.
Ingredients: pseudoephedrine sulfate; azatadine maleate
Dosage Form: Sustained-release tablet; pseudoephedrine sulfate, 120 mg and azatadine maleate, 1 mg
Use: For the relief of nasal and upper respiratory congestion

Minor Side Effects: Anxiety; blurred vision; constipation; diarrhea; dizziness; drowsiness; dry mouth; headache; insomnia; irritability; nausea; rash; reduced sweating; sedation; stomach upset; weakness

Major Side Effects: Abdominal cramps; breathing difficulties; chest pain; confusion; difficulty in urinating; headache; high or low blood pressure; loss of coordination; palpitations; sore throat; unusual bleeding or bruising

Contraindications: This drug should not be used to treat asthma or symptoms of lower respiratory infections. This drug should not be taken by persons allergic to it or to other antihistamines. If you are allergic to antihistamines, check with your doctor or pharmacist before taking this drug. • This drug should not be used by persons with narrow-angle glaucoma, urinary retention, hyperthyroidism, severe hypertension, or severe heart disease or by persons concurrently taking monoamine oxidase inhibitors (ask your pharmacist if you are unsure). Consult your doctor immediately if this drug has been prescribed for you and any of these conditions applies. • This drug should not be taken by children under 12 years of age. • This drug should be used with extreme caution during pregnancy. Discuss the benefits and risks with your doctor. • Use of this drug by nursing mothers is not recommended.

Warnings: This drug should be used cautiously by persons with peptic ulcer, blood vessel disease, high blood pressure, or diabetes and by persons taking digitalis or oral anticoagulants. If you are unsure of the type or contents of your medications, ask your doctor or pharmacist. • Because this drug causes drowsiness, avoid tasks that require alertness. This drug must be used cautiously by persons over 60 years of age who may be more likely to experience dizziness, sedation, and low blood pressure. To prevent oversedation, avoid the use of alcohol and other drugs having sedative properties.

Comments: Because this is a sustained-release product, the tablets must be swallowed whole; do not crush or chew them. • Never increase your dose or take this drug more frequently than prescribed; a serious overdose could result. • Chew gum or suck on ice chips or a piece of hard candy to reduce mouth dryness. • While taking this drug, do not take any nonprescription medicine for weight control, cough, cold, or sinus problems without first checking with your doctor or pharmacist. • Because this drug reduces sweating, avoid excessive work or exercise in hot weather. • If this drug causes stomach upset, take it with food.

Tri-Phen-Chlor decongestant and antihistamine (Rugby Laboratories), see Naldecon decongestant and antihistamine.

Triple-Gen ophthalmic antibiotic (Goldline Laboratories), see Cortisporin ophthalmic antibiotic.

triple ophthalmic antibiotic (various manufacturers), see Cortisporin ophthalmic antibiotic.

Tri-Vi-Sol vitamin supplement (Mead Johnson Nutritional), see Poly-Vi-Flor vitamin and fluoride supplement (comments).

Truphylline bronchodilator (G & W Laboratories, Inc.), see aminophylline bronchodilator.

Tussi-Organidin antitussive and expectorant

Manufacturer: Wallace Laboratories
Ingredients: codeine phosphate; iodinated glycerol

Equivalent Products: Iophen-C, various manufacturers; Oridol-C, LuChem; Tussi-R-Gen, Goldline Laboratories

Dosage Form: Liquid (content per 5 ml teaspoon): codeine phosphate, 10 mg and iodinated glycerol, 30 mg

Use: Symptomatic relief of cough

Minor Side Effects: Acne flare-up; blurred vision; constipation; dizziness; drowsiness; headache; nausea; stomach upset; vomiting

Major Side Effects: Breathing difficulties; difficulty swallowing; euphoria; impaired coordination; rash; thyroid gland enlargement

Contraindications: This drug should not be used by pregnant or nursing women, newborns, or persons sensitive (allergic) to codeine or iodides. Call your doctor immediately if any of these conditions applies.

Warnings: This drug should be used cautiously by persons with a history or any evidence of thyroid disease and by children with cystic fibrosis. Be sure your doctor knows if either of these conditions applies. • This drug interacts with lithium and antithyroid drugs. If you are currently taking any drugs of these types, consult your doctor about their use. If you are unsure about the type or contents of your medications, ask your doctor or pharmacist. • If you develop a rash while taking this medication, stop using it and call your doctor; you may be sensitive to the drug. • This drug may cause a flare-up of acne in adolescents. • This drug may cause drowsiness; avoid tasks requiring alertness, such as driving or operating machinery. To avoid oversedation, avoid alcohol and other central nervous system depressants while taking this drug. • Codeine has the potential for abuse and must be used with caution. Do not take this drug more frequently than prescribed, and do not increase the dose without consulting your doctor. Prolonged or excessive use of products containing codeine may be habit-forming.

Comments: If you need an expectorant, you need more moisture in your environment. Use of a vaporizer or humidifier may be helpful. Also, drink nine to ten glasses of water daily. • While taking this medication, do not take any nonprescription items for weight control, coughs, colds, or sinus problems without first checking with your doctor or pharmacist.

Tussi-R-Gen antitussive and expectorant (Goldline Laboratories), see Tussi-Organidin antitussive and expectorant.

Tusstat antihistamine (Century Pharmaceuticals, Inc.), see Benadryl antihistamine.

Tylenol with Codeine analgesic (McNeil Pharmaceutical), see acetaminophen with codeine analgesic.

Tylox analgesic (McNeil Pharmaceutical), see Percocet analgesic.

Ty-Pap with Codeine analgesic (Major Pharmaceuticals), see acetaminophen with codeine analgesic.

Ty-Tab analgesic (Major Pharmaceuticals), see acetaminophen with codeine analgesic.

Ultracef antibiotic (Bristol Laboratories), see Duricef antibiotic.

Uniphyl bronchodilator (The Purdue Frederick Company), see theophylline bronchodilator.

Urodine analgesic (various manufacturers), see Pyridium analgesic.

Urogesic analgesic (Edwards Pharmacal), see Pyridium analgesic.

Uroplus DS and Uroplus SS antibacterials (Shionogi USA), see Bactrim and Bactrim DS antibacterials.

Utimox antibiotic (Parke-Davis), see amoxicillin antibiotic.

Valdrene antihistamine (The Vale Chemical Company), see Benadryl antihistamine.

Valisone topical steroid hormone

Manufacturer: Schering Corp.
Ingredient: betamethasone valerate
Equivalent Products: betamethasone valerate, various manufacturers; Betatrex, Savage Laboratories; Beta-Val, Lemmon Company; Valnac, NMC Laboratories, Inc.
Dosage Forms: Cream: 0.01%; 0.1%. Lotion: 0.1%. Ointment: 0.1%
Use: Relief of skin inflammation associated with conditions such as dermatitis, eczema, and poison ivy
Minor Side Effects: Acne; burning sensation; dryness; irritation of the affected area; itching; rash
Major Side Effects: Blistering; increased hair growth; loss of skin color; secondary infection; skin wasting
Contraindications: This drug should not be used by people who are allergic to it or by those with severe circulatory system disorders or infections of the skin. This drug should not be used in the ear if the eardrum is perforated. Consult your doctor immediately if this drug has been prescribed for you and any of these conditions applies.
Warnings: If irritation develops when using this drug, immediately discontinue use and notify your doctor. • This drug should be used with caution during pregnancy. • These products are not for use in the eyes or other mucous membranes. • Systemic absorption of this drug will be increased if extensive areas of the body are treated, particularly if occlusive bandages are used. Therefore, suitable precautions should be taken under this circumstance and under long-term use, particularly in children and infants; consult your doctor. If this drug is being used in the diaper area, avoid tight-fitting diapers or plastic pants. • This drug should not be used in the presence of infection.
Comments: Use this drug exactly as prescribed. Do not use it more often or for a longer period than your doctor prescribed. • If the affected area is extremely dry or is scaling, the skin may be moistened before applying the medication by soaking in water or by applying water with a clean cloth. The ointment form is probably better for dry skin. • A mild, temporary stinging sensation may occur after this medication is applied. If this persists, contact your doctor. • Do not use this product with an occlusive wrap unless your doctor directs you to do so. If it is necessary for you to use this drug under a wrap, follow your doctor's instructions exactly; do not leave the wrap in place longer than specified. • If the condition being treated worsens while using this drug, notify your doctor.

Valium antianxiety

Manufacturer: Roche Products Inc.

Ingredient: diazepam

Equivalent Products: diazepam, various manufacturers; Valrelease, Roche Laboratories; Vazepam, Major Pharmaceuticals

Dosage Forms: Sustained-release capsule: 15 mg (yellow) (see Comments). Tablet: 2 mg (white); 5 mg (yellow); 10 mg (blue)

Uses: Relief of anxiety, nervousness, tension, muscle spasms, and symptoms of withdrawal from alcohol addiction

Minor Side Effects: Confusion; constipation; depression; diarrhea; dizziness; drowsiness; dry mouth; fatigue; headache; heartburn; increased salivation; loss of appetite; nausea; sweating; vomiting; weakness

Major Side Effects: Blurred vision; breathing difficulties; difficulty in urinating; double vision; excitement; fever; hallucinations; jaundice; low blood pressure; menstrual irregularities; palpitations; rash; slurred speech; sore throat; stimulation; tremors; uncoordinated movements

Contraindications: This drug should not be given to children under six months of age. • This drug should not be taken by persons with certain types of glaucoma or by people who are allergic to it. Consult your doctor immediately if either condition applies to you.

Warnings: This drug is not recommended for use by people with severe mental illness. • This drug should be used cautiously by people with epilepsy, respiratory problems, myasthenia gravis, porphyria, a history of drug abuse, or impaired liver or kidney function; by pregnant women; by children; and by the elderly or debilitated. Be sure your doctor knows if any of these conditions applies to you. • This drug may cause drowsiness; avoid tasks that require alertness. If the drowsiness becomes severe or if you are lethargic, contact your doctor. There are other drugs that are similar in action to this one that may or may not be as debilitating; talk to your doctor about the alternatives. • This drug should not be taken simultaneously with alcohol or other central nervous system depressants; serious adverse reactions may develop. • This drug should be used cautiously in conjunction with cimetidine, oral anticoagulants, and phenytoin. • Do not stop taking this drug without informing your doctor. If you have been taking the drug regularly and wish to discontinue use, you must decrease the dose gradually, following your doctor's instructions. • This drug has the potential for abuse and must be used with caution. Tolerance may develop quickly; do not increase the dose without first consulting your doctor. • Persons taking this drug for prolonged periods should have periodic blood counts and liver function tests.

Comments: This drug currently is used by many people to relieve nervousness. It is effective for this purpose, but it is important to try to remove the cause of the anxiety as well. • Notify your doctor if you develop signs of jaundice (yellow skin or eyes; dark urine). • Chew gum or suck on ice chips or a piece of hard candy to reduce mouth dryness. • To lessen stomach upset, take with food or a full glass of water. • The sustained-release form must be swallowed whole; do not crush or chew the capsule. • The sustained-release form of this drug is available under the name Valrelease.

Valnac topical steroid hormone (NMC Laboratories, Inc.), see Valisone topical steroid hormone.

Valrelease antianxiety (Roche Laboratories), see Valium antianxiety.

Vamate antianxiety (Major Pharmaceuticals), see Atarax antianxiety.

Vanceril antiasthmatic

Manufacturer: Schering Corp.
Ingredient: beclomethasone dipropionate
Equivalent Product: Beclovent, Glaxo, Inc.
Dosage Form: Pressurized inhaler for oral use (content per one actuation from mouthpiece): 42 mcg
Use: Control of chronic asthma
Minor Side Effects: Bronchospasm; coughing; dry mouth; hoarseness; rash
Major Side Effects: Breathing difficulties; depression; muscle aches and pains; nosebleeds; sore throat or infections of the mouth or throat; weakness
Contraindications: This drug is a steroid. It should not be used in the primary treatment of severe asthma attacks where intensive measures are required. • This drug should not be used by people who are allergic to it or by those who have reacted adversely to other steroids.
Warnings: If you have been taking oral steroids to control your asthma, conversion to therapy with this inhaled drug will have to be accomplished slowly. You will have to exercise special caution if you develop an infection, need to have surgery, or experience other trauma. Talk with your doctor about this transition, and make sure you understand what you must do. You should carry a card with you that explains how your asthma is being treated in case an emergency arises and you are unable to explain it yourself. • Pregnant women, nursing mothers, women of childbearing age, and children under the age of six should use this drug with caution. Consult your doctor immediately if this drug has been prescribed for you and any of these conditions applies. • This drug is not for rapid relief of bronchospasm. If you have a bronchospasm and your dilator drugs do not help, call your doctor. • The dosage of this drug should be monitored very carefully. Taking more of this drug than is recommended will probably not give you more relief over the long term. • This drug may have to be discontinued if localized infections occur.
Comments: Use this drug exactly as prescribed. Do not use it more often than prescribed. Full benefit from this drug may not be apparent for two to four weeks. • Shake the canister well before use. • Your pharmacist should dispense patient instructions with this drug that explain administration technique. • If you use a bronchodilator with this drug, use the bronchodilator first, wait a few minutes, then use this drug. This use has been shown to be the most effective and to have the least potential for toxicity. • The contents of one canister of this drug should provide at least 200 oral inhalations. • This drug is sealed in the canister under pressure. Do not puncture the canister. Do not store the canister near heat or an open flame. • Rinsing your mouth after inhalation of this drug is advised in order to reduce irritation and dryness of mouth and throat. • This drug is not useful during acute asthma attacks. It is used to prevent attacks. • If you develop mouth sores or a sore throat while taking this medication, call your doctor.

Vapocet analgesic (Major Pharmaceuticals), see Vicodin analgesic.

Vasominic T.D. decongestant and antihistamine (A.V.P. Pharmaceuticals, Inc.), see Naldecon decongestant and antihistamine.

Vasotec antihypertensive

Manufacturer: Merck Sharp & Dohme
Ingredient: enalapril maleate
Dosage Form: Tablet: 2.5 mg (yellow); 5 mg (white); 10 mg (red); 20 mg (peach)
Uses: Treatment of high blood pressure; management of heart failure
Minor Side Effects: Cough; diarrhea; dizziness; fatigue; headache; insomnia; nausea; stomach upset; sweating
Major Side Effects: Breathing difficulties; chest pain; fever; impotence; itching; low blood pressure; muscle cramps; nervousness; palpitations; rash; sore throat; swelling of face, lips, and tongue; tingling in fingers and toes; vomiting
Contraindication: This drug should not be used by persons who are allergic to it. Remind your doctor that you have such an allergy if this drug has been prescribed for you.
Warnings: This drug should be used cautiously by pregnant women, nursing mothers, persons with kidney disease, and diabetics. Be sure your doctor knows if any of these conditions applies to you. • Persons taking this drug in conjunction with other antihypertensive or heart medications should use it cautiously, especially during initial therapy. Dosage adjustments may be required to prevent blood pressure from dropping too low. • This drug must be used cautiously with agents that increase serum potassium, such as spironolactone, triamterene, amiloride, potassium supplements, and salt substitutes containing potassium. If you are currently taking any drugs of these types, consult your doctor about their use. Dosages may need to be adjusted. Your doctor may wish to test your blood periodically to check the potassium level. • It is recommended that persons taking this drug for a prolonged period have periodic blood tests to monitor the effects of therapy. • Contact your doctor immediately if you notice swelling of the face, lips, tongue, or eyes, or have breathing difficulties while taking this drug. Stop using this drug until you talk to your doctor.
Comments: Side effects of this drug are usually mild and transient. During the first few days you may experience light-headedness, which should subside as therapy continues. If light-headedness continues or becomes more pronounced, contact your doctor. • To avoid dizziness or light-headedness when you stand, contract and relax the muscles of your legs for a few minutes before rising. Do this by pushing one foot against the floor while raising the other foot slightly, alternating feet so that you are "pumping" your feet in a pedaling motion. • If this medication makes you dizzy, avoid driving and operating machinery. • Notify your doctor if you develop signs of an infection (sore throat, fever) while taking this drug. • Avoid prolonged work or exercise in hot weather since excessive sweating can intensify the effects of this drug. • Notify your doctor if you develop severe vomiting or diarrhea while taking this drug, since they can lead to dehydration. • If you have high blood pressure, do not take any nonprescription item for weight control, cough, cold, or sinus problems without consulting your doctor or pharmacist; such items can increase blood pressure. • Take this drug as prescribed. Do not skip doses or take extra doses without consulting your doctor. • This drug may be taken with food if stomach upset occurs. • Learn how to monitor your pulse and blood pressure while taking this drug; discuss this with your doctor.

Vazepam antianxiety (Major Pharmaceuticals), see Valium antianxiety.

V-Cillin K antibiotic (Eli Lilly & Co.), see penicillin potassium phenoxymethyl (penicillin VK) antibiotic.

Veetids antibiotic (E. R. Squibb & Sons, Inc.), see penicillin potassium phenoxymethyl (penicillin VK) antibiotic.

Ventolin bronchodilator

Manufacturer: Allen & Hanburys
Ingredient: albuterol
Equivalent Product: Proventil, Schering Corp.
Dosage Forms: Capsules for inhalation (Rotacaps): 200 mcg (light blue/clear). Inhaler (content per actuation): 90 mcg. Syrup (content per 5 ml teaspoon): 2 mg. Tablet: 2 mg (white); 4 mg (white)
Use: Prevention of bronchospasm
Minor Side Effects: Dizziness; dry mouth and throat; headache; hyperactivity; increased appetite; increased blood pressure; insomnia; nausea; nervousness; restlessness; stomach upset; sweating; unusual taste in mouth; weakness
Major Side Effects: Breathing difficulties; chest pain; confusion; difficulty in urinating; flushing; irritability; muscle cramps; palpitations; trembling; vomiting
Contraindication: This drug should not be used by people allergic to it.
Warnings: This drug should be used with caution by people who have diabetes, high blood pressure, heart disease, or thyroid disease and by pregnant or nursing women. Be sure your doctor knows if any of these conditions applies to you. • This drug is not recommended for use in children under two years of age. • This drug has been shown to interact with amphetamines, monoamine oxidase inhibitors, antidepressants, beta blockers, and epinephrine. If you are currently using any drugs of these types, consult your doctor. If you are unsure of the type or contents of your medications, ask your doctor or pharmacist.
Comments: Take this drug as prescribed. Do not take it more often than prescribed without first consulting your doctor. Excessive use of the inhaler may lead to loss of effectiveness or adverse effects. • If two inhalations per dose are prescribed, wait at least one minute between inhalations for maximum effectiveness. • If your symptoms do not improve or if they get worse while using this drug, contact your doctor. • Chew gum or suck on ice chips or a piece of hard candy to reduce mouth dryness. • If stomach upset occurs, take the syrup or tablets with food or milk. • Make sure you know how to use the inhaler form properly. Ask your pharmacist for the instruction sheet on use of the inhaler. The contents of one canister of this drug should provide at least 200 oral inhalations. Keep spray away from eyes. The drug is sealed in the canister under pressure. Store away from heat or open flame. Do not puncture, break, or burn the container. • The Rotacaps are for use in a special inhaler. DO NOT SWALLOW THE CAPSULES. The contents of the capsules are to be inhaled. Make sure your doctor or pharmacist has demonstrated the use of the Rotacaps. • Proventil is also available as a 4 mg extended-release tablet.

verapamil antianginal and antihypertensive (various manufacturers), see Isoptin antianginal and antihypertensive.

Vicodin analgesic

Manufacturer: Knoll Pharmaceutical Company
Ingredients: hydrocodone bitartrate; acetaminophen
Equivalent Products: Amacodone, Trimen Laboratories, Inc.; Anodynos-DHC, Forest Pharmaceuticals, Inc.; Bancap HC, O'Neal, Jones, and Feldman Pharmaceuticals; Co-Gesic, Central Pharmaceuticals, Inc.; Damacet-P, Mason Pharmaceuticals; Dolacet, W. E. Hauck, Inc.; Duradyne DHC, Forest Pharma-

ceuticals, Inc.; Hydrocet, Carnrick Laboratories, Inc.; Hydrogesic, Edwards Pharmacal; Hy-Phen, B. F. Ascher & Company, Inc.; Lorcet-HD, UAD Laboratories, Inc.; Lortab 5, Russ, Inc.; Norcet, Holloway Labs, Inc.; Vapocet, Major Pharmaceuticals; Zydone, Du Pont Pharmaceuticals, Inc.

Dosage Form: Tablet: hydrocodone bitartrate, 5 mg and acetaminophen, 500 mg (white with red stripe)

Use: Relief of moderate to severe pain

Minor Side Effects: Anxiety; constipation; dizziness; drowsiness; euphoria; fatigue; light-headedness; loss of appetite; nausea; sedation; stomach upset; sweating; vomiting; weakness

Major Side Effects: Breathing difficulties; confusion; difficulty in urinating; excitation; fear; hallucinations; jaundice; mood changes; palpitations; rash; restlessness; tremors; unpleasant emotions

Contraindications: This drug should not be used by persons allergic to either of its components or to certain other narcotic analgesics. Consult your doctor immediately if this drug has been prescribed for you and you have such an allergy.

Warnings: This drug should be used cautiously by pregnant women; the elderly; children; persons with liver or kidney disease, Addison's disease, or prostate disease; and in the presence of head injury or acute abdominal conditions. Be sure your doctor knows if any of these conditions applies to you. • This drug interacts with narcotic analgesics, tranquilizers, phenothiazines, sedatives, and hypnotics. If you are currently taking any of these drugs, consult your doctor about their use. If you are unsure of the type or contents of your medications, ask your doctor or pharmacist. • Because this drug causes sedation, it should not be used with other sedative drugs or with alcohol. • Avoid tasks requiring alertness, such as driving a car or operating machinery, while taking this drug. • This drug contains the narcotic hydrocodone; therefore, it has the potential for abuse and must be used with caution. Tolerance may develop quickly. Do not increase your dosage or take this medication more often than prescribed without first consulting your doctor. • Products containing narcotics are usually not used for more than seven to ten days.

Comments: If stomach upset occurs, take this drug with food or milk. • Notify your doctor if you develop signs of jaundice (yellow eyes or skin; dark urine). • Side effects of this drug may be somewhat relieved by lying down. • While taking this medicine, be cautious of taking nonprescription medicines containing acetaminophen.

Vi-Daylin/F vitamin and fluoride supplement (Ross Laboratories), see Poly-Vi-Flor vitamin and fluoride supplement.

Vistaril antianxiety (Pfizer Laboratories Division), see Atarax antianxiety.

warfarin sodium anticoagulant (various manufacturers), see Coumadin anticoagulant.

Wyamycin antibiotic (Wyeth-Ayerst Laboratories), see erythromycin antibiotic.

Wymox antibiotic (Wyeth-Ayerst Laboratories), see amoxicillin antibiotic.

Xanax antianxiety

Manufacturer: The Upjohn Company
Ingredient: alprazolam
Dosage Form: Tablet: 0.25 mg (white); 0.5 mg (peach); 1 mg (lavender)
Uses: Relief of anxiety disorders and anxiety associated with depression
Minor Side Effects: Blurred vision; change in sex drive; constipation; diarrhea; dizziness; drowsiness; dry mouth; fatigue; headache; heartburn; irritability; nervousness; stomach pains; sweating; weakness
Major Side Effects: Breathing difficulties; clumsiness; confusion; depression; difficulty in urinating; hallucinations; jaundice; menstrual changes; nervousness; rapid heartbeat; rash; shakiness; sleeping difficulties; slurred speech; sore throat; uncoordinated movements
Contraindications: This drug should not be used by persons allergic to it or those with acute narrow-angle glaucoma. Consult your doctor immediately if this drug has been prescribed for you and either condition applies. This drug should not be used in the treatment of psychotic disorders.
Warnings: This drug should be used cautiously by pregnant or nursing women, elderly people, children, and people with a history of kidney or liver disease. Be sure your doctor knows if any of these conditions applies to you. • To prevent oversedation, avoid the use of alcohol or other drugs with sedative properties. • This drug may cause drowsiness; avoid tasks that require alertness. • Do not stop taking this drug suddenly without first consulting your doctor. If you have been taking this drug for a long time, your dosage should gradually be reduced, according to your doctor's directions. • This drug should be used cautiously with psychotropic medications, pain medications, anticonvulsants, antihistamines, alcohol, or other central nervous system depressants. If you are currently taking any drugs of these types, consult your doctor about their use. If you are unsure of the type or contents of your medications, ask your doctor or pharmacist. • This drug has the potential for abuse and must be used with caution. Tolerance may develop; do not increase the dose of this medication without first consulting your doctor. • If you are taking this drug for an extended duration, your doctor may require you to have periodic blood and liver-function tests.
Comments: This drug is currently used by many people to relieve anxiety. Although it is effective for this purpose, it is important to try to remove the cause of the anxiety as well. • Chew gum or suck on ice chips or a piece of hard candy to reduce mouth dryness. • To lessen stomach upset, take this medication with food or with a full glass of water. • The full effects of this drug may not become apparent for three to four days. • Notify your doctor if you develop signs of jaundice (yellow eyes or skin; dark urine).

Zantac antisecretory

Manufacturer: Glaxo, Inc.
Ingredient: ranitidine
Dosage Form: Tablet: 150 mg (white); 300 mg (yellow)
Uses: Treatment of ulcers and hypersecretory conditions; prevention of recurrent ulcers
Minor Side Effects: Constipation; decreased sexual ability; depression; diarrhea; dizziness; headache; insomnia; nausea; sedation; stomach upset
Major Side Effects: Agitation; blood disorders; confusion; impotence; muscle aches; palpitations; rash; weakness; weak pulse
Contraindication: This drug should not be taken by anyone who is allergic to it. Consult your doctor if you have such an allergy.

Warnings: This drug must be used with caution by pregnant or nursing women, elderly people, and people with liver or kidney diseases. If this drug has been prescribed for you and any of these conditions applies, consult your doctor. • Safety of this drug for use in children has not yet been established; therefore, it is not recommended for children under 12. • This drug has not been shown to affect the concurrent use of other medications. However, check with your doctor or pharmacist before taking any other drugs.

Comments: To ensure best results, this drug must be taken continuously for as long as your doctor prescribes, even if you feel better. • This drug may be used in conjunction with antacids to relieve pain. For maximum effect, stagger the doses of Zantac and antacids by at least two hours. • This drug is very similar in action to Tagamet and Pepcid. Talk to your doctor about these medications to determine the least expensive alternative.

Zaroxolyn diuretic and antihypertensive

Manufacturer: Pennwalt Pharmaceutical Division
Ingredient: metolazone
Equivalent Products: Diulo, Searle & Co.; Microx, Pennwalt Pharmaceutical Division
Dosage Form: Tablet: 2.5 mg (pink); 5 mg (blue); 10 mg (yellow); see Comments
Uses: Treatment of high blood pressure; removal of fluid from body tissues
Minor Side Effects: Bloating; chills; constipation; diarrhea; dizziness; drowsiness; fatigue; headache; heartburn; loss of appetite; nausea; rash; restlessness; sensitivity to sunlight; stomach upset; vomiting; weakness
Major Side Effects: Blood disorders; blurred vision; breathing difficulties; chest pain; clotting disorders; cramps; dehydration; dry mouth; fainting; fever; jaundice; low blood pressure; mood changes; muscle spasm; palpitations; rash; sore throat; tingling in the fingers and toes
Contraindications: This drug should not be used by people who are allergic to it or by those with anuria (inability to urinate) or liver disease. If this drug has been prescribed for you and any of these conditions applies, call your doctor at once.
Warnings: If you are allergic to sulfa drugs or thiazide diuretics (such as Diuril), you may also be allergic to this drug. Talk to your doctor before you take this drug. • This drug may cause a serious loss of potassium from the body, so it is often prescribed along with a potassium supplement. • This drug is not recommended for use by children. • Nursing mothers who must take this drug should stop nursing. • This drug should be used cautiously by pregnant women and by people with diabetes, kidney disease, or gout. Be sure your doctor knows if any of these conditions applies to you. • Remind your doctor that you are taking this drug if you are scheduled for surgery. • Persons taking this drug along with other high blood pressure medications may need to have their dosages carefully monitored. It may be necessary to reduce the dose of the other drug(s). • This drug should be used cautiously with digitalis, nonsteroidal anti-inflammatory drugs, and lithium. • Periodic laboratory tests should be performed while you are taking this drug. • This drug may affect kidney function tests. Be sure your doctor knows you are taking this drug if you are scheduled for such tests. • While taking this product, limit your consumption of alcoholic beverages in order to prevent dizziness or light-headedness.
Comments: If you have high blood pressure, do not take any nonprescription item for weight control, cough, cold, or sinus problems without first checking with your doctor; such medications may contain ingredients that can increase blood pressure. • Try to avoid taking this drug at bedtime. • This product causes frequent urination. Expect this effect; do not be alarmed. • This drug must

be taken exactly as directed. Do not take extra doses or skip a dose without first consulting your doctor. • Watch for signs of potassium loss (dry mouth, thirst, weakness, muscle pain or cramps, nausea, or vomiting), and call your doctor if any occur. To help prevent this loss, you can take this product with a glass of fresh or frozen orange juice, or eat a banana every day. The use of a salt substitute also helps prevent potassium loss. Do not change your diet, however, without consulting your doctor. Too much potassium can also be dangerous. Your doctor may want to check your blood potassium levels periodically while you are taking this drug. • If you are taking digitalis in addition to this drug, watch carefully for symptoms of increased digitalis toxicity (e.g., nausea, blurred vision, palpitations), and notify your doctor immediately if they occur. • Notify your doctor if you develop signs of jaundice (yellow eyes or skin; dark urine). • To avoid dizziness or light-headedness when you stand, contract and relax the muscles of your legs for a few minutes before rising. Do this by pushing one foot against the floor while raising the other foot slightly, alternating feet so that you are "pumping" your legs in a pedaling motion. The light-headed feeling is more likely to occur in persons who combine this drug with other high blood pressure drugs, alcohol, sedatives, or narcotics. • If this drug causes stomach upset, take it with food or milk. • Learn how to monitor your pulse and blood pressure while taking this medication; discuss this with your doctor. • Microx is only available in a 0.5 mg tablet.

Zaxopam antianxiety and sedative (Quantum Pharmics), see Serax antianxiety and sedative.

Zovirax antiviral

Manufacturer: Burroughs Wellcome Co.
Ingredient: acyclovir
Dosage Forms: Capsule: 200 mg (blue). Ointment: 5%
Uses: Management of genital herpes and herpes infections of the skin
Minor Side Effects: Capsule: Bad taste in mouth; dizziness; fatigue; headache; loss of appetite; nausea; rash; vomiting. Ointment: Temporary pain, burning, stinging, itching, or rash after application
Major Side Effects: Blood disorders; muscle cramps; sore throat
Contraindication: This drug should not be used by anyone who is allergic to it. Consult your doctor immediately if this drug has been prescribed for you and you have such an allergy.
Warnings: The ointment is intended for use on the skin only and should not be used in the eyes. • This drug should be used with extreme caution during pregnancy; discuss the benefits and risks with your doctor. • Nursing women should also use Zovirax with caution, since it is not known whether the drug passes into breast milk. • Use of this drug in children is not recommended.
Comments: This drug will not cure or prevent a herpes infection but may relieve pain associated with the viral infection and may shorten its duration. Notify your doctor if the frequency and severity of recurrences does not improve. • Apply this drug as soon as possible after symptoms of a herpes infection begin, and use a rubber glove to apply the ointment in order to avoid spreading the infection. Avoid sexual intercourse when visible lesions are present. • To achieve full effect, this drug must be used as prescribed. The ointment is usually applied six times a day for a one week period. Continue taking this drug for the prescribed period, even if symptoms disappear before that time. Do not use more than is prescribed. • The ointment may cause temporary burning, itching, and stinging. Notify your doctor if these symptoms worsen or persist. • This drug should be stored in a cool, dry place. • Patient information is available on this drug. Ask your pharmacist.

Zurinol antigout drug (Major Pharmaceuticals), see Zyloprim antigout drug.

Zydone analgesic (Du Pont Pharmaceuticals, Inc.), see Vicodin analgesic.

Zyloprim antigout drug

Manufacturer: Burroughs Wellcome Co.

Ingredient: allopurinol

Equivalent Products: allopurinol, various manufacturers; Lopurin, Boots Pharmaceuticals, Inc.; Zurinol, Major Pharmaceuticals

Dosage Form: Tablet: 100 mg (white); 300 mg (peach)

Use: Treatment of gout

Minor Side Effects: Diarrhea; drowsiness; nausea; stomach upset; vomiting

Major Side Effects: Blood disorders; bruising; chills; fatigue; fever; kidney or liver damage; loss of hair; muscle ache; numbness or tingling sensations; paleness; rash; sore throat; visual disturbances

Contraindications: This drug should not be used by children, with the exception of those children with cancer; by nursing mothers; or by persons who have had a severe reaction to it. Consult your doctor immediately if this drug has been prescribed for you and any of these conditions applies.

Warnings: This drug should be discontinued at the first sign of skin rash or any sign of adverse reaction. Notify your doctor immediately if reactions occur. • This drug should be used with caution by pregnant women; persons with blood disease, liver disease, or kidney disease; and people receiving other antigout drugs. Be sure your doctor knows if any of these conditions applies to you. • Some investigators have reported an increase in gout attacks during the early stages of use of this drug. • Drowsiness may occur as a result of using this drug; avoid tasks that require alertness. • Periodic determination of liver and kidney function and complete blood counts should be performed during therapy with this drug, especially during the first few months. • This drug should be used cautiously in conjunction with ampicillin, azathioprine, cyclophosphamide, mercaptopurine, oral anticoagulants, theophylline, or thiazides. If you are currently taking any drugs of these types, consult your doctor about their use. If you are unsure about the type or contents of your medications, ask your doctor or pharmacist. • Avoid large doses of vitamin C while taking this drug. The combination may increase the risk of kidney stone formation.

Comments: It is common for persons beginning to take this drug to also take colchicine for the first three months. Colchicine helps minimize painful attacks of gout. • If one tablet of this drug is prescribed three times a day, ask your doctor if a single dose (either three 100 mg tablets or one 300 mg tablet) can be taken as a convenience. • The effects of therapy with this drug may not be apparent for at least two weeks. • Drink at least eight glasses of water each day to help minimize the formation of kidney stones. • While you are on this drug, do not drink alcohol without first checking with your doctor. • To lessen stomach upset, take this drug with food. Take each dose with a full glass of water.

Glossary

adrenergic—a substance that mimics the effects of adrenaline; stimulates the part of the nervous system that controls involuntary actions such as blood vessel contraction, sweating, etc.; used in the treatment of low blood pressure, asthma, shock, glaucoma, and respiratory congestion

adverse reaction—an undesirable, even dangerous effect cased by the use of a drug

allergy—an unusual physical response to a foreign substance; allergic symptoms (such as nasal congestion, itchy eyes, certain rashes, and sneezing) are caused by the release of histamine

amphetamine—a substance that acts as a central nervous system stimulant; increases blood pressure and reduces appetite; used as an anorectic and to treat hyperkinesis

analgesic—having pain-relieving properties; a pain-relieving substance; may be narcotic

anesthetic—causing loss of feeling and sensation; a substance that causes loss of feeling and sensation

angina—chest pain or discomfort caused by a lack of oxygen to the heart muscle

anorectic—a substance that decreases the appetite; usually a sympathomimetic amine, an amphetamine, or a related drug

antacid—a drug that neutralizes excess acidity, usually of the stomach; most frequently used to relieve gastrointestinal distress and to treat peptic ulcers

anthelmintic—an anti-infective used to kill worms infecting the body

antianginal—a substance used to relieve or prevent the chest pain known as angina

antiarrhythmic—a drug that improves abnormal heart rhythms

antibacterial—a drug that destroys or prevents the growth of certain bacteria

antibiotic—a drug that destroys or prevents the growth of bacteria and/or fungi; can be derived from a mold or produced synthetically

anticholinergic drug—a drug that blocks the passage of certain nervous impulses; used to treat Parkinson's disease, to relieve motion sickness, to reduce acid production in the stomach, to relieve spasms of the intestines, and to treat diarrhea

anticoagulant—a substance that prevents the clotting of blood; "blood-thinner"

anticonvulsant—a substance used to treat or prevent seizures or convulsions

antidepressant—a substance used to treat symptoms of depression; drugs currently used as antidepressants are generally tricyclic antidepressants, monoamine oxidase inhibitors, or amphetamines

antidiabetic—a drug used to treat diabetes mellitus that is not controlled by diet and exercise alone

antidiarrheal—a drug used to treat diarrhea; may work by altering the contents of the bowel or by slowing the action of the bowel

antidote—a substance that counteracts or stops the action of ingested poison

antiemetic—an agent that prevents or relieves nausea and vomiting

antiflatulent—a drug used to relieve intestinal gas

antifungal—a drug that destroys and prevents the growth and reproduction of fungi

antihistamine—a drug used to relieve the symptoms of an allergy; works by blocking the effects of histamine

antihyperlipidemic—a drug used in conjunction with diet to reduce elevated serum (blood) cholesterol and/or triglyceride levels, which are associated with an increased risk of coronary heart disease

antihypertensive—a drug that counteracts or reduces high blood pressure

anti-infective—an agent used to treat an infection by microorganisms (bacteria, viruses, or fungi), protozoa, or worms

anti-inflammatory—a drug that counteracts or suppresses inflammation; aspirin has anti-inflammatory properties

antinauseant—a drug used to relieve nausea; most antinauseants work by blocking the transmission of nerve impulses that stimulate vomiting; antiemetic

antispasmodic—a drug that relieves spasms (violent, involuntary muscular contractions or sudden constrictions of a passage or canal); antispasmodics are typically used to treat dysfunctions of the gastrointestinal tract, the gallbladder, or the urinary system

antitussive—a drug used to relieve coughing; may be narcotic

barbiturates—a class of drugs used as sedatives or hypnotics; can be addictive

beta blocker—an adrenergic used to slow the heart rate, reduce blood pressure, prevent the chest pain known as angina, and relieve migraine headaches

bronchodilator—a drug used to help breathing; works by relaxing bronchial muscles, thereby expanding the air passages of the lungs

central nervous system depressant—a drug that acts on the brain to decrease energy and concentration

central nervous system stimulant—a drug that acts on the brain to increase energy and alertness

contraindications—conditions for which a drug should not be used; conditions in which the benefits of a given drug would be outweighed by its negative effects

decongestant—a drug that relieves congestion in the upper respiratory system; sympathomimetic amines are used as decongestants

deficiency—an insufficient supply of an element or elements necessary for health; scurvy, which is caused by a lack of vitamin C, is an example of a deficiency disease

dependence—habituation to the use of a drug; may be used to refer to either a physical or a psychological need for the substance

digitalis—a drug used to improve heart rhythm or increase the output of the heart in heart failure; slows the heart rate and increases the force of contraction

diuretic—a drug that acts on the kidneys to cause an increase in urine flow; often used in the treatment of high blood pressure; also called water pill

emetic—a substance that causes vomiting

expectorant—a drug used to increase the secretion of mucus in the respiratory system, thus making it easier to "bring up" phlegm from the lungs

gastric—pertaining to the stomach

generic—not protected by trademark

histamine—a substance produced by the body in an allergic reaction; causes dilation of blood vessels, constriction of smooth muscles in the lungs, and the stimulation of gastric secretions

hormone—a chemical substance produced by glands in the body; regulates the action of certain organs

hypersensitive—characterized by an abnormal or excessive response to a substance; allergy

hypnotic—a drug that is used to induce sleep

immunity—resistance to a specific infection

indications—uses for a drug that are approved by the government

inflammation—a localized condition characterized by redness, itching, swelling, pain, and heat

keratolytic—an agent that softens and promotes peeling of the outer layer of the skin

mineral—an inorganic element found in foods; a variety of minerals, including iron and calcium, are necessary for normal body function

monoamine oxidase (MAO) inhibitor—a drug used to treat severe depression; acts by inhibiting the production of enzymes called monoamine oxidases

narcotic—a drug derived from the opium poppy; used to relieve pain and coughing; addictive

otic—pertaining to the ear

over-the-counter (OTC) drug—a nonprescription medication; a drug that can be purchased without a prescription

palpitations—rapid heartbeats; a feeling of throbbing in the chest

pediculicide—a preparation used to treat a person infested with lice

phenothiazine—a drug used to relieve certain psychological disorders; also used as an antinauseant

salicylates—a class of drugs prepared from the salts of salicylic acid; the most commonly used pain relievers in the U.S.

scabicide—a preparation used to treat a person infested with scabies

scabies—an infection caused by the itch mite; marked by intense itching and skin damage from scratching

sedative—a drug given to reduce nervousness and promote calm, thereby inducing sleep

side effect—any effect from a drug other than that for which the drug is taken; minor side effects are usually expected and are not usually life-threatening; major side effects are rare and signal the need for a doctor's attention

smooth muscle relaxant—a drug that causes the relaxation of smooth muscle tissue (i.e., muscle tissue, such as that in the lungs, stomach, and bladder, that performs functions not under voluntary control)

steroid—any one of a group of compounds secreted primarily by the adrenal glands; used to treat allergic or inflammatory reactions

sulfa drug—an antibacterial drug belonging to the chemical group sulfonamides

superinfection—an infection that occurs during the treatment of another infection

sympathomimetic amine—a drug that raises blood pressure, acts as a decongestant, improves air passage into the lungs, and decreases the appetite

symptom—any subjective evidence of disease; pain, for example, is a symptom

thyroid preparation—a drug used to correct thyroid hormone deficiency; may be natural or synthetic; affects the biochemical activity of all body tissues and increases the rate of cellular metabolism

topical—applied directly on the skin rather than taken orally, injected, or administered in other ways

toxic—poisonous, harmful, possibly lethal

tranquilizer—a drug that, when taken in normal doses, calms part of the brain without affecting clarity of mind or consciousness

tricyclic antidepressant—a drug used to suppress symptoms of depression; differs slightly in chemical structure from the phenothiazines

uricosuric—a drug that promotes the excretion of uric acid in the urine; used to prevent gout attacks

vaccine—a medication containing weakened or killed germs that stimulates the body to develop an immunity to those germs

vasoconstrictor—a drug that constricts blood vessels, thereby increasing blood pressure and decreasing blood flow

vasodilator—a drug that expands blood vessels to increase blood flow or to lower blood pressure

vitamin—a natural element present in foods that is vital to normal body functions

Index

antiulcer, 35
  Carafate, 65
  See also antisecretory
Antivert antinauseant, 54
  antiviral, 28
  amantadine HCl, 49, 200
  Symadine, 200
  Symmetrel, 200
  Zovirax, 232
Antrizine antinauseant, 54
Anucort steroid-hormone-containing
    anorectal product, 54
Anugard-HC steroid-hormone-
    containing anorectal product, 54
Anumed HC steroid-hormone-
    containing anorectal product, 54
Anusol-HC steroid-hormone-
    containing anorectal product, 54
Anxanil antianxiety, 55
Aquaphyllin bronchodilator, 55, 210
Aquatensen diuretic and
    antihypertensive, 55, 90
Armour thyroid hormone, 55, 212
Asmalix bronchodilator, 55, 210
Aspirin with Codeine analgesic, 55, 89
Atarax antianxiety, 55
Ativan antianxiety and sedative, 56
Atozine antianxiety, 55, 57
Augmentin antibiotic, 57
Azo-Standard analgesic, 58, 186

B

B-A-C #3 analgesic, 58, 96
Bacticort Suspension ophthalmic
    preparation, 58, 74
Bactrim and Bactrim DS antibacterials,
    58
Bancap HC analgesic, 59, 228
Banex-LA decongestant and
    expectorant, 59, 91
Barbita sedative and hypnotic, 59, 175
Baridium analgesic, 59, 186
Beclovent antiasthmatic, 59, 226
Beepen VK antibiotic, 59, 169
Belix antihistamine, 59
belladonna alkaloids with
    phenobarbital sedative and
    anticholinergic, 59, 86
Benadryl antihistamine, 59
Benaphen antihistamine, 59, 60
Bentyl antispasmodic, 60
beta blocker, 30-31
  Blocadren, 62
  Corgard, 73

Inderal, 110, 184
Ipran, 114, 184
Lopressor, 126
propranolol, 184
Tenormin, 208
betamethasone valerate topical steroid
    hormone, 61, 224
Betapen-VK antibiotic, 61, 69
Betatrex topical steroid hormone, 61,
    224
Beta-Val topical steroid hormone, 61,
    224
Bethaprim DS and Bethaprim SS
    antibacterials, 58, 61
Bexophene analgesic, 61, 79
birth control pills. *See* oral
    contraceptives
Blocadren beta blocker, 62
blood disorders, drug-induced, 27
blood pressure drug. *See*
    antihypertensive; diuretic and
    antihypertensive
blood thinner. *See* anticoagulant
Brethine bronchodilator, 62
Bricanyl bronchodilator, 62, 63
bronchodilator, 37
  Accurbron, 42, 210
  Aerolate, 43, 210
  Alupent, 49
  aminophylline, 50
  Amoline, 50, 52
  Aquaphyllin, 55, 210
  Asmalix, 55, 210
  Brethine, 62
  Bricanyl, 62, 63
  Bronkodyl, 63, 210
  Constant-T, 73, 210
  Elixicon, 89, 210
  Elixomin, 89, 210
  Elixophyllin, 89, 210
  Lanophyllin, 120, 210
  Lixolin, 125, 210
  Lodrane, 125, 210
  Metaprel, 49, 136
  Phyllocontin, 50, 176
  Proventil, 185, 228
  Quibron-T, 187, 210
  Respbid, 189, 210
  Slo-bid, 197, 210
  Slo-Phyllin, 197, 210
  Somophyllin, 50, 197
  Somophyllin-DS, 50, 197
  Somophyllin-T, 197, 210
  Sustaire, 200, 210
  Theo-24, 210
  Theobid, 210

Lo-Trol antidiarrheal, 125, 129
Low-Quel antidiarrheal, 125, 129
Lozol diuretic and antihypertensive, 129
Ludiomil antidepressant, 130
Luramide diuretic and antihypertensive, 121, 131

M

Macrodantin antibacterial, 131, 152
Malatal sedative and anticholinergic, 86, 131
Mallergan VC with Codeine expectorant, 131, 174
Marnal analgesic, 95, 131
Maxolon gastrointestinal stimulant, 131, 188
Maxzide diuretic and antihypertensive, 131
meclizine hydrochloride antinauseant, 54, 132
meclofenamate anti-inflammatory, 132
Meclomen anti-inflammatory, 132
Medipren anti-inflammatory, 108, 133
Medrol steroid hormone, 133
Mellaril antipsychotic, 135
Meprolone steroid hormone, 134, 136
Metaprel bronchodilator, 49, 136
methyclothiazide diuretic and antihypertensive, 90, 136
methyldopa and hydrochlorothiazide diuretic and antihypertensive, 47, 136
methyldopa antihypertensive, 46, 136
methylphenidate hydrochloride central nervous system stimulant, 136, 191
methylprednisolone steroid hormone, 134, 136
Meticorten steroid hormone, 136, 179
Metizol antimicrobial and antiparasitic, 96, 136
metoclopramide gastrointestinal stimulant, 136, 188
metronidazole antimicrobial and antiparasitic, 97, 136
Metryl antimicrobial and antiparasitic, 97, 136
Mevacor antihyperlipidemic, 136
Micro-K potassium chloride replacement, 137, 178
Micronase oral antidiabetic, 137
Microx diuretic and antihypertensive, 138, 231

Mictrin diuretic and antihypertensive, 103, 138
Midol 200 anti-inflammatory, 108, 138
Millazine antipsychotic, 135, 139
mineral, 38
Minipress antihypertensive, 139
Minizide antihypertensive, 139
Minocin antibiotic, 140
Mitran antianxiety, 123, 140
Moduretic diuretic and antihypertensive, 140
Monistat antifungal agent, 141
monoamine oxidase inhibitor, 34
Motrin anti-inflammatory, 108, 142
muscle relaxant, 33, 37
muscle relaxant and analgesic Flexeril, 97
Myapap with Codeine analgesic, 42, 142
Mycelex antifungal agent, 128, 142
Mycelex-G antifungal agent, 100, 142
Mycogen II topical steroid hormone and anti-infective, 142
Mycolog II topical steroid hormone and anti-infective, 142
Mycostatin antifungal agent, 143
Myco-Triacet II topical steroid hormone and anti-infective, 142, 144
Mykacet topical steroid hormone and anti-infective, 142, 144
My-K Elixir potassium chloride replacement, 144, 178
Mykinac antifungal agent, 143, 144
Mytrex topical steroid hormone and anti-infective, 142, 144

N

Naldecon decongestant and antihistamine, 144
Naldelate decongestant and antihistamine, 144, 145
Nalfon anti-inflammatory, 145
Nalgest decongestant and antihistamine, 144, 146
Napamide antiarrhythmic, 146, 159
Naprosyn anti-inflammatory, 147
narcotic, 32
Nasalcrom respiratory inhalant, 114, 147
Nasalide topical steroid, 148
Navane antipsychotic, 148
Neocidin ophthalmic antibiotic preparation, 149, 150

Restoril sedative and hypnotic, 189
Retin-A acne preparation, 190
Rhinolar-EX 12 antihistamine and
     decongestant, 165, 190
Rhythmin antiarrhythmic, 183, 190
Ritalin central nervous system
     stimulant, 191
Robicillin VK antibiotic, 169, 191
Robimycin antibiotic, 93, 192
Robitet antibiotic, 192, 209
Ronase oral antidiabetic, 192, 217
Roxicet analgesic, 170, 192
Roxiprin analgesic, 171, 192
R-Tannate antihistamine and
     decongestant, 192
Rufen anti-inflammatory, 108, 192
Rum-K potassium chloride
     replacement, 178, 192
Ru-Tuss II antihistamine and
     decongestant, 165, 192
Ru-Vert-M antinauseant, 54, 192
Rymed-TR decongestant and
     expectorant, 91, 192
Rynatan antihistamine and
     decongestant, 192

S

salicylate, 32
Scabene pediculicide and scabicide,
     119, 193
sedative, 33-34
sedative and anticholinergic
     belladonna alkaloids with
          phenobarbital, 59, 86
     Donnamor, 85, 86
     Donnapine, 85, 86
     Donna-Sed, 85, 86
     Donnatal, 86
     Hyosophen, 86, 107
     Malatal, 86, 131
     Relaxadon, 86, 189
     Spaslin, 86, 197
     Spasmolin, 86, 198
     Spasmophen, 86, 198
     Spasquid, 86, 198
     Susano, 86, 200
sedative and hypnotic
     Barbita, 59, 175
     Dalmane, 77
     Durapam, 77, 87
     flurazepam, 77, 98
     Halcion, 101
     phenobarbital, 175
     Razepam, 188, 189

Restoril, 189
Solfoton, 175, 197
Temaz, 189, 206
temazepam, 189, 206
Seldane antihistamine, 193
Septra and Septra DS antibacterial,
     58, 194
Serax antianxiety and sedative, 194
sex hormones, 36
     See also estrogen; progesterone
side effects, 21-27
Sinemet antiparkinson drug, 195
Sinequan antidepressant and
     antianxiety, 196
Slo-bid bronchodilator, 197, 210
Slo-Phyllin bronchodilator, 197, 210
Slow-K potassium chloride
     replacement, 178, 197
smoking deterrent
     Nicorette, 150
smooth muscle relaxant, 37
SMZ-TMP antibacterial, 58, 197
Sofarin anticoagulant, 76, 197
Solfoton sedative and hypnotic, 175,
     197
Somophyllin bronchodilator, 50, 197
Somophyllin-DF bronchodilator, 50,
     197
Somophyllin-T bronchodilator, 197,
     210
Sorbitrate antianginal, 116, 197
Spaslin sedative and anticholinergic,
     86, 197
Spasmolin sedative and
     anticholinergic, 86, 198
Spasmophen sedative and
     anticholinergic, 86, 198
Spasquid sedative and anticholinergic,
     86, 198
Spironazide diuretic and
     antihypertensive, 44, 198
spironolactone diuretic and
     antihypertensive, 45, 198
spironolactone with
     hydrochlorothiazide diuretic and
     antihypertensive, 44, 198
Spirozide diuretic and
     antihypertensive, 44, 198
S-P-T thyroid hormone, 198, 212
Stelazine antipsychotic, 198
Sterapred steroid hormone, 179, 199
Steroid
     Anucort, 54
     Anugard-HC, 54
     Anumed HC, 54
     Anusol-HC, 54

V

vaccines, 28
vaginal anti-infective. *See* anti-
infective
vaginal medication administration, 18
Valdrene antihistamine, 59, 224
Valisone topical steroid hormone, 224
Valium antianxiety, 225
Valnac topical steroid hormone, 224,
225
Valrelease antianxiety, 225
Vamate antianxiety, 55, 226
Vanceril antiasthmatic, 226
Vapocet analgesic, 226, 229
Vasominic T.D. decongestant and
antihistamine, 144, 226
Vasotec antihypertensive, 227
Vazepam antianxiety, 225, 227
V-Cillin K antibiotic, 169, 227
Veetids antibiotic, 169, 228
Ventolin bronchodilator, 228
verapamil antianginal and
antihypertensive, 114, 228
Vicodin analgesic, 228
Vi-Daylin/F vitamin and fluoride
supplement, 176, 229
Vistaril antianxiety, 55, 229
vitamin and fluoride supplement
Florvite, 98, 176
Polytabs/F, 176
Poly-Vi-Flor, 176
Poly-Vi-Sol, 177
Poly-Vitamins with Fluoride, 176,
177
Polyvite with Fluoride Drops, 176,
177
Vi-Daylin/F, 176, 229
vitamin-mineral supplement
Prenatal-1, 181, 199
Prenatal 1 mg+Iron, 181, 199
Stuartnatal 1+1, 199
vitamin supplement, 38

W

warfarin sodium anticoagulant, 76, 229
water pills. *See* diuretic; diuretic and
antihypertensive
Wyamycin antibiotic, 93, 229
Wymox antibiotic, 52, 229

X

Xanax antianxiety, 230

Z

Zantac antisecretory, 230
Zaroxolyn diuretic and
antihypertensive, 231
Zaxopam antianxiety and sedative,
194, 232
Zovirax antiviral, 232
Zurinol antigout drug, 233
Zydone analgesic, 229, 233
Zyloprim antigout drug, 233